OXFORD HANDBOOK OF
Gastrointestinal Nursing

T0202119

Published and forthcoming Oxford Handbooks in Nursing

Oxford Handbook of Adult Nursing 2e
Edited by Maria Flynn and Dave Mercer

Oxford Handbook of Cancer Nursing, 2e
Edited by Mike Tadman and Dave
Roberts

Oxford Handbook of Cardiac Nursing, 3e
Edited by Kate Olson

Oxford Handbook of Children's and
Young People's Nursing, 2e
Edited by Edward Alan Glasper, Gillian
McEwing, and Jim Richardson

Oxford Handbook of Clinical Skills in
Adult Nursing, 2e
Edited by Frank Coffey, Alison Wells, and
Mark Fores

Oxford Handbook of Clinical Skills for
Children's and Young People's Nursing
Paula Dawson, Louise Cook, Laura-Jane
Holliday, and Helen Reddy

Oxford Handbook of Critical Care
Nursing, 2e
Sheila Adam and Sue Osborne

Oxford Handbook of Dental Nursing
Elizabeth Boon, Rebecca Parr, Dayananda
Samarawickrama, and Kevin Seymour

Oxford Handbook of Diabetes Nursing
Lorraine Avery, Joanne Buchanan, Anita
Thynne

Oxford Handbook of Emergency
Nursing, 2e
Edited by Robert Crouch, Alan Charters,
Mary Dawood, and Paula Bennett

Oxford Handbook of Gastrointestinal
Nursing, 2e
Edited by Jennie Burch and Brigitte
Collins

Oxford Handbook of Learning and
Intellectual Disability Nursing
Edited by Bob Gates and Owen Barr

Oxford Handbook of Mental Health
Nursing, 2e
Edited by Patrick Callaghan and
Catherine Gamble

Oxford Handbook of Midwifery, 3e
Janet Medforth, Susan Battersby, Maggie
Evans, Beverley Marsh, and Angela
Walker

Oxford Handbook of Musculoskeletal
Nursing
Edited by Susan Oliver

Oxford Handbook of Neuroscience
Nursing 2e
Edited by Sue Woodward and Catheryne
Waterhouse

Oxford Handbook of Nursing Older
People, 2e
Edited by Marie Honey, Annette Jinks,
and Lauren Hanson

Oxford Handbook of Trauma and
Orthopaedic Nursing 2e
Rebecca Jester, Julie Santy, and Jean
Rogers

Oxford Handbook of Perioperative
Practice
Suzanne Hughes and Andy Mardell

Oxford Handbook of Prescribing for
Nurses and Allied Health Professionals
Sue Beckwith and Penny Franklin

Oxford Handbook of Primary Care and
Community Nursing 3e
Edited by Judy Brook, Caroline McGraw,
and Val Thurtle

Oxford Handbook of Renal Nursing
Edited by Althea Mahon, Karen Jenkins,
and Lisa Burnapp

Oxford Handbook of Respiratory
Nursing
Terry Robinson and Jane Scullion

Oxford Handbook of Surgical Nursing
Edited by Alison Smith, Maria Kisiel, and
Mark Radford

Oxford Handbook of Women's Health
Nursing, 2e
Edited by Sunanda Gupta, Debra
Holloway, and Ali Kubba

OXFORD HANDBOOK OF

Gastrointestinal Nursing

SECOND EDITION

Jennie Burch
Head of St Mark's Nurse Education,
St Mark's Hospital,
Harrow, UK

Brigitte Collins
Global Clinical Education Manager,
MacGregor Healthcare Ltd,
Macmerry,
East Lothian, UK

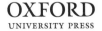

OXFORD
UNIVERSITY PRESS

Great Clarendon Street, Oxford, OX2 6DP,
United Kingdom

Oxford University Press is a department of the University of Oxford.
It furthers the University's objective of excellence in research, scholarship,
and education by publishing worldwide. Oxford is a registered trade mark of
Oxford University Press in the UK and in certain other countries

First Edition published in 2008
Second Edition published in 2021

Impression: 1

Published in the United States of America by Oxford University Press
198 Madison Avenue, New York, NY 10016, United States of America

British Library Cataloguing in Publication Data
Data available

Library of Congress Control Number: 2020943967

ISBN 978–0–19–883317–8

DOI: 10.1093/med/9780198833178.001.0001

Printed and bound in China by
C&C Offset Printing Co., Ltd.

Preface

The first edition of the *Oxford Handbook of Gastrointestinal Nursing* was published more than 10 years ago. The opportunity to produce a second edition has arisen. Each chapter has been updated and summarizes gut function and gives an overview of what is considered as best practice. The handbook is intended to provide a pocket-size resource allowing healthcare professionals easy access to anatomy, physiology, investigations, and common conditions and problems, regarding the gastrointestinal tract with details of further reading, including online information, where applicable.

Jennie Burch and Brigitte Collins
December 2019

Foreword to the second edition

It gives me great pleasure to see this *Handbook* being updated in this second edition. The nursing role in helping people with gastrointestinal disorders has continued to develop in the decade since the first edition, and this is fully reflected in the content of this new edition. This *Handbook* provides an excellent quick reference guide for both the specialist nurse working specifically with patients with gut disorders and the generalist nurse whose patients happen to have gastrointestinal symptoms.

This is a rapidly developing speciality, with many advances in understanding of gastrointestinal disorders and in their investigation, treatment, and management. Nurses working in both hospital and community settings need to consider the gut health of all of their patients.

A range of patients with various illnesses and disorders or taking a variety of medications will experience gut issues or side effects. These can be as bothersome as the primary disease, if not at times even more so. Additionally, many patients presenting with a variety of problems may have pre-existing gastrointestinal disorders, or will be at risk of gastrointestinal problems if their gut health is not proactively managed. The more we understand about the gut, the more we come to appreciate its central role in health. There are now strong suggestions that the gut microbiota is a major determinant of health and dysbiosis, and is a factor in many major health problems, such as depression, dementia, and diabetes. Gone are the days when we could give a broad-spectrum antibiotic without considering its effect on gut ecology, or manage a major illness such as cancer or an injury without attention to long-term gut consequences.

Nurses in all settings need the basic understanding of the gut contained in this volume. Many will want to refer to it regularly when encountering patients with gut problems as a primary or secondary health issue. The editors have done a great job of updating the text and providing links to sources of further information. I commend it to all nurses.

Christine Norton
Professor of Clinical Nursing Research, King's College London
January 2020

Contents

Symbols and abbreviations

↑	increase
↓	decrease
~	approximately
∴	therefore
♂	male
♀	female
➔	cross-reference
5-ASA	5-aminosalicylic acid
5-FU	5-fluorouracil
ACBS	Advisory Committee on Borderline Substances
ACE	antegrade continence enema
AFLP	acute fatty liver of pregnancy
AFP	α-fetoprotein
ALT	alanine aminotransferase
AMA	anti-mitochondrial antibody
ANA	antinuclear antibody
APER	abdominoperineal excision of the rectum
ASMA	anti-smooth-muscle antibody
AST	aspartate aminotransferase
BMD	bone mineral density
BMI	body mass index
BMR	basal metabolic rate
BSG	British Society of Gastroenterology
Bx	biopsy
CAM	complementary and alternative medicine
CBD	common bile duct
CD	Crohn's disease
CEA	carcinoembryonic antigen
CJD	Creutzfeldt–Jakob disease
CMV	cytomegalovirus
COSHH	Control of Substances Hazardous to Health
CPD	continuing professional development
CRP	C-reactive protein
CS	Caesarian section
CT	computed tomography
DAC	dispensing appliance contractor
DBE	double-balloon enteroscopy

DEXA	dual-energy X-ray absorptiometry
DN	district nurse
DOH	Department of Health
DRV	dietary reference value
EAR	estimated average requirement (nutrients)
EAS	external anal sphincter
ECF	enterocutaneous fistula
ECG	electrocardiogram
ELAPE	extralevator abdominoperineal excision
EMG	electromyography
EN	enteral nutrition
ENT	ear, nose, and throat
ERAS	enhanced recovery after surgery
ERCP	endoscopic retrograde cholangiopancreatography
ESR	erythrocyte sedimentation rate
EUA	examination under anaesthesia
FAP	familial adenomatous polyposis
FBC	full blood count
FI	faecal incontinence
FOBT	faecal occult blood test
g	gram(s)
GI	gastrointestinal
GIST	gastrointestinal stromal tumour
GIT	gastrointestinal tract
GORD	gastro-oesophageal reflux disease
GP	general practitioner
GTN	glycerine trinitrate
h	hour(s)
H&E	haematoxylin and eosin
HAV	hepatitis A virus
HBV	hepatitis B virus
HCC	hepatocellular carcinoma
HCV	hepatitis C virus
HDV	hepatitis D virus
HEN	home enteral nutrition
HETF	home enteral tube feeding
HEV	hepatitis E virus

HIDA	hepatobiliary iminodiacetic acid	NHS	National Health Service
HIV	human immunodeficiency virus	NICE	National Institute for Health and Clinical Excellence (formerly National Institute for Clinical Excellence)
HNPCC	hereditary non-polyposis colorectal cancer		
HPV	human papilloma virus	NJ	nasojejunal
HRT	hormone replacement therapy	NMC	Nursing and Midwifery Council
HSE	Health and Safety Executive	NSAID	non-steroidal anti-inflammatory drug
HV	health visitor		
IAS	internal anal sphincter	NSP	non-starch polysaccharide
IBD	inflammatory bowel disease	NST	nutrition support team
IBS	irritable bowel syndrome	OGD	oesophageal gastroduodenoscopy
IF	intestinal failure		
IM	intramuscular	OGIB	obscure gastrointestinal bleeding
IPAA	ileo-pouch anal anastomosis		
ISO	International Organization for Standardization	PAC-SYM	patient assessment of constipation symptoms
IV	intravenous	PABA	para-amino benzoic acid
IVF	in vitro fertilization	PBC	primary biliary cirrhosis
IVH	intravenous hyperalimentation	PCA	patient-controlled anaesthesia
JP	juvenile polyposis	PCR	polymerase chain reaction
L	litre(s)	PCT	primary care trust
LD	learning disabilities	PE	push enteroscopy
LIFT	ligation of the intersphincteric fistula tract	PEC	percutaneous endoscopic colostomy
LOCM	low-osmolar contrast media	PEG	percutaneous endoscopic gastrostomy
LRNI	lower reference nutrient intake		
MAP	MYH-associated polyposis	PEG-J	percutaneous endoscopic gastro-jejunostomy
MC&S	microscopy, culture, and sensitivity	PEJ	percutaneous endoscopic jejunostomy
mcg	microgram(s)	PG	pyoderma gangrenosum
MDT	multidisciplinary team	PICC	peripherally inserted central catheter
mg	milligram(s)		
min	minute(s)	PJS	Peutz–Jeghers syndrome
ml	millilitre(s)	PMARSI	peristomal medical adhesive related skin injury
MMC	migrating myoelectric complex		
MRI	magnetic resonance imaging	PMASD	peristomal moisture associated skin damage
MRSA	methicillin-resistant Staphylococcus aureus		
		PME	partial mesorectal excision
MS	multiple sclerosis	PN	parenteral nutrition
MSI	microsatellite instability	PNE	peripheral nerve evaluation
NAFLD	non-alcoholic fatty liver disease	PPC	prescription prepayment certificate
NASH	non-alcoholic steatohepatitis	PPI	proton pump inhibitor
NBM	nil by mouth	PR	per rectum
NCD	nutrition-related non-communicable disease	PROM	patient-reported outcome measure
NCJ	needle catheter jejunostomy	PTML	pudendal terminal motor latency
ND	nasoduodenal	PV	per vagina
NHL	non-Hodgkin lymphoma	RAIR	recto-anal inhibitory reflex

RIG	radiologically inserted gastrostomy		TAMIS	transanal minimally invasive surgery
RLQ	right lower quadrant		TAP	transverse abdominis plane
RN	registered nurse		TEA	Thoracic epidural analgesia
RNI	reference nutrient intake		TENS	transcutaneous electrical nerve stimulation
s	second(s)		TIPS	transjugular intrahepatic porto-systemic shunt
SC	subcutaneous			
SCFA	short-chain fatty acid		TME	total mesorectal excision
SCI	spinal cord injury		TPMT	thiopurine metyl transferase
SCN	stoma care nurse		TTS	through the scope
SG	surgical gastrostomy		U&Es	urea and electrolytes
SI	safe intake		UC	ulcerative colitis
SJ	surgical jejunostomy		VAAFT	video assisted anal fistula treatment
SNS	sacral nerve stimulation			
SPN	supplementary parenteral nutrition		VC	virtual colonoscopy
			vCJD	variant Creutzfeldt–Jakob disease
SSRI	selective serotonin-reuptake inhibitor			
			w/v	weight/volume
STI	sexually transmitted infection		WBC	white cell count
TAI	transanal irrigation		WCRF	World Cancer Research Fund

Chapter 1

Anatomy and physiology of the gastrointestinal tract

Gut overview

The gastrointestinal (GI) tract (Fig. 1.1) is a hollow tube passing from the mouth to the anus. There are several names for the GI tract, including the alimentary canal or gut. The GI tract is about 7–11 metres long but appears shorter due to the creases in the gut wall. There are many organs making up the GI tract:
- Mouth
- Pharynx
- Oesophagus
- Stomach
- Small bowel
- Large bowel.

There are also a number of accessory organs that help breakdown ingested food:
- Teeth
- Tongue
- Salivary glands
- Gall bladder
- Pancreas
- Liver.

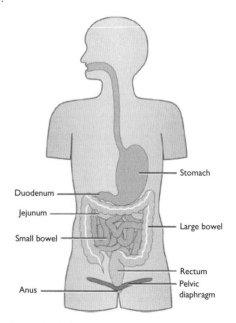

Fig. 1.1 The gastrointestinal tract.
Reproduced with kind permission © Burdett Institute 2008.

The main function of the GI tract is to make ingested nutrients available for the body to use. There are five main processes involved in the functioning of the GI tract:
- Ingestion
- Propulsion
- Digestion
- Absorption
- Elimination.

Ingestion
This is another term for eating—taking food into the body.

Propulsion
Ingested food is moved through the GI tract, initially by swallowing (voluntary action) and progressing to peristalsis, an involuntary action. In peristalsis, the gut wall contracts and pushes the food bolus or waste further along the GI tract; the muscles then relax and contract again. This combination of contracting and relaxing helps to break down the food and propels it forward. Peristalsis occurs in the oesophagus, stomach, small bowel, and large bowel.

Digestion
Ingested food is broken down into smaller parts in two ways: chemically and mechanically. In the mouth, the teeth chew the food, breaking it into smaller parts, and mix it with saliva (mechanical breakdown). The saliva begins to digest the food (chemical breakdown). The stomach churns the food (mechanical breakdown), and acid and digestive enzymes are secreted to breakdown it down chemically. Segmentation contractions in the small bowel mix the food with the digestive enzymes and break it down (mechanical breakdown), with peristalsis moving food further along the GI tract. There is further chemical breakdown of the food by bile, which is made in the liver (❷ pp. 15–6) and stored in the gall bladder (❷ p. 14), and pancreatic juice from the pancreas (❷ p. 14).

Absorption
The nutrients from the diet are taken from the GI tract into the blood or lymph. Additionally, the 7 litres of secretions (❷ p. 6) produced by the body and added to the GI tract are absorbed. Nutrients, electrolytes, and water are absorbed in the small bowel. Electrolytes and water are absorbed in the colon.

Elimination
This is the passage of faeces, out of the body via the anus, past the anal sphincters that control defaecation (❷ p. 446).

Further reading
Waugh A and Grant A (2018). *Ross & Wilson Anatomy and Physiology in Health and Illness*. 13th ed. Elsevier. Cambridge.

Gut structure

There are four main layers of tissue in the GI tract, these are:
- Serosa
- Muscularis
- Submucosa
- Mucosa.

Serosa

The serosa is the outer layer of the GI tract (except the oesophagus) and the largest serous membrane of the body. In the abdominal cavity the serosa comprises:
- Parietal peritoneum—lines the abdominopelvic cavity
- Visceral peritoneum—covers the gut and other organs
- Peritoneal cavity—space between the layers
- Folds—binds organs to each other and the abdominal wall.

Muscularis

The muscle layer that surrounds the submucosa is termed the muscularis. There are longitudinal and circular smooth muscles in the GI. This layer is responsible for peristalsis and segmentation. Thicker areas of circular muscles also form the sphincters.

Submucosa

The submucosa is formed from connective tissue. The blood vessels, lymphatics, and enteric nervous system that supply the wall of the GI tract are found in this layer, and due its elasticity, organs such as the stomach (→ p. 9) can stretch and regain their shape.

Mucosa

Finally, the mucosa, the inner most part of the GI tract, is lined with epithelial cells that renew every 4–7 days. This layer varies somewhat in different areas of the GI tract. Mucus is secreted into the stomach, small bowel, and large bowel to protect the GI tract from digestive enzymes and lubricate passage of food. In the stomach and small bowel, there are endocrine cells that secrete hormones into the bowel lumen. Also, in the small bowel the inner surface is covered with villi and microvilli that increase the surface area about 20-fold to vastly increase absorptive capacity from the bowel lumen. The lamina propria is part of the mucosa and is made from connective tissue; it is responsible for absorption and defence from bacteria and other pathogens.

Abdominal cavity and pelvic cavity

In the main, the GI tract is within the abdominal cavity. The thoracic cavity is separated from the abdominal cavity by the diaphragm. The abdominal cavity contains the stomach, small and large intestine, gall bladder, pancreas, and liver, and other organs such as the spleen. There is no physical separation between the abdominal cavity and the pelvic cavity. The pelvic cavity contains the rectum and other organs such as the urinary bladder.

The abdominal and pelvic cavities are lined with serous membranes. The largest membrane within the abdomen and pelvis is the peritoneum. The peritoneum is formed from the parietal peritoneum and visceral peritoneum, which are joined. The parietal peritoneum lines the body walls and the visceral peritoneum covers the organs. The space between the parietal peritoneum and the visceral peritoneum is the peritoneal cavity, which contains fluid that enables the membranes to slide and allows movement within the abdominal cavity. Thus mobile organs, such as the small bowel, are able to move as the body moves. Digestive organs within the peritoneal cavity are termed intraperitoneal, and those that are posterior to the peritoneum, such as the pancreas and duodenum, are termed retroperitoneal organs.

Within the abdominal cavity, there are parts of the peritoneum that are folded: this is called the mesentery. The mesentery holds parts of the digestive tract in place. Additionally, the mesentery is a passage for blood vessels, lymphatics, and nerves to reach the digestive viscera.

Gut nerves, hormones, secretions, and blood supply

Enteric nervous system

Enteric nerves are mediators of movement and sensation in the gut. Gut motility is mostly controlled by the enteric nervous system, with stimulation or inhibition by the central autonomic nervous system. This is why the GI tract continues to work after complete spinal cord injury, albeit more slowly and often with constipation. Local reflexes are mostly in response to distension, modified by the luminal content of the gut.

Autonomic nervous system

The gut is also supplied by the autonomic (involuntary) part of the central nervous system. Sympathetic nerves slow down gut motility and close sphincters. This is useful when gut activity is not desirable, such as in relation to 'fight or flight'. Parasympathetic nerves stimulate motility and open sphincters. Digestion occurs best when the body is relatively at rest.

Hormones

Many hormones control secretions within the gut. Three important examples are:
• Cholecystokinin—released in the duodenum and jejunum when fat is present. The function is to inhibit stomach activity and stimulate release of bile by the gall bladder.
• Secretin—released from the duodenum. The function is to inhibit motility in response to acid from the stomach.
• Gastric inhibitory peptide—released in the small bowel in response to the presence of fats, carbohydrate, and amino acids. The result is to inhibit the stomach and allow time for digestion and absorption in the small bowel, before the release of more gastric contents.

Secretions

There are about 7 litres of secretions that enter the GI tract every day; predominantly in the upper gut, up to and including the duodenum. This is made up from saliva (0.5–1.5 litres), gastric juices (2–3 litres), and pancreas and gall bladder (1.5–2 litres).

Blood supply

The blood supply to the GI tract is via the abdominal aorta: the splanchnic circulation. The arterial blood supply to the stomach is through the coeliac artery. The blood drains via the hepatic portal vein. The blood supply for the liver is via the portal circulation, with 70% of blood supply being carried to the liver from the small bowel. This blood contains nutrients, amongst other substances. The three hepatic veins drain into the vena cava. The other 30% of the blood supply is taken to the liver via the hepatic artery; 25% of the cardiac output goes to the liver.

Motility

In general, meals empty from the stomach within 2–3 h, with liquids emptying faster than solids. Most food residue reaches the colon within 6 h.

Mouth, pharynx, oesophagus, and stomach

Mouth

The mouth is the first part of the GI tract. External to the mouth are the lips and cheeks. Within the mouth are the palate, teeth, and tongue. The palate separates the oral and nasal cavities. The teeth are used for mastication (chewing). The tongue is used for taste and speech, and is involved in mastication and swallowing. The lining of the mouth is made up of epithelial cells. The mouth produces saliva from three sets of salivary glands: the parotid glands are located between the ears and the jaw, the submandibular glands under the jaw, and the sublingual glands under the tongue. Saliva lubricates and begins digestion. The salivary glands produce ptyalin, a type of amylase, which breakdowns starch, and an antibacterial agent.

The mouth receives food and drink. Digestion begins in the mouth by mechanical and chemical means: ingested food is masticated and mixed with saliva and formed into a food bolus. When the food bolus is voluntarily swallowed, it will pass into the pharynx (⊃ p. 8).

Pharynx

The pharynx, also termed the throat, is funnel shaped and connects the mouth and oesophagus. The pharynx also joins the nasal cavity to the larynx, part of the respiratory system. These two areas are separated by the epiglottis, a flap of tissue that prevents food getting into the larynx and airway.

Oesophagus

The oesophagus is a muscular tube about 25 cm long and a little under 2 cm in diameter. It begins at the pharynx and ends at the stomach, at the cardiac sphincter, and is situated behind the trachea and close to the greater vessels and left atrium of the heart. It passes through the diaphragm as it travels to the stomach. The upper portion of the oesophagus is formed of striated muscle to aid the swallowing reflex (voluntary decision), while the lower two-thirds is formed of smooth muscle to move food towards the stomach by peristalsis (involuntary). The muscles of the oesophagus contract and relax to move food down to the stomach. Peristalsis is effective and food will pass to the stomach, even if the person is lying down.

The inner lining of the oesophagus is epithelial tissue, the function of which is to protect the oesophagus. Protection of the oesophagus is also aided by the mucus produced from the mucous glands.

Food and fluid are swallowed from the mouth, and pass into the pharynx, the oesophagus, and to the stomach. There are sphincters at the top and bottom of the oesophagus. The upper sphincter is closed except during the swallowing, when it opens to allow food to enter the oesophagus. The lower or cardiac sphincter prevents partially digested food from re-entering the oesophagus.

If the oesophagus is involved in the vomiting reflex, the peristaltic action is reversed.

Stomach

The stomach is a hollow, J-shaped, sac-like organ that lies within the abdomen. Its function is mechanical churning, storage, and digestion of ingested food. The stomach is joined to the oesophagus ⊃ p. 8) at the top and the duodenum (⊃ p. 10) at the bottom. The sphincters prevent unregulated flow from the stomach into the bowel (pyloric sphincter) or backflow from the stomach to the oesophagus (cardiac sphincter). The main part of the stomach is termed the body, the top is the fundus, and the lower aspect is the antrum (Fig. 1.2). The mucosa covers coarse folds (rugae) with smoother antral mucosa. The muscles of the stomach wall enable it to perform the mechanical digestion of churning and also allow for expansion. Additionally, there is chemical digestion by substances secreted into the stomach. These include hydrochloric acid (HCl) which is produced in the parietal cells, pepsin produced in the chief cells, and mucus made by the goblet cells. These gastric secretions are stimulated by either the presence of food or the anticipation of food. Once food is broken down the pyloric sphincter will allow passage of the semiliquid (chyme) into the duodenum.

Liquids generally leave the stomach faster than solids, with most meals leaving the stomach within 2–3 h.

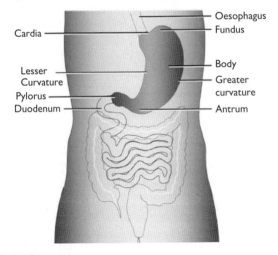

Fig. 1.2 The stomach.
Reproduced with kind permission © Burdett Institute 2008.

Small bowel, colon, rectum, and anus

Small bowel

The small bowel, also termed the small intestine, is a long, hollow tube (see Fig. 1.3). The small bowel varies in length from about 3 to 9 m, and is usually longer in ♂ than ♀. The inner surface is deeply folded and covered in villi that, in turn, are covered in microvilli, to dramatically increase the surface area and increase the absorptive ability. There are three sections to the small bowel: duodenum, jejunum, and ileum.

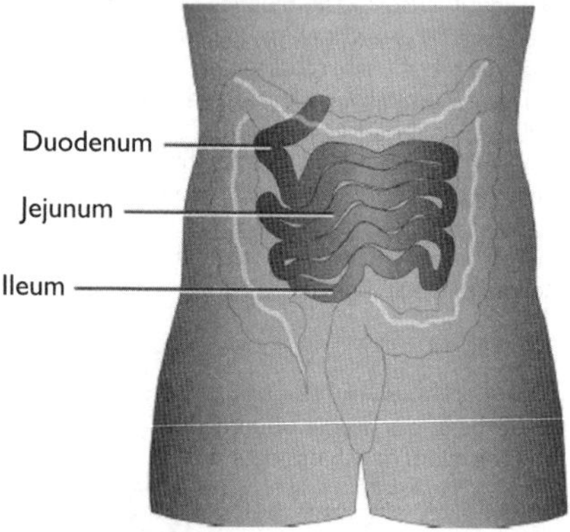

Fig. 1.3 Duodenum, jejunum, and ileum.

Reproduced with kind permission © Burdett Institute 2008.

Duodenum

The duodenum directly follows from the stomach (➲ p. 9) onto the jejunum and is a hollow tube about 20 cm long. Pancreatic juice (from the pancreas) and bile (from the gall bladder) are secreted into the duodenum. Within the duodenum, further breakdown of ingested food occurs by activity of pancreatic enzymes, specifically polypeptides (into peptides), polysaccharides (into monosaccharides and disaccharides), and triglycerides (into glycerol and free fatty acids). Biliary secretions (bile) make lipids soluble.

Jejunum

The jejunum follows the duodenum and precedes the ileum. At the brush border of the jejunum (formed by microvilli) simple sugars and amino acids are absorbed. Lipids are absorbed in the jejunum and ileum.

Ileum

The ileum varies in length from 2 to 4 m and follows the jejunum, although there is no definite demarcation between the two. It ends at the ileocaecal valve, which joins the small bowel to the caecum, and has a pH of neutral to alkaline. Digestion and absorption continue in the ileum. Bile salts are mainly absorbed from the last 100 cm of the ileum, and vitamin B_{12} from the terminal ileum (last 60 cm).

Colon

The colon is a tubular structure about 1.5 m long in the average adult. It starts at the ileocaecal valve and ends at the anal verge. The sections of the colon are caecum (attached here is the appendix), ascending colon, transverse colon, descending colon, and sigmoid colon passing to the rectum. The area of the colon that joins the ascending and transverse colon is termed the hepatic flexure as it passes near the liver. The junction joining the transverse and descending colon is termed the splenic flexure as it passes the spleen.

The inner lining of the colon differs from the small bowel as there are no villi. The colonic mucosa consists of tightly packed crypts, lined with goblet cells. The average lifespan of the colonic cells is 3–5 days. The function of the colon is:

- To concentrate faeces by removal of water and electrolytes
- Storage and evacuation of faeces
- Fermentation of undigested sugars.

Most food residue will reach the colon within 6 h.

Rectum and anus

The rectum follows the sigmoid colon and ends at the anal canal. The rectum has three sections. The rectum accepts stools, and once a level of filling is reached, it stimulates a conscious sensation. Overfilling of the rectum can result in overdistension or inflammation.

The anus is about 3–5 cm in length, and shorter in women. Proximally, the anus is similar to the colon and distally it is formed of squamous epithelium, similar to the skin. Within the anus is the dentate line, the transition zone where the colonic mucosa and the anal mucosa meet. There are three blood-filled anal (haemorrhoidal) cushions.

There are two anal sphincters, internal (IAS) and external (EAS), which circle the anus.

Anal sphincters

There are two anal sphincters—sleeves of muscle, separated by a layer of longitudinal muscle—which circle the anus: the internal (IAS) and external (EAS) anal sphincters (Fig.1.4).

Internal anal sphincter

- Smooth (involuntary) muscle, which is 2–3 mm thick (thickens with age) and 2–3 cm long
- Continuous with circular smooth muscle wall of the rectum
- Extends along the proximal (upper) two-thirds of the anal canal
- Responsible for passive retention of stools at rest (contributes 80% of resting anal pressure)
- Subject to idiopathic degeneration with age and disruption by anal trauma (e.g. following anal surgery or abuse).

External anal sphincter
- Voluntary (striated) muscle comprising three sections, which is 3–5 cm long—longer in ♂ than ♀
- Inserts into the pelvic floor (puborectalis) proximally and extends to the subcutaneous level distally
- ♀ have a natural 'defect' in the upper anterior EAS, above the level where the puborectalis meets the EAS
- Responsible for resisting defaecation during the recto-anal inhibitory reflex (RAIR)—functions as the 'brakes' for defaecation, allowing voluntary retention of stool
- Subject to trauma—especially during difficult childbirth.

Longitudinal anal sphincter muscle

The longitudinal anal sphincter muscle is found between the IAS and EAS and is continuous with the outer longitudinal muscle of the gut wall and is more prominent in ♂ than ♀. Its function is unclear, but the muscle probably 'splints' the anus during defaecation to enable shortening of the sphincter and facilitate stool expulsion.

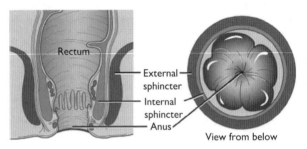

Rectum

External sphincter

Internal sphincter

Anus

View from below

Fig. 1.4 Rectum, anus, and anal sphincters.
Reproduced with kind permission © Burdett Institute 2008.

Accessory organs

Pancreas

The pancreas is situated below the stomach, with one end by the spleen and the other end at the duodenum. The pancreas is a large gland about 12 cm long and 25 mm in depth, formed of the body, head, and tail. The central pancreatic duct passes through the middle of the pancreas and joins the common bile duct, and subsequently opens into the duodenum at the ampulla of Vater. There are about 1.5 litres of pancreatic juices secreted each day into the duodenum.

The pancreas has both exocrine and endocrine functions.

Endocrine function

The pancreas secretes two hormones, insulin and glucagon from the islets of Langerhans, into the blood stream to control blood sugar levels. Insulin is secreted when blood glucose levels increase, whereas glucagon is secreted in response to hypoglycaemia. Epinephrine (another hormone) also affects pancreatic secretion.

Exocrine function

The pancreas produces digestive enzymes that are synthesized and secreted. Secretion is stimulated by hormonal signals, when food enters the duodenum from the stomach. These clear, colourless secretions (about 1.5 litres daily) are rich in enzymes and contain bicarbonate that helps neutralize the acidic chyme, which enters the duodenum from the stomach. Additionally, the enzymes digest fat (pancreatic lipase), proteins (trypsin and chymotrypsin), and carbohydrates (amylase). Pancreatic juice is highly irritant to the skin.

Gall bladder

The gall bladder (Fig. 1.5) is a small pear-shaped sac, about 3 cm by 7 cm, and can contain about 30–50 ml of bile. The three parts of the gall bladder are the fundus, body, and neck. The gall bladder inner surface is enlarged by the presence of the rugae (folds) and it is covered in columnar epithelium and a layer of smooth muscle. The gall bladder is situated beneath the liver and is connected to the cystic duct. The cystic duct joins the hepatic ducts from the liver and become the common bile duct which leads to the duodenum.

The function of the gall bladder is to store and concentrate (up to 10-fold) the bile, produced by the liver. Secretion of the bile occurs by contraction of the smooth muscle of the gall bladder wall, into the common bile duct and the duodenum.

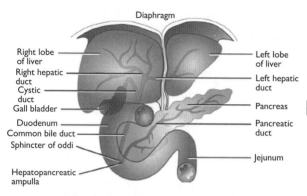

Fig. 1.5 Structure of the biliary system.
Reproduced with kind permission © Burdett Institute 2008.

Liver

The liver is a large (1–2 kg), smooth, convex organ covered in a fibrous capsule, and is smaller in ♀ than ♂. The liver is situated in the right upper quadrant of the abdominal cavity, under the diaphragm, within the rib cage (protection). The liver moves during respiration. The liver has eight segments and a left and right lobe (Fig.1.6). The tissue can regenerate up to two-thirds of its weight, if needed following damage.

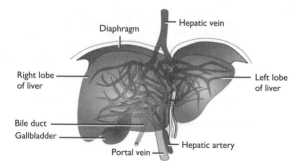

Fig. 1.6 Liver structures.
Reproduced with kind permission © Burdett Institute 2008.

The portal circulation enables nutrients and other substances that are absorbed through the gut to pass via the liver into the systemic circulation. The portal veins carry 70% of the nutrient-rich blood supply to the liver, directly from the small intestine. The three hepatic veins drain into the vena cava. The hepatic artery carries 30% of the blood supply to the liver and 25% of the cardiac output goes to the liver.

There are many functions of the liver but the main one is to process the nutrients absorbed from the small intestine. Additionally:

- Bile is produced and excreted to digest fats
- Excretion of bilirubin and cholesterol
- Metabolism of carbohydrates, proteins, and fats
- Synthesis of plasma proteins, such as albumin and clotting factors
- Glucose homeostasis—conversion of blood glucose to glycogen for storage and back to glucose when energy is needed. This maintains a stable blood glucose
- Metabolism of drugs and hormones—oxidation (change due to addition of oxygen), conjugation, and elimination through secretion of bile or via the kidneys
- Detoxification of micro-organisms and toxic substances that have been absorbed from the gut to stop transfer to the general blood circulation
- Storage of minerals, vitamin B_{12}, and the fat-soluble vitamins A, D, E, and K
- Manufacture of substances needed for blood coagulation and other proteins
- Destruction of worn-out red blood cells.

Bile

Bile is produced by the liver; up to a litre daily is synthesized. Bile is 97% water plus bile salts (made from cholesterol in the liver), bile pigment, mostly bilirubin (breakdown product of red blood cells), and excess cholesterol excreted from the body. The pH of bile is about 7.6–8.0. Bile is a green-brown, viscous liquid. It does not contain digestive enzymes but its function is to emulsify fats and enable absorption of fat-soluble vitamins and iron. Additionally, it deodorizes faeces and colours them brown.

Bile is transferred via the hepatic ducts to the common hepatic duct: there are over 2 km of bile ducts within the liver. Bile is released in response to food, specifically fat, being released from the stomach into the duodenum. The common hepatic duct joins with pancreatic duct at the ampulla of Vater to empty into the duodenum via the sphincter of Oddi.

Mouth, pharynx, oesophagus, and stomach

Achalasia

Achalasia is a rare condition of the muscles of the oesophagus. The muscles in the oesophagus fail to open adequately to enable passage from the oesophagus into the stomach.

Symptoms

Not everyone who has achalasia will have symptoms, but most will report food becoming stuck in the oesophagus and regurgitation or dysphagia (⊃ p. 24). Other symptoms include choking, coughing, symptoms associated with gastro-oesophageal reflux disease (GORD) (⊃ pp. 36–7), weight loss, and drooling. Symptoms gradually worsen, often over several years.

Causes

The cause is not totally understood but may be due to nerve damage in the oesophagus. Alternatively, achalasia may be the result of a viral infection or an autoimmune disease. Rarely, it may be familial.

Investigations

- Chest X-rays
- Manometry (⊃ p. 223)
- Barium swallow (⊃ p. 218)
- Oesophageal gastroduodenoscopy(⊃ p. 250).

Treatment

There is no cure for achalasia. Treatment is to relieve symptoms and improve swallowing. Treatment includes:
- Medication, such as calcium channel blockers (⊃ p. 416), neurotoxins (⊃ p. 424) and vasodilators
- Endoscopic balloon dilation of the cardiac sphincter—repeated dilation may be necessary
- Surgery (Heller's myotomy) to cut the muscle fibres of the cardiac sphincter
- Rarely a resection of part of the oesophagus is necessary.

Side effects

The side effects of surgery and balloon dilation include reflux (⊃ pp. 36–7) and heartburn. Initially there may be chest pain, resolved by drinking cold water.

Barrett's oesophagus

Barrett's oesophagus can occur as a result of repeated GORD (➲ pp. 36–7) that results in cellular changes.

Symptoms

Repeated heartburn, GORD (➲ pp. 36–7), and dyspepsia (➲ pp. 22–3), but the disease can be symptom-free.

Incidence

Fewer than 1 in 100 people in the UK have Barrett's oesophagus. About 1 in 10 people with GORD will develop Barrett's oesophagus. More ♂ are affected than ♀ and the disease can occur at any age, but is more common in people aged over 50 years.

Causes

GORD can result in acidic damage and cause changes to the cells lining the oesophagus. There are greater risks of reflux for people who are:
• Overweight
• Smokers
• Drink too much alcohol
• Eat spicy foods
• Eat fatty foods
• Have a hiatus hernia (➲ p. 44).

Treatment

Treatment aims to reduce reflux and control symptoms. Treatment can include medication to control GORD, such as antacids (➲ p. 407), or Halo® 360 ablation procedure, surgery—fundoplication. The Halo® 360 ablation procedure is an endoscopic procedure, whereby the entire Barrett's oesophagus is treated by radiofrequency energy to remove the lining of the oesophagus. Endoscopic mucosal resection (EMR) is used to remove the affected area and radiofrequency ablation (RFA) is used to destroy abnormal cells. Surgery may be used to resect the affected part of the oesophagus.

Prevention

Lifestyle changes can reduce acid reflux, for example losing weight, stopping smoking, drinking less alcohol, eating smaller, regular meals, and avoiding foods that give symptoms, and not eating within 3 h of sleep.

Prognosis

Potentially over a period of time (10–20 years) about 1 in 10–20 people with Barrett's oesophagus will develop oesophageal cancer; thus, the disease is termed precancerous and requires surveillance.

Further reading

NICE (2018). Barrett's oesophagus overview. https://pathways.nice.org.uk/pathways/barretts-oesophagus (Accessed 14/10/2018).

Cleft lip and palate

The meaning of cleft is a gap or split, in this condition, in the upper lip and/or the palate, present from birth. A cleft lip may affect one or both sides. The length of the cleft can be small or reach the nose. A cleft palate may be a small opening at the back of the mouth or run to the front.

A cleft lip or palate occurs in the womb when the upper lip and/or palate fail to fuse during development. It is usually diagnosed on the mid-pregnancy anomaly scan, although it can be difficult to detect on a routine ultrasound scan. If a cleft lip and/or palate are unidentified prior to birth, it is normally picked up within days of birth and may be linked with other birth defects.

Incidence

Cleft lip and palate is the most common facial defect in the UK: it affects about one baby in every 700 born. The incidence of a parent who is born with a cleft lip or palate having a child with a cleft lip or plate is about 5% for each child.

Problems

- Difficulty in feeding as it is not possible to make a good seal with the mouth on the breast or bottle
- Hearing problems—some babies encounter more ear infections or glue ear
- Dental problems—teeth develop incorrectly and can be at a higher risk of tooth decay
- Speech problems—if the cleft palate is not repaired speech can be unclear or nasal-sounding as the child grows older.

Causes

The exact reason for a cleft lip and palate are unknown but is associated with:
- Genetics
- Obesity, smoking, drinking, or a lack of folic acid during pregnancy
- Antiepileptic medications and steroids (➲ p. 428) during early pregnancy may increase the incidence of the baby having a cleft lip and palate.

Treatment

Surgical repair at a specialist centre will generally improve the problems listed. In addition to speech and language therapy, surgery is usually performed at about 3–6 months-old for a cleft lip and a cleft palate at 6–12 months.

If feeding is a problem, there are specifically designed bottles or different methods of positioning the baby to assist breast feeding.

Glue ear can be treated by grommets to drain the fluid.

Careful oral hygiene is necessary. Braces may be necessary to treat problems with the teeth.

Prognosis

The majority of babies born with a cleft lip or palate will have a normal life.

Dumping syndrome

Dumping syndrome occurs when rapid gastric emptying occurs, moving food into the next part of the gastro-intestinal (GI) tract, i.e. the duodenum (➔ p. 10). This means that the jejunum fills too quickly with undigested food from the stomach. Dumping syndrome can be defined as 'early dumping', occurring within 30 min of eating. Alternatively, 'late dumping' occurs about 2–3 h after eating. Many patients have both forms of the syndrome.

Symptoms

- Nausea
- Vomiting
- Bloating
- Cramp
- Diarrhoea
- Sweating
- Dizziness
- Fatigue
- Palpitations.

Causes

Dumping syndrome occurs following some types of gastric surgery, such as a gastrectomy and gastric bypass surgery. Dumping syndrome is also seen in patients with gastrin-secreting tumours in the pancreas. Early dumping occurs as a result of rapid hypertonic load in the small intestine. Late dumping occurs as a result of rapid carbohydrate absorption, which stimulates the pancreas to release excessive amounts of insulin into the bloodstream, causing hypoglycaemia.

Treatment

It is important for the nurse to provide advice and support to patients as symptoms can be frightening. Dietary advice includes:

- Eating smaller, more frequent meals
- ↓carbohydrate intake (especially simple carbohydrates)
- ↑ fibre intake
- Drink before or after meals, rather than during meals.

In hospital and at home consider enabling consumption of snacks between meals. Refer to a dietitian for specific advice. Surgical revision is an option if conservative treatment fails.

Dyspepsia

Dyspepsia is more commonly termed indigestion. Dyspepsia is not usually serious and is generally self-treated.

Symptoms

Dyspepsia is a collection of symptoms that occur after eating and/or drinking and can include:
- Feeling nauseous
- Belching
- Passing flatus
- Burning feeling in the chest (heartburn)
- Food or fluid returning up to the mouth
- Bloating.

Causes

Dyspepsia occurs when the stomach or oesophageal lining is irritated by the stomach acids. Dyspepsia can be a functional disorder without pathology, despite symptoms, and may be the result of smoking, medication, or alcohol. It can occur in the latter stages of pregnancy due to hormonal changes and the baby pressing on the stomach. Other causes can include:
- Ulcers—gastric (➔ pp. 30–1) or duodenal
- Gastric cancer (➔ pp. 26–7)
- Oesophagitis (➔ p. 56)
- Gastritis (➔ pp. 32–3)
- Duodenitis
- Cholelithiasis
- Hiatus hernia (➔ p. 44)
- GORD (➔ pp. 36–7)
- Helicobacter pylori infections (➔ p. 42).

Treatment

There are many simple things that can be tried to reduce the effects of dyspepsia. This can include:
- Reducing caffeine such as tea, coffee, and/or cola
- Reducing alcohol consumption
- Stopping smoking
- Sleeping more upright to prevent reflux
- Losing weight
- Stopping rich, spicy, and/or fatty foods
- Not eating within 4 h of sleeping
- Stopping medications such as ibuprofen (➔ p. 406) or aspirin (➔ p. 406).

Taking medication can also reduce or stop symptoms. Dyspepsia can be reduced by taking antacids (➔ p. 407).

It might be necessary to seek help from a healthcare professional for urgent investigation, if:
- Symptoms persist
- There is pain
- Aged 55 years or more
- There is unintentional weight loss

- There is also dysphagia
- There is recurrent vomiting
- There is iron-deficiency anaemia
- Bleeding is noted in vomit or stool.

Further reading

NICE (2018). Managing uninvestigated dyspepsia in adults. https://pathways.nice.org.uk/pathways/
    dyspepsia-and-gastro-oesophageal-reflux-disease/helicobacter-pylori-testing-and-eradication-in-
    adults#path=view%3A/pathways/dyspepsia-and-gastro-oesophageal-reflux-disease/managing-
    uninvestigated-dyspepsia-in-adults.xml&content=view-index (Accessed 14/10/2018).
NICE (2018). Managing functional dyspepsia in adults https://pathways.nice.org.uk/pathways/
    dyspepsia-and-gastro-oesophageal-reflux-disease/helicobacter-pylori-testing-and-eradication-in-
    adults#path=view%3A/pathways/dyspepsia-and-gastro-oesophageal-reflux-disease/managing-
    functional-dyspepsia-in-adults.xml&content=view-index (Accessed 14/10/2018).

Dysphagia

Difficulty in swallowing is termed dysphagia: this can mean different things. For some people there is a total inability to swallow; others cannot swallow liquids; and for some it can be certain foods that are difficult to swallow.

Symptoms

Signs of dysphagia include:
- Coughing, choking, or gurgling voice when eating and/or drinking
- Bringing up food, possibly through the nose
- Feeling that food is stuck in the throat
- Constant saliva production.

Dysphagia can lead to weight loss due to problems eating. It may also result in recurrent chest infections as a result of aspiration.

Causes

Dysphagia is a symptom of an underlying disease, including:
- Stroke
- Head injury
- Multiple sclerosis
- Dementia
- Malignancy—mouth (**Ɔ** p. 46), pharynx, oesophagus (**Ɔ** p. 50)
- Stricture—malignant or benign in the oesophagus
- Pharyngeal pouch
- Oesophagitis
- Oesophageal candidiasis
- Extrinsic pressure from lung cancer or aortic aneurysm
- Achalasia (**Ɔ** p. 18)
- Oesophageal spasm (**Ɔ** p. 54)
- GORD (**Ɔ** pp. 36–7).

Incidence

The incidence is not fully understood but seems to occur with at least half of cases following a stroke.

Treatment

Treatment will vary depending on the cause of the dysphagia and the type of symptoms reported; a cure may not be possible. Treatment includes:
- Thickening fluids
- Softer foods
- Speech and language therapy
- Feed via a nasogastric tube or percutaneous endoscopic gastrostomy tube
- Strictures—may be dilated or stented
- Medications such as proton pump inhibitors (PPIs) (**Ɔ** p. 427) can be used for dysphagia (**Ɔ** p. 24) to improve symptoms of indigestion caused by the strictured or scarred oesophagus. Botox (**Ɔ** p. 424) can be used to treat achalasia (**Ɔ** p. 18) to paralyse the tightened muscles of the oesophagus.

Gastric cancer

There are several different types of gastric cancer. Most (95%) develop in the cells that line the stomach and are adenocarcinomas. Less common types of stomach cancer include:
- Gastric lymphoma—developing in the lymphatic tissue
- Gastrointestinal stromal tumours (GISTs)—developing in the muscle or connective tissue of the stomach wall.

Incidence

Incidence ↓ worldwide. Gastric cancer is a fairly uncommon type of cancer but more than 6,000 people are diagnosed and over 4,000 people die each year in the UK.

Symptoms

Initial symptoms of gastric cancer are easy to mistake for other less serious conditions and thus are easily missed. Initial symptoms include:
- Persistent heartburn
- Trapped wind
- Frequent belching
- Feeling bloated after meals
- Abdominal pain
- Dyspepsia.

Symptoms of advanced gastric cancer can include:
- Melaena
- Iron-deficiency anaemia
- Blood in the stool
- Loss of appetite
- Unintentional weight loss.

Causes

There are a number of risk factors associated with gastric cancer:
- Being male
- Being over 55 years old
- Smoking
- Chronic gastritis (→ pp. 32–3)
- H. pylori (→ p. 42)
- Chronic gastric ulcers (→ pp. 30–1)
- Previous gastric surgery.
- Gastric adenomatous polyps
- Family history of gastric cancer
- Low socio-economic status
- Diets diet low in fibre
- Diets high in processed food, salt, pickled foods, smoked foods, or red meat
- Epstein Barr virus.

Investigations

To confirm the diagnosis:
- Upper GI endoscopy with biopsies
- Barium meal.

To assess suitability for surgery:
- Computed tomography (CT) scan
- Possibly a laparoscopy.

Treatment

Treatment is coordinated by a specialist multidisciplinary team, including a specialist nurse and dietitian. Early and long-term support includes psychosocial support and symptom control, and it is essential to ensure adequate nutrition.

Early disease can be cured with a gastrectomy or partial gastrectomy. After a gastrectomy, dietitians are required as the altered anatomy affects nutritional intake: small frequent meals are advocated. Postoperative management also includes prevention, identification, and management of dumping syndrome (➔ p. 21).

Palliative surgery is indicated for obstruction, pain, and excessive bleeding. Additionally, chemotherapy or radiotherapy can be used as adjunct therapy. Drugs, such as PPIs (➔ p. 427) and H_2 receptor antagonists (➔ p. 420) are effective for pain relief.

Prognosis

Prognosis for stomach cancer depends on factors such as age, general health, and any spread of the cancer. As stomach cancer is frequently diagnosed in the later stages, the prognosis is often poor.

Gastric polyps

Gastric polyps are a mass of cells that form on the stomach lining. Gastric polyps are often an incidental finding on endoscopy. The most common polyps (70%) are hyperplastic (regenerative) and of no consequence. Adenomatous polyps in the stomach are unusual but have malignant potential.

Symptoms

The majority of patients are asymptomatic. Occasionally polyps bleed, presenting as haematemesis (➲ p. 43) or melaena. Rarely, large pedunculated polyps can obstruct the pylorus, leading to nausea, abdominal bloating, and vomiting (± projectile).

Investigation

Upper GI endoscopy (➲ p. 250) is indicated, if symptoms exist, to elicit the cause. Histological assessment of all polyps is essential because early gastric cancers can look insignificant.

Treatment

Removal or resection of adenomatous polyps is essential. Otherwise, treatment is related to symptomology and may include a polypectomy (polyp removal). Also provide reassurance regarding natural history and progression.

Gastric ulcers

Gastric ulcers, also known as stomach ulcers or peptic ulcers, are open sores that develop on the lining of the stomach.

Symptoms

Some patients might be asymptomatic, if the ulcer is drug-induced or an iron-deficiency ulcer. Other symptoms include:
* Pain—related to meals and relieved by antacids; described as a burning or gnawing pain in the centre of the abdomen
* Nausea and vomiting
* Weight loss
* Bleeding—haematemesis (➲ p. 43) and melaena
* Perforation—presents in one-third of patients
* Indigestion.

Incidence

Gastric ulcers are less common than duodenal ulcers. Identification and eradication of *H. pylori* has led to a sharp ↓ in acute hospital admissions from ulcer disease.

Causes

Gastric ulcers more common in the people aged over 60 and men. *H. pylori* infection causes 70–80% of gastric ulcers (➲ pp. 30–1). Other risk factors include:
* Non-steroidal anti-inflammatory drugs (NSAIDs) (➲ p. 406)
* Corticosteroids (➲ p. 428)
* Chronic antral gastritis (➲ pp. 32–3)
* Smoking
* Heavy alcohol use
* Environmental stress (e.g. intensive care setting or burns).

There is little evidence that stress or certain foods might cause stomach ulcers.

Investigations

An upper GI endoscopy is needed to identify the ulcer and enable accurate histological assessment. The endoscopy is repeated 8 weeks after treatment to confirm healing or if there is a symptom relapse. A barium meal will show the ulcer crater, but endoscopic assessment is still required.

Carcinoma should be excluded in the first instance and suspected if there is a failure of the ulcer to heal despite compliance with treatment.

Treatment

- Stop NSAIDs (➔ p. 406)
- Treat the ulcer—PPI (➔ p. 427)
- Eradication therapy for *H. pylori* if present (➔ p. 42)
- Stop smoking
- ↓ alcohol intake
- Dietary advice—avoid foods exacerbating symptoms, ensure a good nutritional intake, and take regular meals.

Urgent medical assistance is needed if there is blood in the vomit, melaena, or the sharp pain worsens.

Further reading

NICE (2018). Managing peptic ulcer disease in adults https://pathways.nice.org.uk/pathways/
dyspepsia-and-gastro-oesophageal-reflux-disease/helicobacter-pylori-testing-and-eradication-in-
adults#path=view%3A/pathways/dyspepsia-and-gastro-oesophageal-reflux-disease/managing-
peptic-ulcer-disease-in-adults.xml&content=view-index (Accessed 14/10/2018).

Gastritis

Gastritis is an inflammation of the gastric mucosa, as a response to injury, and is usually classified as 'acute' or 'chronic'. Gastritis can be isolated to one area of the stomach, such as the antrum, body, or fundus, or affect all of the stomach—'pan' (total) gastritis.

Symptoms

Gastritis is often asymptomatic, but might present with symptoms of:
- Dyspepsia (➲ pp. 22–3)
- Retching
- Haematemesis (erosive gastritis) (➲ p. 43)
- Chronic dull pain
- Early satiety (fullness)
- Anorexia.

Chronic inflammation (in the presence of intestinal metaplasia) could precede early gastric cancer but is not in itself a pre-malignant condition.

Causes

- Drugs (mainly NSAIDs)
- Excessive alcohol
- Cocaine usage
- Severe stress (e.g. major surgery, trauma, or burns)
- Infection (e.g. H. pylori)
- Post-gastrectomy (bile reflux: alkaline toxicity)
- Crohn's disease (rare)
- HIV/AIDS
- Parasitic infection
- Connective tissue disorders
- Autoimmune atrophic (antibodies attack healthy mucosa, with resultant gradual thinning of mucosa and destruction of glands). Can lead to interference with production of vitamin B_{12} and pernicious anaemia
- Chronic inflammation is common in developing countries or individuals of low socio-economic status (association with H. pylori)
- Prevalence ↑ with age.

Investigation

- A stool test—to exclude infection
- A breath test (➲ p. 219)—to exclude H. pylori
- Upper GI endoscopy (➲ p. 250)—to exclude other causes
- Histology—confirms inflammation, activity, atrophy, intestinal metaplasia, and H. pylori.

Treatment

Treatment is not required if asymptomatic. If symptomatic, treat the underlying cause. Treatment can be over-the-counter medication, such as antacids (→ p. 407) to neutralize acid within the stomach.

- Avoid risk factors (e.g. NSAIDs (→ p. 406) and alcohol)
- *H. pylori* eradication and appropriate drug treatment (→ p. 42)
- Medications include antacids (→ p. 407), H_2 receptor antagonists (→ p. 420), and PPIs (→ p. 427)
- Bile reflux post-gastrectomy: sucralfate 1 g four times a day
- Rarely Roux-en-Y surgery is needed.

Patients should be advised to contact a healthcare professional if symptoms last a week or more, or there is blood in the vomit or faeces. Advice to relieve symptoms can include:

- Eating smaller, more frequent meals
- Avoiding irritating foods such as spicy, acidic, or fried foods
- Avoiding or cutting down on alcohol.

Gastroenteritis

Gastroenteritis is a very common condition, commonly termed food poisoning, gastric flu, or stomach flu. Food poisoning is a notifiable disease in the UK.

Symptoms

Symptoms usually commence within a few days of eating infected food and can be acute in their onset and short in duration. Symptoms include:
- Nausea and vomiting
- Diarrhoea
- Abdominal cramps
- Abdominal pain
- Pyrexia of 38°C or more
- Feeling generally unwell, feeling tired, or having aches and chills.

Causes

The cause of gastroenteritis is ingestion of bacteria, viruses, or toxins. In about half of cases, no specific cause is found. Patient groups that are more susceptible to gastroenteritis are the elderly or very young, people who are immunocompromised, or who have no spleen. It should be noted that excessive alcohol intake can mimic infective causes.

Assessment

Assess for:
- Recent history of travel
- Eating known susceptible food types (e.g. seafood, chicken, reheated food, or take-aways)
- Excessive antibiotic use
- More than one person affected (e.g. families, schools, or institutions)
- History of swimming or other water sports
- Bloody diarrhoea
- Aching joints
- Headaches.

Investigation

A stool specimen should be sent for microscopy, culture, and sensitivity (MC&S), and *Clostridium difficile* toxin.

If an outbreak is suspected (e.g. in a school), food sample analysis is recommended.

Gastroenteritis when uncomplicated and quickly resolved might not need investigation.

If diarrhoea is persistent or is associated with bleeding, refer to a gastroenterologist for endoscopic assessment.

Treatment

Gastroenteritis is rarely serious and symptoms will usually resolve within a week, without the need for hospitalization. However, people who are affected should not attend work or school until asymptomatic for 48 h. Treatment is dependent on the cause. Antidiarrhoeal medication (⊃ p. 411) and antiemetic agents (⊃ p. 412) should be used with caution if symptom control is required, as they could mask other conditions.

In-patients should be isolated until an infective cause is excluded.

Ensure adequate fluid intake—consider oral rehydration fluids if diarrhoea is severe and intravenous (IV) fluids if the patient is dehydrated.

Prevention

The nurse can provide patient education on basic hygiene, such as hand-washing. Advice can include food preparation to ensure that food is:
• Cooked or reheated thoroughly
• Stored correctly
• Not left 'out' for too long
• Not touched by people without washing their hands
• Not eaten after the 'use by' date

Furthermore, educate patients about travel: that when abroad to be cautious of ice cubes and salads and consider drinking bottled water and peeling fruit.

Gastro-oesophageal reflux disease

Gastro-oesophageal reflux disease, also GORD or GERD, is repeated episodes of acid reflux, where stomach acid enters the oesophagus and damages its lining.

Symptoms

There are two main symptoms heartburn (a retrosternal burning sensation) and an unpleasant sour taste in the mouth. Additional symptoms include:
- Recurrent hiccup
- Belching
- Regurgitation of bile or food
- Excessive salivation
- Pain on swallowing (odynophagia)
- Dysphagia
- Chest pain
- Hoarse voice
- Halitosis
- Bloating
- Nausea

Symptoms can be exacerbated by:
- Eating
- Lying down
- Bending forward
- Hiatus hernia (**⊃** p. 44)
- Obesity
- Smoking
- Alcohol
- Tight clothing
- Large meals, especially late at night
- Pregnancy
- *H. pylori*
- Medications such as tricyclic antidepressants (**⊃** p. 410), nitrates (**⊃** p. 425), anticholinergics (**⊃** p. 409), and bisphosphonates.

Causes

The cause of acid reflux is due to a dysfunctional lower oesophageal sphincter which allows back flow of acid into the oesophagus.

Treatment

Treatment for GORD can include medication related to the symptoms. The nurses can advise that medication can be used as required rather than continually once symptoms are controlled. The nurse can advise patients to:
- Avoid smoking
- Lose weight
- Eat small, frequent meals
- Raise the bed head
- Avoid food or drink that triggers symptoms
- Not eat within 4 h of sleeping
- Avoid tight-waisted clothes
- Avoid excessive alcohol intake.

If symptoms continue for 3 or more weeks or are associated with unintentional weight loss or dysphagia, it may be advisable to see advice rather than treatments.

In very severe cases, surgery may be considered, such as fundoplication.

Children

Children (up to two years old) should be assessed by a healthcare professional, such as a paediatrician if they present with:

- Haematemesis
- Melaena
- Dysphagia.

Further reading

NICE (2018). Managing gastro-oesophageal reflux disease in adults. https://pathways.nice.org.uk/pathways/dyspepsia-and-gastro-oesophageal-reflux-disease/helicobacter-pylori-testing-and-eradication-in-adults#path=view%3A/pathways/dyspepsia-and-gastro-oesophageal-reflux-disease/managing-gastro-oesophageal-reflux-disease-in-adults.xml&content=view-index (Accessed 14/10/2018).

NICE (2019). GORD in children. https://cks.nice.org.uk/gord-in-children (Accessed 14/10/2018).

Gastroparesis

Gastroparesis is a chronic condition where the stomach cannot empty itself properly, with the passage of food being slower than usual.

Symptoms

Symptoms can be mild to severe, tend to be intermittent and include:
- Early satiety (fullness)
- Feeling sick (nausea) and vomiting may lead to dehydration
- Loss of appetite
- Weight loss
- Malnutrition
- Bloating
- Abdominal pain or discomfort
- GORD
- Unpredictable blood sugars in people with diabetes.

Causes

Often there is no obvious cause; it is then termed idiopathic gastroparesis. Gastroparesis can be the result of problems with nerves and muscles controlling the emptying of the stomach. Other causes include:
- Poorly controlled diabetes
- Bariatric surgery
- Gastrectomy
- Medication such as opioids (→ p. 406) and antidepressants (→ p. 410)
- Scleroderma
- Parkinson's disease
- Amyloidosis.

Investigations

- Barium X-ray
- Gastric emptying scan using scintigraphy: food containing a very small amount of a radioactive substance is ingested with a subsequent scan
- Capsule endoscopy (→ p. 245)
- Endoscopy (→ p. 236).

Treatment

There is no cure for gastroparesis but symptoms can be reduced/resolved with dietary changes such as:
- Eating small, frequent meals
- Eating soft and liquid foods that are easier to digest
- Chewing food well before swallowing
- Drinking non-fizzy liquids with meals
- Avoiding or reducing certain foods such as high-fibre and foods high in fat.

Other treatments include:
- Gastroelectrical stimulation—surgical implantation of a battery-operated device, to deliver electrical impulses to stimulate the muscles involved in controlling the passage of food through the stomach
- Botulinum toxin (→ p. 424) can be injected into the pyloric sphincter (→ p. 9) through an endoscope, to relax the valve
- Medications that may be prescribed to help improve symptoms include antiemetics (→ p. 412) and antibiotics (→ p. 408).

It might be necessary to find alternative feeding methods, such as:
• A nasojejunal tube (temporary feeding tube)
• A feeding jejunostomy inserted through the abdominal wall (permanent feeding tube)
• Parenteral nutrition
• Some people benefit from a gastroenterostomy or gastrojejunostomy to release gas and relieve bloating).

Advice that should be provided to diabetics is to check blood glucose levels frequently after eating.

Further reading

NICE (2014) Gastroelectrical stimulation for gastroparesis. https://www.nice.org.uk/Guidance/IPG489 (Accessed 20/7/2020).

Halitosis

Halitosis is malodourous breath.

Cause

The usual cause of halitosis is poor oral hygiene, resulting in a build-up of bacteria in the mouth that produce toxins.

If bad breath persists it might also be a sign of gum disease or tooth decay, although halitosis can simply be a result of strong foods such as garlic. Smoking and alcohol can also cause bad breath, as can being ill or some medication. Alternatively, crash diets can lead to ketones being formed, which can then be smelt on the breath.

Incidence

It is thought that about a quarter of people regularly have halitosis.

Treatment

Improving oral hygiene will cure and prevent bad breath in most cases. This should include brushing teeth and gums, flossing, and cleaning the tongue.

Hand, foot, and mouth disease

Hand, foot, and mouth disease is a common childhood illness, but it may also affect adults. The disease is usually self-limiting and will resolve within 7–10 days. This disease is not related to foot and mouth (found in farm animals). Hand, foot, and mouth disease is contagious, mainly within the first 5 days of symptoms.

Symptoms

The initial symptoms of hand, foot and mouth disease include:
- Sore throat
- Pyrexia above 38°C
- Not wanting to eat.

Followed a few days later with:
- Ulcers—mouth and tongue
- Rash.

These red spots develop into blisters on the hands and feet, painful with grey centres. Symptoms are usually worse in adults than children.

Treatment

There is no treatment. To help resolve symptoms advise:
- Drinking to avoid dehydration
- Avoiding acidic drinks
- Eating soft food
- Avoiding hot food and drinks
- Avoiding spicy food
- Analgesia to ease sore mouth, throat, or ulcers

Prevention

Hand, foot, and mouth disease is contagious: easily passed on through coughs, sneezes, and faeces. Thus, hand washing and careful toileting is essential and washing soiled clothes on a hot wash.

Helicobacter pylori (H. pylori)

Helicobacter pylori, more commonly termed *H. pylori*, are spiral bacteria that colonize the stomach, mainly in the antrum. It is the causal agent in 90–95% of duodenal ulcers and 70–80% of gastric ulcers. *H. pylori* is listed as a grade 1 carcinogen, because gastric cancer can occur if infection leads to gastritis, atrophy, and metaplasia.

Symptoms

Various strains of *H. pylori* exist; host factors and the bacterial strain determine the outcome of infection (the patient could remain asymptomatic). Symptoms include:

- Aching or burning abdominal pain; worse when hungry
- Nausea
- Frequent belching
- Bloating
- Anorexia
- Unintentional weight loss.

Causes

H. pylori is strongly linked to social deprivation in childhood and is higher in insanitary overcrowded conditions.

Investigations

- Blood tests to detect antibodies via GP
- Simple colorimetric (CLO) test is performed on endoscopic biopsies
- Breath test is used to confirm the success of treatment
- Carbon-13 urea breath test or stool antigen test.

Treatment

Eradication therapy is combined therapy with a PPI (→ p. 427) and a combination of antibiotics (→ p. 408). Most standard regimens are successful in up to 90% of cases. Successful eradication should be confirmed (by urease breath test) if symptoms are continued or recurrent in ulceration with history of bleeding.

Further reading

NICE (2018). *Helicobacter pylori* testing and eradication in adults. https://pathways.nice.org.uk/ pathways/dyspepsia-and-gastro-oesophageal-reflux-disease/helicobacter-pylori-testing-and-eradication-in-adults (Accessed 14/10/2018).

Haematemesis

Haematemesis is vomiting of fresh or altered (coffee-ground) blood. It is the commonest of gastroenterology emergencies. There is an increased risk with age.

Causes

- Peptic (gastric or duodenal) ulcers (➋ p. 30–1)
- NSAIDs (➋ p. 406)
- Oesophageal and gastric varices (➋ p. 443)
- Mallory–Weiss tear (➋ p. 45)
- Oesophagitis (➋ p. 56)
- Gastric cancer (➋ p. 26–7)
- Angiodysplasia.

Assessment

Assess cause and severity. Obtain history, including drug history especially use of NSAIDs (➋ p. 406) and alcohol use. Observe vomitus. This may need to be completed after the initial treatment.

Assess the risk of re-bleed and death, using the Rockall risk score.

Investigation

Undertake an oesophageal gastroduodenoscopy (OGD) to establish the site of bleeding.

Treatment

Initial treatment is resuscitation and fluid replacement.

Use endoscopic therapy to stop bleeding or medication. Patients require reassurance. If vomiting and/or haematemesis are prolonged, patient needs observation and the quantity and consistency of the vomitus monitoring as well as monitoring of vital signs. If there is severe bleeding or re-bleeding surgery may be indicated. The risk of bleeding can be predicted using the Rockall risk scoring system.

Prevention

Stop NSAIDs (➋ p. 406).

Further reading

Vreeburg EM, Terwee CB, Snel P, et al. (1999). Validation of the Rockall risk scoring system in upper gastrointestinal bleeding. *Gut* 44: 331–5.

Hiatus hernia

A hiatus hernia is herniation of the proximal stomach through the diaphragm into the thorax. The hernia is sliding in the majority of cases (80%), where the gastro-oesophageal junction moves up into the chest (Fig. 2.1). It is otherwise termed rolling, with the gastro-oesophageal junction remaining in the abdomen with a portion of the stomach herniating into the chest.

Symptoms

For half of people symptoms are similar to GORD.

Incidence

A hiatus hernia is common, more so in obesity.

Investigations

Barium swallow is used to ascertain the type and size of the hiatus hernia. Often diagnosed when investigating symptoms of GORD and dyspepsia (➲ p. 22–3).

Treatment

Treatment is used for symptom management. Surgery is only indicated if symptoms are severe and are uncontrolled with conservative treatment and there is a risk of strangulation. Education and reassurance are necessary on lifestyle changes to manage reflux symptoms. Other education can include referral for smoking cessation and weight-loss programmes.

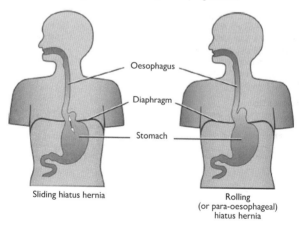

Sliding hiatus hernia

Rolling
(or para-oesophageal)
hiatus hernia

Fig. 2.1 Sliding hiatus hernia and rolling hiatus hernia.
Reproduced with kind permission © Burdett Institute 2008.

Mallory–Weiss tears

A Mallory-Weiss tear is a mucosal tear in the oesophagus, most commonly at the gastro-oesophageal junction.

Symptoms

The symptoms are haematemesis after forceful vomiting.

Causes

In younger patients, Mallory–Weiss tears are often provoked by alcohol.

Investigations

Endoscopy might not reveal the site of the tear but will exclude other diagnoses.

Treatment

The majority of cases will resolve with conservative management. Patients require reassurance. If vomiting and/or haematemesis is prolonged, patient's needs observation and the quantity and consistency of the vomitus monitoring as well as monitoring of vital signs.

Mouth cancer

Mouth cancer, is also termed oral cancer and is a tumour in the lining of the mouth, tongue, inside the cheeks, palate, lips, or gums. Less commonly a mouth cancer can be a tumour of the salivary glands, tonsils, or pharynx. Mouth cancer is most commonly (90%) a squamous cell carcinoma. Less commonly seen are adenocarcinomas in the salivary glands. Sarcomas grow from abnormalities in the bone, cartilage, muscle, or other body tissue. Lymphomas can also develop in the mouth.

Symptoms

- Mouth ulcers that are unhealed within 3 weeks
- Persistent lumps in the mouth or neck
- Persistent numbness or sensations on the lip or tongue
- White/red patches on the mouth lining
- Changes in speech
- Unexplained loose teeth.

Causes

More men than women are affected and there is an increased risk associated with:

- Alcohol
- Heavy smoking.

Most people diagnosed with mouth cancer are aged 50–74 years old. Human papilloma virus (HPV) is associated with the majority of cases.

Incidence

In the UK, each year about 7000 people are diagnosed with mouth cancer; this is about 2% of all cancers. The incidence worldwide is much greater, with mouth cancer being the sixth most common cancer.

Treatment

The three main treatments for mouth cancer are surgery, radiotherapy, or chemotherapy. Treatment is most commonly surgery plus radiotherapy.

Side effects

Mouth cancer and its treatment can cause many problems including changes in the appearance of the mouth, speech, and dysphagia (◆ p. 24). The latter can potentially result in aspiration pneumonia if food enters the airways.

Prevention

To prevent mouth cancer from developing or to prevent recurrence after treatment:

- Stop smoking
- Drink alcohol within recommended limits
- Eating a healthy diet
- Regular dental check-ups.

Prognosis

Prognosis is better for cancer of the lip, tongue, or oral cavity. About 60% of people with mouth cancer will live for 5 years.

Mouth ulcers

A mouth ulcer is usually seen on the inside the mouth, cheeks, or lips, and can also occur under the tongue. Mouth ulcers can be singular or multiple. If there are multiple mouth ulcers, consider a differential diagnosis of hand, foot, and mouth disease (◆ p. 41) or oral lichen planus (◆ p. 57). Mouth ulcers are not contagious. Mouth ulcers are common and generally resolve within 1–2 weeks; a mouth ulcer that lasts longer can be a sign of mouth cancer. Although, mouth ulcers are rarely serious; if they become more red and painful, there may be an infection that will require antibiotic treatment.

Causes

The cause of a mouth ulcer may be related to hormonal changes, such as from pregnancy or from a familial predisposition. Mouth ulcers may be the result of inflammatory bowel disease (◆ p. 368–9), coeliac disease (◆ p. 64–5), or Behcet's disease. Alternatively, there may be a deficiency in vitamin B_{12} or iron. Furthermore, mouth ulcers may be as a result of some medications.

Medications that may lead to the formation of mouth ulcers include some NSAIDs, beta-blockers, or nicorandil.

Treatment

Treatment can be used to increase ulcer healing, prevent infection, or reduce pain. These treatments can include antimicrobial mouthwash, mouthwash with analgesia, and/or corticosteroid lozenges. When a mouth ulcer is present it is ideal to:

- Use a soft toothbrush
- Drink cool drinks using a straw
- Eat soft foods
- Have regular dental check-ups
- Eat a healthy diet
- Avoid spicy or salty foods
- Avoid rough or crunchy food
- Avoid hot drinks
- Avoid acidic food or drinks
- Avoid chewing gum.

Prevention

To prevent mouth ulcers, it is ideal to prevent mouth irritation, such as by avoiding:

- Biting the inside of the cheek
- Poorly fitting braces, dentures
- Broken, rough teeth
- Burning the mouth with hot food or drink
- Allergy or food intolerance.

Mucositis

Mucositis is painful, inflamed mucosa inside the mouth or gut.

Symptoms

Symptoms of mucositis in the mouth include:
- Dry lips
- Mouth ulcers
- Sore, dry mouth
- Dysphagia.

Symptoms of mucositis in the gut include:

- Diarrhoea
- Pain on defaecation
- Rectal bleeding.

Causes

Mucositis is a common side effect of chemotherapy and radiotherapy. Mucositis often occurs within 2 weeks of commencing treatment and resolves within a few weeks of treatment ending.

Treatment

Treatment includes:
- Analgesia
- Mouthwash
- Saliva substitute sprays or gels
- Antidiarrhoeal medication (Ⓔ p. 411).

Prevention

To prevent or ease mucositis, advise patients to:
- Have good mouth hygiene
- Eat soft, moist foods
- Drink plenty of cold fluids
- Suck on ice
- Chew sugar-free gum.

Additionally, advise patients to avoid:
- Smoking
- Drinking hot, fizzy, or alcoholic drinks
- Eating hot, spicy or acidic foods.

Nausea and vomiting

Vomiting is a protective mechanism to expel potentially harmful substances from the stomach. Vomiting is often preceded by nausea but both can occur in isolation and may not always be protective in nature, and possibly also due to nerves or self-induced. To aid expulsion, muscle contractions increase intra-abdominal and intrathoracic pressure. Vomiting can result in:

• Anorexia, weight loss, and electrolyte imbalance
• Aspiration of vomit
• Oesophageal tears
• Acid damage to teeth (chronic vomiting).

Causes

• Abdominal—gastroenteritis (● p. 34–5), peptic ulcer (● p. 30–1), pyloric stenosis (● p. 60), intestinal obstruction (● p. 87), pancreatitis (● p. 182), cholecystitis (● p. 192–3), appendicitis (● p. 86), and constipation (● p. 458–9)
• Irritation—bacterial infection, viral infection, food poisoning, and gastric surgery
• Metabolic—diabetic ketoacidosis, hypercalcaemia, hyponatraemia, and uraemia
• Drug—opioids (● p. 406), chemotherapy, anaesthetic agents, antibiotics (● p. 408), and more
• Cerebral—increased intracranial pressure and migraine
• Vestibular—motion sickness and Ménière's disease
• Endocrine—pregnancy, Addison's disease
• Other—severe pain, non-ulcer dyspepsia (● p. 22–3), bulimia (● p. 309), self-induced, unpleasant odours, offensive sight, and anxiety

Investigations

• Bloods to investigate any electrolyte imbalance
• Endoscopy
• Pregnancy test.

Treatment

Treatment is to treat the underlying cause and antiemetics (● p. 412). Caution should be used with antiemetics as this may delay diagnosis. Care includes careful observation for signs of dehydration; including reduced urine output and dry tongue. Psychological support may be necessary for chronic vomiting.

Additionally it is essential to prevent spread of the infection. This can be achieved with good hand and toileting hygiene.

Oesophageal cancer

Oesophageal cancer is a tumour affecting the oesophagus (gullet). Most commonly adenocarcinoma but also squamous cell carcinoma. Adenocarcinomas develop in the glandular cells, which produce mucus in the lining of the oesophagus, most commonly in the lower section of the oesophagus. Squamous cell carcinomas form in the lining of the oesophagus, and carcinomas of this type originate in the upper or middle section of the oesophagus.

Symptoms

Small tumours tend not to give symptoms. Symptoms can include:
* Difficulty in swallowing
* Persistent indigestion (over 3 weeks)
* Vomiting soon after eating
* Loss of appetite and weight loss
* Pain or discomfort in the upper abdomen, chest, or back
* Persistent cough.

Causes

The exact aetiology is unknown; risk factors include:
* Persistent GORD (⊃ p. 36–7)
* Smoking
* Prolonged, excessive alcohol consumption
* Being overweight or obese
* A diet low in fruit and fibre
* Barrett's oesophagus.

Incidence

Oesophageal cancer most commonly affects more men than women, aged 60–80 years old.

Treatment

Treating oesophageal cancer can include surgery, chemotherapy, and/or radiotherapy. Dietetic input is necessary due to problems with gaining adequate nutrition.

Prevention

Stopping smoking, drinking alcohol within recommended limits, having a healthy body weight, and a healthy diet will reduce the risk of developing oesophageal cancer.

Prognosis

Cure is more likely if the oesophageal cancer is diagnosed at an early stage. Unfortunately, due to the lack of symptoms in early cancers, early diagnosis is rarely made.

Oesophageal diverticula

Oesophageal diverticula (singular is diverticulum) are pouches in the oesophagus, occurring in a variety of areas, most commonly the mid-oesophagus. Diverticula in the upper oesophagus can be termed Zenker's diverticulum (or pharyngeal pouch) and are above the upper oesophageal sphincter. As well as in the mid-oesophagus, a diverticulum can occur above the lower oesophageal (cardiac) sphincter; the latter is termed epiphrenic diverticulum.

Symptoms

There are often no symptoms with an oesophageal diverticulum, although, Zenker's diverticulum can potentially cause dysphagia and aspiration into the respiratory tract.

Causes

The cause is unclear in many situations. It may be the result of abnormal motility and an incoordination of sphincter relaxation.

Investigation

A barium swallow (➲ p. 218) can be used, whereas an OGD is contraindicated due to the risk of entering and perforating the diverticula.

Treatment

Treatment is used to address the symptoms. Surgical excision or revision of the diverticula pouch is advocated.

Oesophageal obstruction

An oesophageal obstruction is a blockage within the oesophagus (➲ p. 8).

Symptoms

Symptoms can be sudden and include complete dysphagia (➲ p. 24) to solids and liquids.

Causes

An obstruction can occur when there is an oesophageal stricture or it can be the result of ingested foreign bodies such as fish bones—additionally tumour, rings, or webs (➲ p. 53).

Investigations

- Bloods (looking for anaemia or dehydration)
- Upper GI endoscopy
- Chest X-ray (looking for obstruction or aspiration).

Treatment

Treatment can be to remove the blockage by endoscopic procedure if safe to do so. Surgery may be necessary for foreign bodies that cannot be endoscopically removed, when they may pose a threat if left to pass from the body, such as batteries, whereas some objects, such as a coin, might pass out without problem. It is important for the nurse to provide support and reassurance in the acute phase.

For people with a known stricture, it is important to advise patients to avoid foods that may cause a blockage. It is also important to advise people with a stricture to wear dentures (if used), chew foods well, and eat little and often.

Oesophageal rings and webs

The Schatzki ring is the main type of oesophageal ring that has symmetrical submucosal fibrous thickening and occurs in the lower third of the oesophagus and at the gastro-oesophageal junction. An oesophageal web can occur at any location along the oesophagus, usually in the upper third, and is not circumferential.

Symptoms

Oesophageal rings and webs can be symptomless and these are without significance. Symptoms include intermittent dysphagia (➔ p. 24) to solids and occasionally bolus obstruction. It is important to exclude other causes, such as a malignant stricture.

Causes

A cervical oesophagus is associated with iron-deficiency anaemia (Paterson–Brown–Kelly syndrome).

Investigations

• OGD
• Barium swallow
• Manometry.

Treatment

If asymptomatic, no treatment is required. Often, the diagnostic endoscopy can be therapeutic in disrupting the web or ring.

If dysphagia persists, oesophageal dilatation is indicated. In Paterson–Brown–Kelly syndrome, webs regress spontaneously after treatment for iron-deficiency anaemia.

Symptomatic patients may benefit from nutritional advice. This includes eating little and often, sitting upright when eating, chewing food carefully, and sipping fizzy drinks to relieve obstruction. Additionally, patients are often 'afraid' to eat: this can be assisted with reassurance and explanation about the condition.

Oesophageal spasm

Oesophageal spasm is disorder of normal peristalsis (⊃ p. 3) of the oesophagus. There may be diffuse oesophageal spasm described as uncoordinated contractions of the oesophageal muscles. Alternatively, there may be nutcracker oesophagus where contractions are extra-long or strong.

Symptoms

Episodic dysphagia (⊃ p. 24) and angina-like chest pain. Although symptoms can occur without warning, they frequently are provoked by ingesting fluids of extreme temperatures. About half of patients also have symptoms of GORD (⊃ p. 36–7).

Causes

Symptoms are caused by high-amplitude aperistaltic oesophageal contractions.

Investigations

• OGD is used to exclude other pathology; but may reveal multiple, simultaneous ring contractions
• Barium swallow infrequently reveals a corkscrew appearance which is classic of oesophageal spasm
• Manometry—if results are positive then it is diagnostic but negative results do not exclude oesophageal spasm

Treatment

Medication is commonly used, such as calcium channel blockers (⊃ p. 416), tricyclic antidepressants (⊃ p. 410), and nitrates (⊃ p. 425) to help relax the smooth muscle. Dilatation is only used on severe cases but results are unpredictable.

Nurses should provide advice and reassurance as symptoms are frightening. Advice includes avoidance of extreme temperatures of oral fluids. Eating little and often can also help and sitting up after meals aids passage of food to the stomach. Reassurance includes explanation that symptoms are not cardiac in origin.

Oesophageal varices

Oesophageal varices are dilated veins or newly formed venous pathways in the lower third of the oesophagus. These veins are fragile and easily damaged, potentially resulting in a large, severe haematemesis. Varices progress over time, but if associated with alcohol they can regress if alcohol is avoided.

Symptoms

There may be no symptoms but varices can present with a large, fresh bleed. Symptoms may include:

- Anaemia—if there is a slow bleeding
- Vomiting with large volumes of blood
- Melaena
- Light-headedness
- Loss of consciousness (in severe cases).

Causes

There are many reasons that varices may occur including:

- Liver cirrhosis—the most common cause, secondary to alcohol abuse
- Primary biliary cirrhosis
- Chronic acute hepatitis
- Portal vein thrombosis, such as malignancy or pancreatitis
- Portal hypertension—people have up to 50% risk of varices, up to half will have bleeding varices
- Right-sided heart failure
- Schistosomiasis—a parasitic infection that damages the liver, lungs, intestine, and bladder.

Treatment

Initial treatment for bleeding varices includes fluid resuscitation or blood transfusion.

Other treatments include therapies to reduce portal venous pressure through medication and endoscopic therapy to stop the bleeding by banding.

Concerns

Encephalopathy can occur with alcohol abuse: ensure that patients are able to consent to treatment and understand any advice provided.

Oesophagitis

Oesophagitis is inflamed mucosa of the oesophagus.

Symptoms

Symptoms can include:
• Heartburn
• An unpleasant sour taste in the mouth
• Recurrent hiccup
• Belching
• Regurgitation of bile or food
• Excessive salivation
• Pain on swallowing (odynophagia)
• Dysphagia
• Chest pain
• Hoarse voice
• Halitosis
• Bloating
• Nausea.

Causes

Prolonged exposure to refluxed gastric contents.

Treatment

There are a number of potential treatments for oesophagitis:
• PPIs (⊃ p. 427)
• Stopping smoking
• Avoiding food or drinks that cause symptoms
• Avoid NSAIDs (⊃ p. 406)
• Maintain a normal body mass index (BMI) (⊃ p. 306)

Potential complications

If oesophagitis is left untreated, scarring and strictures may occur or there may be progression to Barrett's oesophagus or cancer.

Oral lichen planus

Oral lichen planus is a rash on the inside of the mouth. Oral lichen planus is not contagious and does not usually return once symptoms resolve.

Symptoms

Symptoms of oral lichen planus include white patches on the gums, tongue, or inside of the cheeks associated with a burning and stinging in the mouth, particularly when eating or drinking. Other symptoms can include clusters of shiny, raised, purple-red marks on the limbs or torso, bald patches on the scalp, and nails that are rough with grooves. Not all people have all of the symptoms.

Treatment

Oral lichen planus can last for several months. Mouthwash or sprays can resolve burning or sore mucosa. Also, it is advisable to:
• Ensure healthy gums by cleaning the teeth twice daily
• Avoiding salty or spicy foods
• Avoiding acidic food or drinks
• Avoid alcohol and mouthwash with alcohol.

Treatment for lichen planus on the skin can be used to treat symptoms of itching or to control the rash. Lichen planus on the skin will usually resolve without treatment within 6–9 months. In severe or non-resolving cases, treatment might include 'light therapy' or other medication, such as steroids (◆ p. 428).

Treatment for lichen planus on the skin may require steroids in severe or non-resolving cases.

Oral thrush

Oral thrush is a common yeast infection caused by *Candida* (fungus). Oral thrush is common in babies and again in later life with people wearing dentures. Oral thrush is usually harmless. It can be spread from one body part to another or passed from a baby to the mother.

Symptoms

Oral thrush is red mucosa in the mouth with white patches; additionally there are red spots that can bleed if wiped. Other symptoms that can occur in adults include:
• Cracks in the corner of the mouth
• Changes in taste
• An unpleasant taste in the mouth
• Sore tongue and gums
• Difficulty eating and drinking.

Other symptoms in babies include:
• Not wanting to feed
• Nappy rash.

Causes

Thrush is linked to:
• Long-term use of antibiotics
• Asthma inhalers
• Chemotherapy.

Treatment

Treatment, such as an antifungal (➔ p. 413) is often needed to resolve oral thrush. Medications are available over the counter.

Prevention

To prevent oral thrush:
• Careful oral hygiene is required, including gums and tongue
• Rinsing mouth after eating
• Ensure regular check-ups if diabetic
• Do not wear dentures at night
• Ensure dentures fit well
• Do not smoke
• Sterilize dummies and bottles regularly (for babies).

Pharyngitis

Pharyngitis, more commonly termed a sore throat, is a commonly encountered problem that is usually self-limiting, with symptoms gone within a week.

Symptoms

Pharyngitis presents as a sore, dry throat, and discomfort on swallowing. There is often erythema at the back of the mouth. There may also be halitosis (➋ p. 40), a cough, or swollen glands in the neck.

Causes

The most common cause of pharyngitis is a virus or smoking; occasionally, there can be a bacterial infection.

Treatment

Treatment is often self-treatment without the need for nursing intervention. Simple treatment can include gargling, drinking plenty of water, eating soft foods (if eating is painful), and avoiding hot drinks. Avoiding smoking also helps reduce discomfort. Sucking on ice cubes or boiled sweets can relieve symptoms but care must be taken with young children due to the risk of choking. Rest is also advocated.

If these measures do not work patients can be advised to take simple analgesia (➋ p. 406) to relieve the pain of the sore throat and medicated lozenges can be useful.

Treatment should be expedited if:

• Symptoms do not resolve within a week
• Symptoms are encountered frequently
• If the sore throat is associated with a temperature
• There are comorbidities, such as diabetes or chemotherapy.

Treatment by antibiotics (➋ p. 408) will be ineffective unless there is a bacterial infection.

Further reading

NICE (2018). Sore throat (acute): antimicrobial prescribing. https://www.nice.org.uk/guidance/ng84 (Accessed 13/10/2018).

Pyloric stenosis

Pyloric stenosis is often called 'infantile hypertrophic pyloric stenosis'. It comprises hypertrophy and hyperplasia of the pyloric sphincter between the stomach (→ p. 9) and the duodenum (→ p. 10) during the neonatal period. This mainly affects the circular muscles of the pylorus, causing it to become elongated and thickened, and the result is gastric outflow obstruction.

Symptoms

Symptoms usually present between 3 and 6 weeks after birth, although late presentation (6 months) can occur. Symptoms include:
- Projectile vomiting
- A palpable mass in the right upper quadrant of the stomach during feeding
- Dehydration and hunger after vomiting feed
- Electrolyte imbalance can result.

Causes

Affects ♂ more than ♀, with a strong genetic factor.

Investigations

Abdominal ultrasound.

Treatment

Initial treatment is to rehydrate and a nasogastric tube will relieve pressure. Surgery is pyloromyotomy, where the thickened muscle is cut to widen the passage.

Chapter 3

Small bowel

Bacterial overgrowth

Bacterial overgrowth is said to occur if the flora in the upper small bowel resembles that found in the colon. These micro-organisms (mainly anaerobes—bacteroides, lactobacilli, and coliforms) compete for nutrients and might injure the enterocytes.

Symptoms

Bacterial overgrowth may present with:
- Bloating
- Diarrhoea.

In more severe forms it is characterized by:
- Weight loss
- Steatorrhoea
- Vitamin B_{12} deficiency (➔ p. 80–1)
- Hypoproteinaemia.

Causes

Bacterial overgrowth can occur if there is:
- No gastric acid
- Small bowel diverticulae
- Blind loops—out-of-circuit loops of bowel such as jejuno–ileal bypass
- Abnormal motility associated with scleroderma, amyloid myopathy, visceral neuropathy or myopathy, diabetic autonomic neuropathy, or chronic bowel obstruction
- A lack of pancreatic enzymes such as from chronic pancreatitis
- Immunodeficiency syndromes, such as common variable immunodeficiency, combined immunodeficiency diseases, or HIV infection
- Cirrhosis.

Investigations

Bacterial overgrowth is confirmed by aspirating the upper small bowel contents during an endoscopy.

Treatment

A trial of antibiotics (➔ p. 408) is used and the diagnosis is confirmed if the symptoms improve.

Coeliac disease

Coeliac disease is an autoimmune condition, where the body's immune system attacks healthy body tissues instead of opposing infection. It is a common inflammatory disorder of the small intestine associated with a loss of villous height and crypt hypertrophy, leading to malabsorption of nutrients.

Symptoms

The symptoms of coeliac disease include:
- Diarrhoea (malodourous)
- Abdominal pain
- Bloating
- Flatulence
- Indigestion
- Constipation.

Additional symptoms include:
- Fatigue
- Unplanned weight loss.

Causes

Coeliac disease is induced by three types of cereals: wheat (gliadins), barley (hordeins), and rye (secalins).

Additionally, the environment and genetics (10% have a family history) seem to be contributory. There is a genetic mutation called HLA-DQ but this is also present in people without coeliac disease, suggesting that environmental factors are also needed to trigger coeliac disease. Environmental factors include rotavirus infection in childhood and introducing gluten into a baby's diet before the child reaches six months of age.

Furthermore, having other conditions is linked with an increased risk, including:
- Type 1 diabetes
- Thyroid disease
- Ulcerative colitis (€ p. 370)
- Down's syndrome
- Turner's syndrome
- Neurological disorders such as epilepsy.

Incidence

Coeliac disease affects about 1% of the population.

Investigations

- Blood tests—looking for antibodies—not always conclusive
- Oesophageal gastroduodenoscopy (OGD) (€ p. 250) to gain a small bowel biopsy.

After a positive diagnosis, further tests may include:
- Blood tests—to check for deficiencies in vitamins/minerals or anaemia
- Skin biopsy if there is a rash (dermatitis herpetiformis)
- Dual-energy X-ray absorptiometry (DEXA) scan—to check for bone thinning.

Treatment

Symptoms usually improve within weeks of taking a gluten-free diet with dietetic advice to ensure that the diet is balanced—the exception is dermatitis herpetiformis which takes considerably longer to treat successfully. Treatment may also include dietary supplements initially after diagnosis.

Prevention

There are support groups available such as coeliacUK at www.coeliac. org.uk. It is also important to consider the side effects of coeliac disease, namely being more vulnerable to infections. Consider vaccinations including influenza.

Reference

NICE (2015). Coeliac disease: recognition, assessment and management. https://www.nice.org.uk/ guidance/ng20 (Accessed 14 October 2018).

Duodenal ulcers

An ulcer within the duodenum.

Symptoms

Most people are symptom-free but symptoms include:
- Abdominal pain—sometimes referred
- Nausea
- Vomiting
- Bloating.

Symptoms can also include:
- Melaena
- Fatigue.

Causes

Ulceration in the first part of the duodenum is most commonly caused by *Helicobacter pylori* (\maltese p. 42). *H. pylori* produces an enzyme, urease, which catalyses the reaction that converts urea to ammonia and carbon dioxide. Ammonia causes an alkaline environment; the gastric antrum responds to this by secreting ↑ gastrin, which causes the gastric fundus to secrete supraphysiological amounts of gastric acid and pepsinogen. This ↑ in the levels of acid and pepsinogen is thought to cause gastric metaplasia in the duodenum and it might be these areas that ulcerate, possibly owing to further colonization by *H. pylori*.

Other causes include:
- Non-steroidal anti-inflammatory drugs (NSAIDs) (\maltese p. 406)
- Ileal Crohn's disease (\maltese p. 377)
- Rarely, a gastrinoma—a gastrin-secreting tumour.

Investigations

Investigations for *H. pylori* (\maltese p. 42)

Treatment

Treatment is usually to resolve *H. pylori* (\maltese p. 42) and to use a proton pump inhibitor (PPI) (\maltese p. 427).

Giardiasis

Giardia duodenalis (previously called *Giardia lamblia*) is a protozoan acquired from drinking water contaminated with its cysts or by direct faeco-oral contact, resulting in colonization of the upper small bowel that leads to malabsorption.

Symptoms

Symptoms of giardiasis are:

- Acute or chronic malodourous diarrhoea
- Flatulence
- Bloating
- Abdominal pain/cramps
- Burping
- Weight loss.

Investigations

Giardiasis is diagnosed by:

- Duodenal aspiration
- Occasionally biopsy
- The protozoa/cysts can be found in the stool.

Treatment

Treatment is antimicrobials, generally resolving symptoms in about a week. If symptoms do not resolve within a week seek advice.

Dehydration needs to be avoided by drinking lots of fluids—not alcohol. Consider oral rehydration solutions (➲ p. 75), if urine is concentrated.

Prevention

Infection is spread via the faecal–oral route. People should be advised not to attend work/school until 48 h after symptom resolution. Further advice includes:

- Not drinking untreated water, when in developing countries
- Not swimming and ingesting water and avoid swimming pools for 2 weeks after symptoms resolve
- Careful handwashing with soap and water
- Daily cleaning of areas, such as toilet seats and taps, that are touched by an infected person
- Not preparing food for others if infected
- Not sharing of towels
- Not having sexual intercourse, particularly unprotected anal sex.

Lactose intolerance (lactase deficiency)

Lactose intolerance is a common problem where people are unable to digest lactose, a sugar found mainly in milk and dairy products.

There are two main types of lactase deficiency: primary and secondary. Primary lactase deficiency is the most common cause of lactose intolerance worldwide, due to a faulty gene and decreased lactase production. Secondary lactase deficiency is due to a faulty small bowel—this is the most common cause of lactose intolerance in the UK especially in young children and babies. Lactase is found on the small bowel and colon brush border, and it hydrolyses the disaccharide lactose to glucose and galactose. The levels of lactase are high at birth but ↓ with age. Lactase is absent in some adults, especially those of Asian or African Caribbean origin, although lactase activity is usually present in >75% of White people.

Symptoms

Symptoms often occur quickly after ingestion of diet or fluids containing lactose, but severity may depend on the amount consumed and per individual. Symptoms include:
- Flatulence
- Diarrhoea
- Bloating
- Abdominal cramp/pain
- Nausea.

Causes

Lactose intolerance is usually the result of the body not producing enough lactase (lactose intolerance). If unabsorbed lactose is passed from the small bowel to the colon, the bacteria in the colon will ferment and breakdown the lactose which produces fatty acids and gases (carbon dioxide, hydrogen, and methane), that result in the above symptoms.

Causes of secondary lactase deficiency include:
- Gastroenteritis
- Coeliac disease
- Crohn's disease
- Ulcerative colitis
- Chemotherapy
- Antibiotics—long course
- Small bowel surgery.

Investigations

If removing lactose from the diet helps, additional tests may not be necessary. However, possible investigations include:
- Hydrogen breath test
- Small bowel biopsy
- Lactose tolerance test
- Milk tolerance test.

Treatment

There is no cure for lactose intolerance, but symptoms can be controlled by dietary modification, such as avoiding/reducing lactose (symptom dependent). Dietary modification can be done alone or following dietetic advice. Caution is necessary to avoid deficiencies in vitamins, minerals, and calcium.

Lactose intolerance as a result of gastroenteritis is temporary and resolves within a few days or weeks. Other types of lactose intolerance that are not the result of gastroenteritis may be lifelong.

Intestinal failure

Overview

Intestinal failure (IF), previously termed short bowel syndrome, describes people who require specialized replacement regimens of fluids and nutrients. It can be acute or chronic and is due to an inability to maintain health through normal absorption of sufficient nutrients or electrolytes from food and drink. It can occur following a massive resection of the small intestine, in the presence of extensive inflammation, or in motility disorders. IF is rare, with incidence of less than 1 in 100,000 individuals.

IF is a difficult gastrointestinal (GI) condition to manage because, in addition to malabsorption of food and drink, reabsorption of GI secretions can be reduced. Impaired absorption results in large quantities of water and electrolytes being lost, either through a stoma or the rectum. Jejunum–colon patients can adapt over time and can show an improvement in intestinal absorption. People with a jejunostomy will not improve nor ↓ their output with time.

Complex cases of IF should be referred to the national centres. There, care is provided by a multidisciplinary team to manage the difficult medical, surgical, radiological, and nursing needs.

Definition and classification

IF can be described as decreased intestinal absorption that requires macronutrient +/− water and electrolyte supplements to maintain health and/or growth. Without this treatment the person will be undernourished and/or dehydrated. IF can be acute or chronic.

There are three types of IF.
- Type I is acute, short term, and will usually self-limit.
- Type II is acute but prolonged; often in metabolically unstable people.
- Type III is chronic in stable people who require months or years of treatment. This may or may not be reversible.

Type I is reasonably common in the perioperative phase of abdominal surgery when a person is critically ill. Intravenous treatment is required for days or weeks. Type II is less common and is usually accompanied by an intra-abdominal catastrophe such as an enterocutaneous fistula and sepsis. Type II IF may occur after mesenteric ischaemia, volvulus, or abdominal trauma. Type III may evolve from type II and will require management at home with parenteral nutrition.

To survive without parenteral supplements, there are guidelines related to the amount of healthy bowel that is necessary. This is about 50 cm of jejunum and a colon in continuity (joined together) or about 100 cm of jejunum.

Reference

Pironi L et al. (2015). ESPEN endorsed recommendations. Definition and classification of intestinal failure in adults. *Clinical Nutrition* 34(2): 171–80.

Symptoms

IF can lead to:
• Undernutrition
• Depleted sodium levels, potentially losing 100 mmol of sodium per litre of faecal output
• Depleted magnesium levels
• Dehydration.

People with a jejunostomy (Fig. 3.1) have major problems with water and sodium loss from their stoma and lose 100 mmol of sodium per litre of stomal output. They also have problems with hypomagnesaemia, undernutrition, and gallstones.

People with jejunum attached to colon (Fig. 3.1) can incur problems with undernutrition, renal calcium oxalate stones, and gallstones.

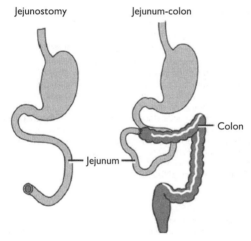

Fig. 3.1 Example of intestinal failure.
Reproduced with kind permission © Burdett Institute 2008.

Causes

The largest cause of IF historically was Crohn's disease (→ p. 377). The number of people with IF and Crohn's disease is decreasing, possibly due to newer treatment modalities. Crohn's disease can lead to massive surgical resections and there may be continuing disease within the remaining bowel.

Acute IF can be the result of:
• Infection—intra-abdominal sepsis or enteritis
• Altered absorption—gastric hypersecretion
• Diseased bowel—Crohn's disease, mucositis
• Motility disorder—prolonged postoperative ileus.

Chronic IF can be the result of:

- An extensive bowel resection—mesenteric infarction, Crohn's disease, trauma
- Diseased bowel—fistula, Crohn's disease, radiation enteritis
- Motility disorder—pseudo-obstruction, scleroderma.

Investigations

To enable effective treatment the residual length of bowel and the intestinal motility need to be determined. Other important factors include:

- An accurate fluid balance of input and output
- Daily body weight (1 kg = 1 L)
- Blood results—urea, electrolytes, albumin; also tests for deficiencies such as magnesium
- Urine sodium concentration.

Treatment

The broad aims of treatment in this complex group of patients are:

- To maintain a fluid and electrolyte balance
- To maintain an adequate nutritional status
- To enable the individual to achieve an acceptable quality of life.

Advice is necessary including about long-term rehabilitation. Accepting the changes that IF can bring may be difficult for many; they might struggle to come to terms with the, often catastrophic, life-changing events that have taken place. Patients and their families need clear and easily understandable information regarding the physiological changes that have taken place so that they can begin to understand the rationale behind the treatment plan, which should aid compliance. The multidisciplinary team may need to refer for additional help, such as from a counsellor, medical social worker, psychologist, or occupational therapist.

A treatment plan is likely to include:

- Oral fluid restriction (500–1000 ml daily)
- Venous access
- If random urine sodium is <20 mmol/l consider intravenous (IV) sodium chloride (0.9%)
- Accurate fluid-balance chart
- IV fluid is calculated from the output from the previous day; it should include:
  - Sodium, potassium, magnesium, and calories, protein, vitamins, and trace elements if they are not being absorbed enterally.

Treatment once a patient is stable may progress to oral intake in addition to IV therapy, with the potential to reduce/stop IV fluids. Oral intake can include:

- A low-fibre diet
- Antidiarrhoeal medication (➔ p. 411) taken 30–60 min before eating
- Separating food and fluid by discouraging drinking with meals
- Limiting oral fluids (non-electrolyte)
- Oral rehydration solution (➔ p. 426)
- Energy-dense and sodium-rich snacks.

Long-term treatment will include:

- Education to ensure a good understanding of bowel function—to aid compliance
- Refer to appropriate team member, such as dietitian
- Train on long-term IV care—if needed
- Regular monitoring to enable detection and correction of abnormalities.

Many people with IF will have undergone numerous investigative procedures and multiple operations, requiring lengthy hospital admissions, usually many months. Patients may be transferred to specialist centres, resulting in them being treated at great distances from their home, family, and friends. It is therefore unsurprising that many patients experience psychosocial difficulties, such as depression, feelings of isolation, loneliness, and low morale. Furthermore, a new body image that may include weight changes, scars, or a stoma requires adjustment. Some people must adapt to a life without eating, with all the social and psychological impacts this implies.

A multidisciplinary team approach, offering support and counselling, is essential for patient recovery and rehabilitation. This will encourage the patient to gradually gain confidence and begin to form relationships that will be effective for recovery and the attainment of goals.

Meckel's diverticulum

Meckel's diverticulum often presents in childhood.

Symptoms

Meckel's diverticulum can be symptomless. Symptoms can include:
- Rectal bleeding
- Peritonitis
- Volvulus (⊃ p. 116)
- Intussusception
- Intestinal blockage
- Necrotic bowel.

Causes

The diverticulum is made of tissues like the stomach that can release acids which results in ulcers that can bleed.

Incidence

Meckel's diverticulum is one of the most common congenital abnormality of the GI tract, affecting about 2% of the population.

Investigations

Investigations include:
- X-ray
- Ultrasound
- Blood test
- Faecal test
- Laparoscopy.

Treatment

Treatment is surgery, which will depend on findings and may include a resection of the diverticulum, ulcerated bowel, or necrotic bowel.

Oral rehydration solution

Oral rehydration solution is commonly termed electrolyte mix (E-mix). It is used to replace losses from loose stool, such as a high-output stoma.

To reduce the additional loss from the gut by consumption of hypotonic fluids, it is necessary to restrict fluids such as water, tea, coffee, and juice. To help aid hydration, it is important to sip a glucose–saline solution (sodium concentration 90–120 mmol/l) and to take antidiarrhoeal (➋ p. 411) or antisecretory (➋ p. 414) drugs to ↓ the high faecal output. Rehydration solutions are described by the World Health Organization (WHO). St Mark's Hospital has devised an oral rehydration solution (Table 3.1).

Table 3.1 Electrolyte mix (E-mix)

Glucose	20g
Sodium chloride	3.5g
Sodium bicarbonate	2.5g
Dissolved in 1 litre of tap water	

The electrolyte mix is better tolerated when kept in the fridge and served chilled. Small amounts of flavourings, such as lime juice, can be added to aid palatability. Rehydration solutions should ideally be sipped throughout the day, interspersed with hypotonic drinks as allowed.

Paralytic ileus

Paralytic ileus occurs when the peristaltic action of the gut is impaired/ceased causing symptoms. A paralytic ileus results in small bowel distention, and impairment of absorption of fluid, electrolytes, and nutrition.

Symptoms

- Usually history of recent abdominal surgery or trauma
- Abdominal distension is often apparent
- Pain is often not a prominent feature
- Vomiting may occur
- No flatus evident.

Causes

- Trauma, surgery
- Intestinal ischaemia
- Sepsis
- Drugs.

Investigation

- Auscultation will reveal absence of bowel sounds
- Plain abdominal X-ray—highlighting loops of bowel
- Gas may be present in large bowel
- Water-soluble contrast agent maybe useful if unclear as to whether obstruction is mechanical or functional.

Treatment

Treat conservatively and resolution is often within a few days to a week.
- Fluid and electrolyte replacement
- Source of sepsis should be eradicated
- Nasogastric tube.

Small bowel infection

Small bowel infections can be viral or bacterial.

Symptoms

Infection of the small bowel rarely causes blood in the stool and, unlike in inflammatory bowel disease, there is not usually an ↑ in the platelet count.

Causes

In children, viral causes are common and include rotavirus, calcivirus, enteric adenovirus, and astrovirus.

In previously healthy adults, bacterial causes might include:
- *Salmonella* spp.
- *Escherichia coli (E. coli)*
- *Vibrio cholera.*

Other organisms that can infect the gut include *Mycobacterium tuberculosis*, which can affect the terminal ileum and be confused with Crohn's disease.

In immunocompromised patients, many organisms can infect the small bowel including:
- *Candida* spp.
- *Cytomegalovirus (CMV)*.

There is also an enteropathy specific to people with HIV.

Investigations

Diagnosis usually depends on stool microscopy and culture.

A small bowel biopsy and/or aspirate might be needed, especially in the immunocompromised.

Treatment

Generally, treatment is to withhold food for 1–2 days but maintain hydration and then gradually reintroduce foods.

Small bowel tumours—benign

Benign tumours of the small bowel are uncommon and include the following:
- Adenomas
- Hamartomas
- Fibromas
- Haemangiomas
- Leomyomas
- Lipomas.

Causes

Periampullary duodenal adenomas are common in patients with familial adenomatous polyposis. Hamartomas occur in juvenile polyposis, Peutz–Jeghers syndrome, and Cronkhite–Canada syndrome. Peutz–Jeghers syndrome is an autosomal dominant inherited condition.

Symptoms

Peutz-Jeghers syndrome in children may be associated with small, dark spots on the lips and mouth, and around the anus. These spots often fade with age. The syndrome is also characterized by the development of non-cancerous growths, particularly in the stomach and intestine. These can result in bowel obstruction, intussusception, chronic bleeding, and abdominal pain. There is also an increased risk of developing cancers of the GI tract, pancreas (Ɔ p. 14), cervix, testes, ovary, and breast.

Investigations

Regular screening of the small bowel +/– polyp removal.

Treatment

Treatment is determined by symptomology and may include removal of the polyp.

Small bowel tumours—malignant

There are four main types of malignant tumour:
• Adenocarcinoma—the most common type of small bowel cancer, usually within the duodenum. Adenocarcinoma can develop from adenomatous polyps.
• Sarcoma—can develop in the supportive tissues of the body, e.g. Kaposi's sarcoma. Leiomyosarcomas grow in the muscle wall of the ileum. A GI stromal tumour (GIST) can develop in any part of the small bowel.
• Neuroendocrine (carcinoid)—commonly in terminal ileum.
• Lymphoma—usually a non-Hodgkin lymphoma (NHL). Tumours can be primary or secondary.

More rarely fibrosarcoma, leiomyosarcoma, or metastatic tumours may occur.

Symptoms
• Abdominal cramps
• Diarrhoea
• Nausea
• Vomiting
• Weight loss
• Bleeding—melaena, anaemia.

Cause
The cause is often unknown, although patients with Crohn's disease, coeliac disease, and Peutz–Jeghers syndrome might be at ↑ risk.

Incidence
Small bowel cancers are rare, accounting for less than 1% of new cancers. Small bowel cancers mainly affect people in their early 80s with more men than women affected. In the UK about 1600 people are diagnosed with a small bowel cancer each year; the incidence has been increasing since the 1990s. 50% of tumours occur in the duodenum, 30% occur in the jejunum, and 20% occur in the ileum.

Investigations
• Endoscopy (➋ p. 236)
• Biopsy
• Barium X-rays
• CT scans (➋ p. 220)
• Magnetic resonance imaging (MRI) scan (➋ p. 222)
• Ultrasound scans.

Treatment
Surgery is the main treatment and can be a curative resection or palliative bypass, depending on the site of origin and extent of the tumour. Radiotherapy and/or chemotherapy are occasionally used.

Patients who have surgery might require a special diet, supplements, or medicine, depending upon the extent of small bowel resection, requiring nursing or dietetic advice.

Vitamin B$_{12}$ deficiency (folate deficiency anaemia)

A lack of vitamin B$_{12}$ or B$_9$ (folate) causes the body to produce abnormal red blood cells resulting in anaemia. There are other types of anaemia, with dissimilar causes. As folate is water soluble the body can only store enough for about 4 months. The stores of vitamin B$_{12}$ in a healthy person last for 3–7 years, so it takes a long time for a macrocytic anaemia to develop.

Symptoms

There are a number of symptoms that are related to a deficiency in vitamin B$_{12}$ or folate, which generally start gradually and worsen if untreated:
• Anaemia
• Fatigue
• Lethargy
• Paraesthesia (pins and needles)
• Sore mouth—tongue, mouth ulcers
• Muscle weakness
• Breathlessness
• Headaches
• Tinnitus
• Palpitations
• Visual disturbances
• Memory impairment
• Depression
• Weight loss.

For people with longer-term deficiencies the symptoms may include:
• Problems with the nervous system—which may be permanent
• Infertility—temporary
• Cardiac issues, such as heart failure
• Birth defects and pregnancy complications.

Causes

Deficiencies in vitamin B$_{12}$ and folate affect older people: about 10% of people aged over 75 years and about 5% of people aged 65–75.
• Pernicious anaemia—an abnormal immune response that prevents absorption of vitamin B$_{12}$ by preventing the production of intrinsic factor needed to absorb vitamin B$_{12}$ from dietary intake; this is the most common cause of vitamin B$_{12}$ deficiency in the UK
• Lack of dietary intake of vitamins; possibly the result of a vegan diet or long-term poor diet
• Medication—such as antiepileptic and PPIs (◗ p. 427)
• Crohn's disease
• Excision of the terminal ileum where vitamin B$_{12}$ is absorbed, such as for Crohn's disease
• After a gastrectomy
• Coeliac disease
• Excessive urination can deplete folate—secondary to congestive cardiac failure, acute liver damage, or long-term dialysis.

Investigation

Blood tests; however, some people may be symptomatic despite 'normal' levels or symptoms-free despite low levels. Further investigations may be necessary by a specialist such as a haematologist, gastroenterologist, or dietitian.

Treatment

Treatment is usually related to the cause of the deficiency. Deficiencies are also commonly treated with replacement therapy; by diet or medication.

Colon

Abdominal bloating/distension

Abdominal bloating and distension are terms that are often used inter-changeably. However, it has been suggested that the term 'distension' should be reserved for an actual change in girth, whereas the term 'bloating' should be used for the subjective symptom of abdominal enlargement.

Symptoms

Abdominal bloating may occur after meals.

Causes

- Intestinal obstruction
- Megacolon (➐ p. 105)
- Faecal loading
- Ascites
- Coeliac disease (➐ p. 64–5)
- Pancreatic disorders
- Irritable bowel syndrome (IBS) (➐ p. 96–8).

Bloating does not appear to be related to excessive abdominal gas.

Incidence

Bloating is more common in ♀. Up to 75% of patients with IBS and 90% of patients with constipation report bloating.

Treatment

The first step in management is to ensure that an organic cause has been excluded, without over-investigating the patient. Patients often con-sume excessive quantities of fibre and ∴ ↓ fibre intake can be beneficial. Additionally, limiting intake of fizzy drinks, artificial sweeteners, and fat might help. Drugs aimed at altering gas volumes have not provided reliable results. Antispasmodics (➐ p. 409), antidepressants (➐ p. 410), and hypno-therapy might help improve bloating in people with IBS.

Abdominal pain

Acute abdominal pain is a pain of short duration. Pain that persists for many weeks can be seen as chronic pain, once abdominal causes have been excluded.

Causes

There are a number of potential causes of abdominal pain, including:

- Inflammatory bowel disease (IBD) (➲ p. 368–9)
- IBS (➲ p. 96–8)
- Diverticulitis (➲ p. 90–1)
- Idiopathic constipation (➲ p. 458–9)
- Mesenteric ischaemia
- Malignancy.

Treatment

Treatment depends upon the cause of the pain but should include explanation by the nurse of different management techniques. This includes avoidance of precipitating factors that have previously been identified and to limit the adverse impact that pain can have. It is preferable to avoid medications such as opioids (➲ p. 406) and codeine-containing analgesia (➲ p. 406) as these are potentially dangerous and addictive. Treatment might include psychological management as well as more specialist treatments, such as nerve blocks.

Appendicitis

Appendicitis is inflammation of the appendix.

Symptoms

- Abdominal pain/tenderness—classic sign of patient guarding
- Pyrexia
- Nausea
- Vomiting.

Causes

Appendicitis occurs if the opening of the appendix becomes blocked by a build-up of mucus from the caecum. This blockage causes an ↑ in bacterial activity which, in turn, leads to inflammation/infection. This inflammation/infection can spread and cause the appendix to rupture, leading to peritonitis.

Investigations

- Full blood count (FBC)—↑ white blood cell (WBC) count
- Urinalysis
- Abdominal X-ray
- Ultrasound
- Computed tomography (CT) scan.

Treatment

Appendicectomy, removal of the appendix. Antibiotics may be necessary.

Bowel obstruction

Bowel obstruction occurs for many reasons including malignancy: a common cause of bowel obstruction is colonic cancer.

Symptoms

Symptoms of bowel obstruction include:
- Colicky abdominal pain
- Nausea or vomiting, possibly faeculent
- Abdominal distension occurs in 75% of patients
- Changes in bowel motions, varying from absolute constipation to diarrhoea
- Bowel sounds might be hyperactive (borborygmic), tinkling, or absent.

Other symptoms may include:
- Fatigue
- Dehydration
- Anorexia.

Causes

Malignant bowel obstruction is often caused by advanced, recurrent cancer.

Investigations

- Abdominal X-rays (**Ɔ** p. 230)
- CT scans to assess dilated bowel loops, air–fluid levels, and masses (**Ɔ** p. 220)
- Barium study
- Occasionally an endoscopy (**Ɔ** p. 236).

Treatment

Initial treatment includes resuscitation and stabilization of the patient. Intravenous (IV) fluids and a nasogastric tube are often advocated. Medication may be necessary to relieve symptoms, such as:
- Antisecretory (**Ɔ** p. 414)
- Antiemetic (**Ɔ** p. 412).

Stenting of the colon may be undertaken. Surgery can relieve distension and is indicated if the tumour is resectable and the patient's general condition allows it. Surgery may include:
- Resection of the affected bowel
- Stoma formation to decompress the bowel
- Bypass procedure
- Division of adhesions.

Dilated colon

A dilated colon occurs when the colon becomes distended.

Symptoms

Symptoms can include severe, idiopathic constipation usually in children and young adults. There may also be soiling because a faecal bolus in the rectum inhibits anal closure and thus liquid stool seeps around the impaction.

Causes

A dilated colon can present as acute abdomen with a volvulus (➲ p. 116) of the sigmoid or Hirschsprung's disease (➲ p. 398–9).

Investigations

A digital rectal examination (➲ p. 208–9) may reveal a lax anal sphincter, frequently seen with faecal impaction.

An abdominal examination (➲ p. 208–9) may reveal a palpable abdominal mass of faeces.

If a sigmoid volvulus is considered—a contrast enema.

Imaging may reveal a dilated colon ± a dilated rectum.

Treatment

Disimpaction—gentle manual evacuation of the faeces might be needed. Care is required not to damage the anal sphincters, which might already be compromised. This may need to be done under anaesthesia.

As symptoms may be lifelong, it is important to teach patients to manage their own bowels by:

• Keeping the faeces permanently soft: consider laxatives (➲ p. 422–3)
• Encouraging regular defaecation after a meal
• Considering biofeedback to teach muscle coordination
• Encourage daily oral intake of 2500 ml of fluids.

If conservative management fails, surgery to remove the affected bowel could be considered for severe symptoms.

Diverticular disease

Diverticular disease is the presence of diverticula (singular is diverticulum) in the colon that cause symptoms. Diverticulosis is the presence of diverticula which are symptomless. A diverticulum is a small hernia or out-pouch in the bowel wall (see Fig. 4.1). Diverticulitis is inflammation of the diverticula.

Symptoms

Many people are asymptomatic with diverticulosis. When undigested food or faeces collect in the diverticulum, there can be symptoms of diverticular disease including:
• Mild abdominal pain
• Altered bowel habit/stool consistency
• Rectal bleeding.

In an acute episode of diverticulitis, the symptoms include:
• Left lower abdominal pain
• Tenderness on examination
• Low-grade pyrexia
• Tachycardia
• Leucocytosis
• Frequency and/or urgency of urine
• Potentially septic shock in severe cases
• Fewer than 20% of patients develop complications, but these can include perforation, peritonitis, fistulae, strictures, bowel obstruction, and haemorrhage.

Causes

Diverticula often occur at a weak point in the colonic wall, probably due to the pressures within the colon as a result of constipation or a low-fibre diet. Incidence increases with age.

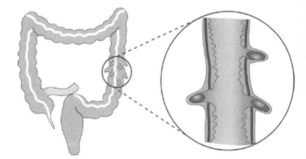

Fig. 4.1 Diverticular disease of the colon.
Reproduced with kind permission © Burdett Institute 2008.

Investigations

- Abdominal examination (➔ p. 210)
- Digital rectal examination (➔ p. 208–9)
- Endoscopy, if safe
- FBC—including haemoglobin, erythrocyte sedimentation rate (ESR), C-reactive protein (CRP), and WBC
- Carcinoembryonic antigen (CEA)—check for concomitant cancer
- Barium enema
- CT scan
- CT pneumocolon—enables more of the internal structure of the bowel to be seen and is less traumatic for older patients.

Treatment

- Dietary advice with an increase in fibre
- ↑ water intake—2 L/day
- Analgesia, if required
- Advice on bowel habit
- Health education.

Blood loss from a bleeding diverticulum is often significant and dramatic and occurs without warning. In acute diverticulitis, consider conservative management, if the patient's condition allows. For emergency surgery, consider pre-operative counselling and siting for a possible stoma. Elective surgery usually results in a segmental colectomy without formation of a stoma.

Surgery, often a Hartmann's procedure (➔ p. 493) may be required if the disease is severe and life threatening. Indications for surgery include:

- Infection
- Perforation
- Peritonitis
- Recurrent diverticulitis
- Paracolic or pelvic abscess
- Sigmoid mass
- Fistulae
- Obstruction
- Stricture
- Major haemorrhage.

Familial adenomatous polyposis

Familial adenomatous polyposis (FAP) has previously been termed adenomatous polyposis coli, familial multiple polyposis, adenomatous polyposis of the colon, Gardner's syndrome, and familial polyposis syndrome. FAP as the name denotes is characterized by the occurrence of a hundred, or more, sometimes thousands of, polyps (colorectal adenomas) in the colon and rectum, usually developing in adolescence. Each polyp has the potential to develop into a carcinoma.

Symptoms

Some people may be symptom free, or there may be the usual symptoms of colorectal cancer (➲ p. 352).

In addition to those in the colon and rectum, there may also be polyps in the stomach (➲ p. 9) and duodenum (➲ p. 10). In the stomach, the gastric polyps mainly do not have a malignant potential, but gastric cancer occasionally occurs.

Furthermore, almost all patients with FAP develop adenomatous polyps in the duodenum, and 10% will develop duodenal carcinoma. Duodenal carcinoma is associated with a poor prognosis but usually occurs in older people with FAP.

Extra-intestinal manifestations (non-gastrointestinal symptoms) include:
• Epidermoid cysts
• Osteomas—harmless bony lumps
• Desmoid tumours—fibrous, soft tissue neoplasms
• Congenital retinal pigmentation
• Abnormal dentition.

Causes

FAP is an autosomal dominantly inherited condition, meaning it is genetically passed down from one parent with a 50% chance of inheritance. FAP is related to the *APC* (adenomatous polyposis coli) gene (on chromosome 5).

Incidence

FAP is rare, occurring in about 1 in every 8,500 live births.

Investigations

In many cases there will be a family history of FAP but not always. Additionally, diagnosis of FAP is based on identification of colorectal adenomas and is often confirmed by genetic testing. It is essential to undertake a detailed extended family history if this is not already known.

Treatment

To avoid cancer, a prophylactic colectomy is advised in teenage years. The operation can be:
• Colectomy with ileorectal anastomosis (IRA) (➲ p. 489)
• Restorative proctocolectomy (RPC) (➲ p. 501)
• Total proctocolectomy with end ileostomy (TPC) (➲ p. 497).

Prevention

To prevent the development of cancer it is advocated that if the rectum is left in situ after colectomy (when an IRA is performed) that the rectum is regularly examined for polyps which should be removed endoscopically; however, if that is not possible, then the rectum can be removed. Polyps can develop in small bowel pouches (RPC) and the pouches require examination regularly. Similarly, a cancer can form on an ileostomy so any growths in this patient group should be considered as a potential cancer until proven otherwise.

On average a cancer will develop by age 39 without a prophylactic colectomy but cancer can occur in teenage years. After removal of the colon, and often the rectum, people with FAP are still at an ↑ risk of cancer of the upper GI and thyroid.

Further reading

Samarasinghe M and Hawkins J (2014). Familial adenomatous polyposis: natural history and care of the patient. *Gastrointestinal Nursing* 12(2): 28–36.

Flatus

Healthy people pass gas from the anus on average between 10 and 20 times/day, releasing ~500–750 ml of air. Contrary to lay belief, age and gender do not influence the frequency of passing flatus.

Causes

- Volume of flatus ↑ if the diet includes large quantities of non-absorbable sugars, such as beans and tropical fruits
- Different individuals' gut flora, in terms of the bacteria's ability to produce gas
- Swallowed air accounts for 80% of flatus—generally odourless nitrogen
- Fermentation of ingested food accounts for 20% of flatus—producing carbon dioxide and methane, the odour of flatus
- Any diarrhoeal illness can cause excess flatus owing to ↑ gut motility
- Lactose intolerance (➔ p. 68–9)
- Coeliac disease (➔ p. 64–5)
- Chronic pancreatitis (➔ p. 184–5)
- Gallstone disease (➔ p. 198–9)
- IBS (➔ p. 96–8).

Treatment

Treatment in general is not necessary, but dietary changes may reduce volumes of flatus.

Irritable bowel syndrome

IBS is a common, chronic disorder that presents with abdominal pain associated with a change in bowel habit, and can be diarrhoea predominant, constipation predominant, or alternating.

Symptoms

There are a number of symptoms that are associated with IBS:
• Abdominal pain/discomfort
• Change in stool frequency or consistency
• Bloating
• Mucus
• Abdominal cramp
• Flatus.

Incidence

IBS often presents in young adults. It affects about one in five adults at some point in their life, although it is thought that many do not present to a healthcare professional, unless symptoms are severe and/or frequent. More ♀ than ♂ present (ratio 2:1), resulting in over 850,000 consultations/year with general practitioners (GPs), who manage the majority of patients. However, IBS accounts for about half of gastroenterology outpatient department consultations.

Causes

The cause of IBS is unknown but is considered to be related to:
• Food intolerance
• Emotional stress and hypersensitivity
• Abnormal peristalsis
• Poorly coordinated signals between the brain and the large bowel
• Post gastroenteritis (possibly due to abnormal levels of gut bacteria).

Diagnosis

Diagnosis of IBS requires a detailed history and physical examination. It can be made, after exclusion of more sinister pathology, if there is abdominal pain/discomfort that is relieved by defaecation or associated with a change in bowel frequency or consistency plus two or more of the following:
• Straining, urgency, incomplete evacuation
• Abdominal bloating, distension, tension, or hardness
• Symptoms worsen after eating
• Passage of mucus.

Other associated symptoms include (but are not diagnostic of IBS):
• Lethargy
• Nausea
• Back ache
• Bladder issues.

Treatment

Treatment will depend upon symptoms and can include dietary changes and medication.

Mild symptoms require:
- Education
- Setting realistic expectations
- Avoidance of alcohol
- Avoidance of caffeine
- ↑ or ↓ of fibre, depending upon symptoms
- Food manipulation to ↓ flatus
- Stress ↓
- Peppermint oil for bloating
- Probiotics may be useful (➔ p. 97).

Moderate/severe symptoms—as above, plus the following:
- Antispasmodics (➔ p. 409)
- Laxatives (➔ p. 422–3) for constipation
- Loperamide (➔ p. 411) for diarrhoea
- Low-dose antidepressants (➔ p. 410) to relieve discomfort
- Exclusion diet (with dietitian supervision).

Dietary advice

The role of food intolerances in IBS is not fully understood. Many people have worse IBS symptoms when they consume certain foods or beverages, including wheat, dairy products, citrus fruits, beans, cabbage, milk, and carbonated drinks. Therefore, dietary modification may be necessary (see ➔ p. 448–9 faecal incontinence/constipation, ➔ p. 204–5), possibly in conjunction with a dietitian. Other tips include:
- Eating regular meals
- Avoid long gaps between meals
- Taking time to eat a meal.

When patients do not respond to the above dietary changes, the next step in dietary modification would be the FODMAP (fermentable oligosaccharides, disaccharides, monosaccharides, and polyols) diet, in conjunction with a dietitian.

Probiotics

Probiotics are bacteria that can beneficially affect health by improving the balance and function of the gut bacteria. They are found in many different forms such as yoghurts, tablets, capsules, and sachets. The general consensus for using probiotics for IBS is to take for 4 weeks and review the effect. Probiotics should only be taken as per manufacturer's recommendation. They are largely safe for healthy people to take. However, anyone who has a disorder of the immune system may be at risk, so should seek professional advice beforehand.

Psychological intervention

Cognitive behavioural therapy

Cognitive behavioural therapy (CBT) is a method used by the individual to reframe and modify negative thoughts. This helps to establish a positive emotional state. As a result, gastrointestinal symptoms experienced in IBS may be reduced.

Hypnotherapy

Hypnotherapy involves progressive relaxation with suggestions of soothing imagery and sensations focused on the person's symptoms. This may be an effective treatment for IBS.

Mindfulness

Mindfulness involves a form of meditation to focus on the present moment experience and letting go of thoughts fixed from the past and the future. Mindfulness can enhance the ability to relax, improve self-esteem and reduce pain.

Further reading

Collins B and Bradshaw E (2016). *Bowel Dysfunction: A Comprehensive Guide for Healthcare Professionals*. Springer Nature, Switzerland.

NICE (2017). Irritable bowel syndrome in adults: diagnosis and management (CG61). www.nice.org.uk/guidance/cg61 (Accessed 30/07/2019).

NICE (2007). Faecal incontinence in adults: management (CG 49) https://www.nice.org.uk/Guidance/CG49 (Accessed 10/07/2020).

www.bda.uk.com/foodfacts/irritable_bowel_syndrome#Probiotics (Accessed 30/07/2019).

www.mayoclinic.org/diseases-conditions/irritable-bowel-syndrome/symptoms-causes/syc 20360016 (Accessed 29/07/2019).

www.ncbi.nlm.nih.gov/pmc/articles/PMC5704118/pdf/jcm-06-00101.pdf   (Accessed   29/07/2019).

www.ncbi.nlm.nih.gov/pmc/articles/PMC2729728/pdf/1472-6882-9-24.pdf   (Accessed   29/07/2019).

www.sciencedirect.com/science/article/abs/pii/S0024320518306180?via%3Dihub (Accessed 29/07/2019).

www.theibsnetwork.org/diet/fodmaps/ (Accessed 29/07/2019).

Ischaemic colitis

Ischaemic colitis is an inflammation of the colon where the blood supply has been compromised.

Signs and symptoms
- Left iliac fossa pain
- Nausea and vomiting
- Loose motion often containing dark blood
- Marked tenderness in left iliac fossa.

Causes
Often there is no known cause, but there are a number of predisposing factors:
- Thrombosis—inferior mesenteric artery thrombosis
- Emboli—mesenteric arterial emboli, cholesterol emboli
- Decreased cardiac output, arrhythmias, or atrial fibrillation
- Shock—sepsis, haemorrhage, hypovolaemia
- Trauma—strangulated hernia or volvulus
- Drugs—oestrogens, immunosuppressive agents, psychotropic agents
- Surgery
- Vasculitis
- Disorders of coagulation
- Colonoscopy (Ɔ p. 246–7)
- Barium enema.

Investigations
- Endoscopy (Ɔ p. 246–7)—may show blue swollen mucosa not showing contact bleeding and sparing the rectum
- Plain abdominal X-ray (Ɔ p. 230)—outlines segment gas
- Barium enema (Ɔ p. 214–15)—shows 'thumb printing' in early phase.

Treatment
Antibiotics.

Surgery is warranted only if evidence of perforation, sepsis, haemorrhage, ischaemic stricture, segmental colitis, continuation of symptoms for more than 2 weeks.

Juvenile polyposis syndrome

Juvenile polyposis syndrome (JPS) is characterized by the development of 'juvenile' (hamartomatous) polyps within the gastrointestinal tract, most commonly the colon, stomach, or duodenum. Polyps termed 'juvenile' can appear visually similar to adenomas; inside there are often multiple, mucin-filled cysts (previously termed retention polyps). Some stalks may not have polyps on them where the polyp has fallen off (auto-amputation)—characteristic of juvenile polyps.

Symptoms

Symptoms of JPS include rectal bleeding and anaemia due to the polyps bleeding and falling off. Sometimes prolapse or defaecation of the polyp can occur onset of JPS might be in early infancy or adulthood, with the average age of onset of symptoms being 9 years.

One small group of people (with *SMAD4* genetic mutation) have hereditary haemorrhagic telangiectasia (HHT), associated with vascular abnormalities. They present with nose bleeds and there is an increased risk of a stroke, particularly under a general anaesthesia.

Congenital abnormalities might occur in conjunction with JPS, including:
- Hydrocephalus
- Pulmonary arteriovenous fistulae
- Undescended testes
- Heart defects
- Genitourinary abnormalities
- Digital clubbing
- Cleft palate
- Larger than usual head (macrocephaly) and hands.

Causes

JPS is an autosomal dominantly inherited condition, meaning it is genetically passed down from one parent with a 50% chance of inheritance. JPS can be caused by a mutation in one of several different genes, including:
- *SMAD4* gene (on chromosome 18)
- *BMPR1A* gene (on chromosome 10)
- *ENG1* gene (on chromosome 9).

Incidence

JPS is rare with an incidence of about 1 in 100,000.

Investigations

There is no genetic testing available for JPS because of the different genes involved. A diagnosis of JPS can be made by meeting one or more of the following criteria:
- Three or more juvenile polyps in the colon or rectum
- Juvenile polyps throughout the GI tract
- Any number of juvenile polyps plus a family history of juvenile polyposis.

Treatment

If there are numerous polyps a colectomy (➔ p. 488–9) may be required. Otherwise removal of polyps is advocated.

Prevention

People with JPS have increased risk of developing cancers outside the gastrointestinal tract.

Further reading

Neale K and Hawkins J (2014). Overview of Peutz-Jeghers and juvenile polyposis syndromes. *Gastrointestinal Nursing* 12(4): 43–7.

Lynch syndrome

Lynch syndrome was previously termed hereditary non-polyposis colo-rectal cancer (HNPCC). Lynch syndrome is characterized by the development of colorectal cancer, endometrial cancer, and other cancers.

Symptoms

Colorectal cancer typically occurs below the age of 50, is more common in men, and in 70% of cases is in the right colon. Women also have a very high risk of endometrial cancer, and an increased risk of ovarian cancer. There are also increased risks of gastric and pancreatic cancers.

Causes

Lynch syndrome is dominantly inherited, meaning it is genetically passed down from one parent with a 50% chance of inheritance. Lynch syndrome is caused by mutations in the mismatch repair genes, *MLH1*, *MSH2*, *MSH6*, and *PMS2*.

Investigations

A detailed history of Lynch syndrome is necessary. People should also be tested for microsatellite instability (MSI).

Treatment

Treatment for Lynch syndrome is a prophylactic colectomy and for women also a total abdominal hysterectomy with bilateral salpingo-oophrectomy.

Prevention

Regular colonoscopy is needed. First-degree relatives should be screened.

Further reading

NICE (2017). Molecular testing strategies for Lynch syndrome in people with colorectal cancer. https://www.nice.org.uk/guidance/dg27 (Accessed 20/7/2020).

Megacolon

There are two categories of megacolon: idiopathic and toxic megacolon. Idiopathic megacolon occurs when there is colonic dilation in addition to pseudo-obstruction, whereas toxic megacolon is a potentially fatal complication of acute, active IBD (➲ p. 368–9) or infectious colitis.

Symptoms

Toxic megacolon is characterized by non-obstructed segmental or total colonic dilation associated with systemic toxicity.

Incidence

Megacolon can affect ♂ and ♀ of all ages.

Causes

- IBD (➲ p. 368–9)
- Infectious colitis
- Ischaemic colitis
- Pseudomembranous colitis.

Investigations

- FBC, urea, and electrolytes, ESR, CRP
- Plain abdominal X-ray (➲ p. 23)
- Stool specimens—ova, parasites, and *Clostridium difficile*
- Ultrasound (➲ p. 227)/CT (➲ p. 220) might aid management
- Colonoscopy (➲ p. 246–7) should usually be avoided owing to the high risk of perforation.

Treatment

Toxic megacolon is an acute emergency and ∴ should be managed in a high-dependency area. Pre- and post-operative considerations include:
- Frequent monitoring
- ↓ severity of underlying inflammation
- Nil by mouth
- Nasogastric tube
- IV corticosteroids (➲ p. 428)
- IV broad-spectrum antibiotics (➲ p. 408)
- Fluid resuscitation/electrolyte depletion
- Stop any anti-motility agents
- Blood transfusion if anaemic
- Repositioning manoeuvres to aid decompression
- Prevention of deep vein thrombosis.

Surgery (subtotal colectomy and end ileostomy) is indicated for:
- Progressive dilatation
- Worsening toxicity
- Failure of medical therapy
- Perforation/haemorrhage.

MYH-associated polyposis

MYH-associated polyposis (MAP) sometimes termed MUTYH-associated polyposis. MAP is characterized by having between ten and hundreds of colorectal adenomas. The adenomas usually develop during young adulthood, with the risk of colorectal cancer.

Symptoms

Symptoms of MAP can include symptoms of colorectal cancer (➋ p. 352). People with MAP are at a significantly increased risk of ovarian, bladder, and skin cancer, often in their 50s.

Causes

MAP is an autosomal recessive inherited condition. This means that both parents need to have the genetic mutation to have a chance to pass the condition on. There are three possible outcomes when two affected parents have a child:

- There is a 25% chance the child will not inherit the mutation, so will not have the condition
- There is a 25% chance the child will be affected by MAP
- There is a 50% chance that the child will be a carrier, but will not have MAP.

Often the parents are unaffected by MAP. The *MYH* gene is located on the short arm of chromosome 1.

Every child born to a person with MAP will be a carrier but may not have the condition, if the other parent is not a carrier.

Investigations

Genetic tests should be considered if people have multiple polyps on endoscopy. Upper GI endoscopy is also needed as there is a risk of duodenal cancer.

Treatment

Treatment is usually a prophylactic colectomy when the number of polyps exceeds 100 or polyps are too large to continue with endoscopic management. The operation can be:

- Colectomy with ileorectal anastomosis (➋ p. 489)
- RPC (➋ p. 501)
- TPC (➋ p. 497).

Prevention

Without intervention, the average age of bowel cancer in patients with MAP is 47 years.

Further reading

Cuthill V and Samarasinghe M (2014). MYH-associated polyposis: natural history and care of the patient. *Gastrointestinal Nursing* 12(3): 20–6.

Peutz–Jeghers syndrome

Peutz-Jeghers syndrome (PJS) is characterized by the development of Peutz-Jeghers polyps within the gut from the stomach to the rectum; these polyps are hamartomas and do not have the same malignant potential as adenomas. The polyps can grow quite large and are often pedunculated (have a stalk).

Symptoms

The small bowel polyps often result in symptoms in babies and very young children. Severe abdominal pain can be caused by peristalsis trying to move the polyp along the intestine, possibly resulting in intussusception (telescoping of a part of the gastrointestinal tract into a lower section) and possible obstruction. This may result in an emergency hospital admission.

Extraintestinal manifestations of PJS include:
• Pigmented lesions on lips, buccal mucosa, and fingers and toes (about 95% of people with PJS develop pigmentation), occurring in childhood often at 2–3 years old
• Increased risk of other cancers, most commonly GI, breast, and pancreatic cancer. Higher risk for female patients, with a cumulative cancer risk of about 70% by 70 years old.

People with a family history of PJS who have a baby with prolonged crying should consider a new diagnosis of PJS in their baby.

Causes

PJS is an autosomal dominantly inherited condition, meaning it is genetically passed down from one parent with a 50% chance of inheritance. PJS is caused by an alteration in the *STK11* (*LKB1*) gene (serine/threonine kinase 11) on chromosome 19.

Incidence

PJS is a rare syndrome with about 1 in 100,000 live births.

Investigations

A clinical diagnosis of PJS can be made when any one of the following are present:
• At least two histologically confirmed PJS polyps
• Any number of PJS polyps in a person with a family history of PJS in a close relative
• Characteristic mucocutaneous pigmentation plus a family history of PJS in close relative
• Any number of PJS polyps in a person who also has characteristic mucocutaneous pigmentation.

Genetic testing of young children suspected of having PJS is advised.

Endoscopic screening is advised in adults. Blood tests looking for anaemia secondary to bleeding polyps.

Treatment

Removal of polyps when identified and avoidance of emergency operations that might result in multiple bowel resections.

Prevention

Due to the ↑ risk of other cancers, such as pancreas and breast, screening or extra vigilance may be required.

Further reading

Neale K and Hawkins J (2014) Overview of Peutz-Jeghers and juvenile polyposis syndromes. *Gastrointestinal Nursing* 12(4), 43–7.

Polyp

A polyp in the bowel is a small growth that does not usually become cancerous. Adenomas may, however, over several years turn into a cancer.

Symptoms

Often bowel polyps are symptomless; larger polyps might present with symptoms:
- Mucus
- Rectal bleeding
- Change in bowel habit
- Abdominal pain.

Causes

The cause of polyps is uncertain but they are more common if there is a family history of polyps or cancer in the bowel, in IBD, in obese people, and in smokers.

Incidence

Bowel polyps are very common with about one in four people having one at some point in their life, though more commonly after the age of 60 years.

Investigation

Polyps are often found during bowel screening (endoscopy) and a CT colonography may be needed.

Treatment

Treatment of a bowel polyp is usually to remove it, commonly during a colonoscopy or surgically. Surgical treatment is usually if the polyp is beginning to change towards being cancerous, if it is large or if there are many polyps.

Prevention

As some types of polyps can recur monitoring may be necessary by endoscopy.

Pseudomembranous colitis

Pseudomembranous colitis is a severe colonic inflammation secondary to overgrowth of *C. difficile*.

Symptoms

- Watery diarrhoea
- Abdominal cramps
- Anorexia
- Fever.

In severe cases:
- Marked leucocytosis
- Hypoalbuminaemia
- Fulminant colitis—2–3% of patients
- Colonic perforation
- Toxic megacolon
- Hypotension
- Electrolyte disturbances
- Prolonged ileus
- Death.

Causes

Pseudomembranous colitis usually occurs as a result of antibiotic therapy, but sporadic cases can occur and older people are more at risk.

Investigation

Stool sample—for the detection of *C. difficile* toxins.

Treatment

Stop the antibiotic and transfer to appropriate antibiotic treatment (⊃ p. 408) for *C. difficile*.

Pseudo-obstruction

Pseudo-obstruction is seen clinically as an intestinal obstruction but without an occluding lesion in the bowel lumen. Acute pseudo-obstruction is termed Ogilvie's syndrome.

Symptoms
- Intestinal obstruction
- Abdominal pain (rarely)
- Distension
- Vomiting
- Weight loss
- Steatorrhoea (chronic only)
- Diarrhoea.

If the oesophagus is involved, there may be no symptoms, or dysphagia, chest pain, regurgitation, reflux, and heartburn may occur. Gastric involvement produces gastroparesis. Colonic involvement usually results in constipation, megacolon, or both.

Causes
Pseudo-obstruction is caused by disorders of the smooth muscle (visceral myopathy), myenteric plexus, or extraintestinal nervous system (visceral neuropathy), causing the intestinal walls to be unable to contract sufficiently to generate peristaltic motion.

Chronic intestinal pseudo-obstruction might be primary or secondary to systemic illnesses, but has multiple causes.

Investigations
The laboratory abnormalities reflect the degree of malabsorption and malnutrition, in addition to the presence of underlying disorders. Patients with diarrhoea usually have steatorrhoea owing to bacterial overgrowth in the small bowel, and often have vitamin B_{12} malabsorption. Mucosal biopsies of the small bowel are of no value in diagnosing this condition.

Plain abdominal X-rays—images might resemble a paralytic ileus or mimic true mechanical obstruction.

Barium contrast studies—in about a third of patients show a distended stomach and delayed gastric emptying. The duodenum is usually, but not invariably, abnormal and can show colonic dilatation and elongation. If extreme, this is classified as a 'megacolon'.

The urinary tract should be studied to look for evidence of megacystitis or megaureters. If there is continuing diagnostic uncertainty, a full-thickness biopsy of the small bowel can be performed.

Treatment

No treatment is curative or halts the natural history of any of the disorders causing intestinal pseudo-obstruction. The treatment goals are to alleviate symptoms and treat any abnormalities. Advice can be given to modify diet, consider frequent, small meals, with a low-fat, lactose-free, low-fibre diet. Supplement drinks are useful, if tolerated. Vitamin and mineral supplements should be prescribed. Dietetic advice may be necessary.

* Bacterial overgrowth—antibiotics
* Drug therapy—metoclopramide (→ p. 412), domperidone (→ p. 412), erythromycin (→ p. 408), octreotide, neostigmine
* Long-term parenteral nutrition might be necessary to maintain patients nutritionally
* Surgery can be considered as a last resort and depends on the area affected
* Small intestinal transplantation has been performed in extreme cases
* Decompression—may be used in acute pseudo-obstruction.

Colonic decompression is performed in one of three ways: transanally (endoscopy), transabdominally, or chemically (neostigmine).

Radiation enteritis and colitis (radiation enteropathy)

Caused by acute or chronic injury to the gut from exposure to therapeutic or supra-therapeutic levels of ionizing radiation.

Symptoms

Acute symptoms include:
- Diarrhoea
- Abdominal discomfort
- Tenesmus
- Rectal bleeding.

Symptoms occur soon after starting radiotherapy, last for the duration of therapy and subside 10–15 days after radiation therapy has stopped.
Chronic symptoms include:
- Constipation
- Altered motility
- Diarrhoea
- Abdominal discomfort
- Tenesmus
- Rectal bleeding
- Adhesions
- Perforation
- Secondary cancer
- Fistula formation
- Faecal incontinence—associated with internal anal sphincter damage.

Risk factors include:
- Concomitant chemotherapy
- High-dose radiation therapy
- Uraemia or diabetes mellitus
- Pelvic inflammatory disease
- Hypertension
- Thin-body habitus
- Abdominal or pelvic surgery
- Accelerated fractionation regimens for delivering radiotherapy.

Causes

Acute radiation induces cell death (apoptosis) resulting in denuding of the intestinal mucosa. Intestinal permeability to bacteria and other antigens is ↑ and diarrhoea results from ↑ fluid and electrolyte loss.

Chronic radiation enteropathy is caused by a progressive occlusive vasculitis, which can affect all layers of the bowel wall. Tissue hypoxia and ischaemia occur, resulting in mucosal atrophy and ulceration, in addition to fibrosis of the muscularis and thickening of the serosa. Stricturing might ensue.

Investigations

- Colonoscopy—demonstrates changes of mucosal or transmural inflammation
- Biopsies—might be inconclusive
- Barium investigations—might be normal or show ulceration, submucosal thickening, single or multiple strictures, adhesions or fistulae, or simply a loss of the normal haustral pattern
- Capsule endoscopy—demonstrates mucosal changes.

Treatment

- Anti-diarrhoeal drugs (⊃ p. 411)
- Biofeedback
- Medications such antibiotics (⊃ p. 408), corticosteroids (⊃ p. 428), antidepressants (⊃ p. 410), and analgesia (⊃ p. 406)
- Bleeding that fails to respond to medical therapy may be treated by direct endoscopic ablative therapy (laser, heater probe, or argon plasma beam).

Consider constipation and faecal loading as the cause of pain.

Volvulus

Sigmoid volvulus occurs when the mesentery lengthens, enabling a dilated sigmoid colon to twist over on itself, causing a mechanical blockage. In some cases, the volvulus can compromise blood supply to the bowel causing ischaemia or necrosis.

Symptoms
- Commonly sudden-onset colicky, lower abdominal pain plus gross abdominal distension and without passage of faeces or flatus
- Alternatively, chronic abdominal distension, constipation with vague lower abdominal discomfort and vomiting
- History of mild symptoms followed by large passage of faeces or flatus
- Vomiting in severe cases
- Pyrexia if perforated
- Colonic ischaemia may present with symptoms of perforation and peritonitis.

Causes
Sigmoid volvulus is rare in children and people from developed countries. Risk factors for a volvulus include:
- Being elderly and male
- Chronic constipation
- Megacolon (➲ p. 105).

Investigations
- Abdominal examination—tympanic, distended abdomen—often non-tender ± palpable mass
- Rectal examination—empty rectum
- Plain abdominal X-ray—single grossly dilated loop of sigmoid colon
- Barium enema—can result in decompression
- CT scan—to assess for bowel wall ischaemia.

Treatment
- Urgent hospitalization.
- Decompression then planned surgery. Decompression can be achieved using an endoscope and flatus tube. Observe for persistent abdominal pain and rectal bleeding—this may indicate ischaemia and requires urgent surgical intervention.
- Surgery is ideally resection of the redundant sigmoid colon ± colostomy if concerned about ischaemia.

Rectum and anus

Anal cancer

Anal cancer, an uncommon cancer, arises from the cells around the anal opening (verge) or within the anal canal up to its junction with the rectum. The position of the cancer and its histology are important considerations. Squamous cell carcinomas account for 80% of anal cancers; these are cancers around the anal opening.

Symptoms

- Bleeding from rectum or anus
- Lump at the anal canal
- Pain
- Persistent or recurrent itching
- Narrowing of stool or other changes in bowel movements
- Abnormal discharge from the anus
- Swollen lymph nodes in the anal or groin areas.

Stages of anal cancer

Stage 0

The cancer is at its earliest stage and is only in the mucosa.

Stage 1

The cancer has grown into the submucosa or muscle but has not spread to the lymph nodes or elsewhere.

Stage 2

The cancer has grown through the muscle wall or through the outer layer of the bowel and may be growing into tissues nearby. The cancer has not spread to the lymph nodes or elsewhere.

Stage 3

The cancer has spread to lymph nodes nearby but has not spread anywhere else in the body.

Stage 4

The cancer has spread to other parts of the body such as the liver or lungs and it may have spread to nearby lymph nodes.

Causes

- Human papillomavirus (HPV-16)
- Sexual activity
- Smoking
- Lowered immunity/HIV infection.

Treatment

Combination therapy, including radiation therapy and chemotherapy, is now gold standard treatment for most anal cancers. Occasionally, very small or early tumours are removed surgically (local excision). Abdominoperineal resection might represent a rescue treatment for partial responders to chemoradiation or in relapsing patients. Control is achieved in 80% of cases.

Post-treatment care

Chemotherapy is generally well tolerated. Perianal skin care is essential during radiotherapy. Anal tissue can also be damaged, causing scar tissue to form and impairing the anal sphincter's function. Reassure the patient about the effectiveness of treatment for anal cancer, although several months are required to assess outcome.

Anal fissure

An anal fissure is a small tear in the mucosa of the anal canal, which most commonly (≥90%) occurs in the posterior anal canal (Fig. 5.1). Anal fissures can be acutely painful, especially during and after defaecation and are often described by patients as 'It feels like passing broken glass.' Defaecation can re-open a fissure. Pain can cause muscle spasm, which exacerbates the pain and leads to chronic lack of blood supply to the area, which, in turn, inhibits healing. A chronic fissure might have a sentinel skin tag at the lower end.

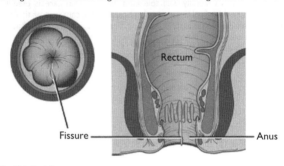

Fig. 5.1 Anal fissure.
Reproduced with kind permission © Burdett Institute 2008.

Symptoms
- Pain, sometimes severe, during bowel movements
- Pain after bowel movements that can last several hours
- Bright red blood on the stool or toilet paper after a bowel movement
- Itching or irritation around the anus
- A visible tear in the skin around the anus.

Causes
Often the cause is unclear but may be due to:
- Anal trauma, e.g. constipation, hard stool, non-relaxing anus, or local injuries
- Diarrhoea
- More common after childbirth (anterior).

For people with multiple fissures consider Crohn's disease (➲ p. 377), syphilis, or anal herpes infection.

Investigations
External inspection with gentle traction of the anal verge. Digital anal examination might be too painful. Proctoscopy can be used to visualize higher fissures (but might be poorly tolerated). Use lidocaine gel.

Treatment

The nurse should provide explanation and reassurance. Advice should include introduction of a high-fibre diet, stool softeners (◆ p. 422–3), analgesia (◆ p. 406), and adequate fluids to keep stool soft and easier to pass without pain. Advise patients to attempt to relax during defaecation; which is not easy. Many patients heal spontaneously, but it can take several weeks. Other medications may be offered such as glycerine trinitrate (GTN) ointment, botox (◆ p. 424), or diltiazem (◆ p. 425).

Surgery

If pharmacological treatment fails, a chronic, troublesome fissure might need surgery, such as a sphincterotomy. A lateral sphincterotomy involves cutting the internal anal sphincter to reduce the muscle pressure and spasm to enable healing. There is a 5–10% risk of flatus or stool incontinence. Midline sphincterotomy and anal stretch are seldom performed because they have a higher risk of incontinence. Rarely, an advancement flap surgery (◆ p. 123) is performed.

Further reading

NICE (2017). Anal fissure. https://cks.nice.org.uk/anal-fissure (Accessed 20/7/2020).

Anal fistula

An anal fistula is an abnormal connection; described as a narrow tunnel with its internal opening originating from the anal glands located between the internal and external sphincter (Fig. 5.2). Glands communicate with the anal canal at the level of the dentate line. If the glands become blocked an abscess can form, which can extend to the surface of the skin. Pus can then track between or transect sphincters, as follows:

• Simple—one track
• Complex—many tracks
• Intersphincteric—between sphincters
• Transphincteric—crosses the sphincter
• Supralevator—extends above the pelvic floor (levator ani muscles)
• Horseshoe—extends around the anus.

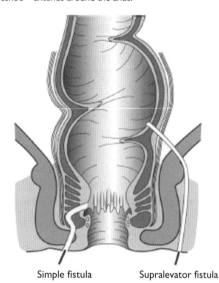

Simple fistula   Supralevator fistula

Fig. 5.2 Anal fistula.
Reproduced with kind permission © Burdett Institute 2008.

Symptoms

Anal fistulae can present with the following symptoms:

• Skin maceration
• Pus, serous fluid, and/or (rarely) discharge of faeces—can be bloody or purulent
• Pruritus ani (⊃ p. 136–7).

Depending on presence and severity of infection:

- Pain
- Swelling
- Tenderness
- Fever
- Unpleasant odour.

Cause

Anal fistula can also be caused by Crohn's disease, previous anal surgery, or tuberculosis.

Investigations

- Visual inspection
- Digital examination—can feel infected tracks but might be painful
- Examination under anaesthesia
- Magnetic resonance imaging (MRI) to define track(s) (➜ p. 222)
- Identify internal and external openings
- If tracks are more extensive, it is harder to eradicate sepsis.

Treatment

The most common treatment for an anal fistula is surgery, although active infection should be addressed first. There are several options:

Lay-open of fistula-in-ano—involves surgically laying open the fistula, which, should be dressed daily to ensure that the wound heals from the inside out by secondary intention. Laying open the fistula can cause faecal incontinence and is not suitable for a fistula that crosses the entire internal and external anal sphincter.

Seton suture—a length of suture material is looped through the fistula, to keep the fistula open and allows pus to drain out. A cutting Seton stitch is gradually tightened to cut through the sphincter, while enabling the track to heal in stages with the aim of preventing faecal incontinence.

Advancement flap—is a procedure in which the internal opening of the fistula is identified and a flap of mucosal tissue is cut around the opening. The flap is lifted to expose the fistula, which is then cleaned and the internal opening is sewn shut. The flap is pulled down over the sewn internal opening and sutured in place. The external opening is cleaned and sutured.

Fibrin glue—involves injecting the fistula with a biodegradable glue which should, in theory, close the fistula from the inside out and let it heal naturally.

Other biomaterials are being tried to achieve healing with or without surgery.

Anal warts (condylomata acuminata)

Perianal manifestation of genital warts ('venereal' warts). The warts affect the areas around the penis, anus, or vagina.

Symptoms

Warts are usually painless, so patients could be asymptomatic carriers; it is common to have no visible warts but still be able to infect other people. Warts can take weeks or months to appear after infection.

• Tiny spots or growths, often as small as a pinhead, which can be near or in the anus
• Single or multiple warts are common and they can occur in various sizes
• Itching
• Bleeding
• Mucus discharge
• Feeling like there is a lump in the anal area.

Cause

Warts are caused by the HPV, of which over 90 types have been identified, many sexually transmitted. HPV types 6 and 11 are the commonest. A person can become infected with HPV without having sexual intercourse. Any direct contact to the anal area (e.g. hand contact, fluids from an infected sexual partner) can cause HPV and anal or genital warts. Anal sex can predispose to anal, rather than genital warts. Immunocompromised patients are at risk. Warts can be associated with HIV infection.

Investigations

• Inspection around the anus, as well as the entire pelvic area including the genitals
• A proctoscope may be performed for inspection of any internal anal warts.

Treatment

If warts are not removed, they can grow larger and multiply. Left untreated, warts may lead to an increased risk of anal cancer in the affected area. Internal anal warts may not respond to topical medications, so surgery may be required. Treatment usually takes place at genitourinary medicine clinics. Warts can take several months of repeated treatments to clear. Warts can spontaneously recur without reinfection. Condoms do not offer full protection if the infected area is not covered.

Treatments include:
• Chemical/topical—podophyllin, trichloroacetic acid, and podophyllotoxin. Avoid in pregnancy
• Laser or electrocautery—to 'burn' the warts
• Cryotherapy (freezing) with liquid nitrogen (spray or application)— might need several treatments
• Surgery—small warts can be removed by local scissor excision under local anaesthetic. Extensive warts might need formal surgical excision. Often done piecemeal to avoid extensive scarring.

Anorectal abscess

An anorectal abscess is a painful condition, which arises from a bacterial infection in one of the anal sinuses. Leads to inflammation and development of a collection of pus near the anus. The most common types of abscesses are perianal and ischiorectal.

Symptoms

There may be a number of symptoms including:
- Acutely tender
- Local erythematous swelling
- Some discharge may be possible.

Ischiorectal abscesses

- Ischiorectal abscesses may take longer to become visible externally
- May have vague pelvic/perianal pain
- Fever
- Skin irritation—swelling, redness and/or tenderness
- Indurated when compared with the other side.

Cause

Although most perianal abscesses are sporadic, certain diseases may increase the risk of developing an abscess.
- Inflammatory bowel disease such as Crohn's disease or ulcerative colitis
- Diabetes
- Diverticulitis
- Pelvic inflammatory disease
- Being the receptive partner in anal sex
- Use of medications, such as prednisone.

Investigations

Digital rectal examination can be painful and may be postponed until examination under anaesthesia is performed, if appropriate. Deep abscesses are often harder to diagnose and may require imaging.

If septic consider blood cultures to identify the relevant bacteria and bloods to assess the severity of the sepsis.

Consider alternative pathology, including fissures or thrombosed haemorrhoids. Sexually transmitted infection can also present with anal lesions and pain. Consider also an anal malignancy.

Test faecal calprotectin, as elevated calprotectin suggests intestinal inflammation and may aid with diagnosis of Crohn's disease.

Treatment

Anal abscesses are rarely treated with antibiotics. Almost all cases will require surgery and preferably managed as follows:
- If evidence of sepsis is seen, treat with antibiotics (❷ p. 408)
- Incise and drain the sepsis under general anaesthesia.

Haemorrhoids

Haemorrhoidal cushions are normal anatomical structures, located within the anal canal, usually occupying the left lateral and right anterior and posterior positions above the dentate line at 3, 7, and 11 o'clock (Fig. 5.3). As these cushions enlarge, they can protrude in the anal lumen and might be visible externally, although the majority are generally internal. Haemorrhoids are not 'varicose veins.'

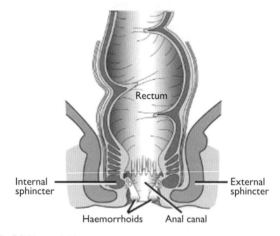

Fig. 5.3 Haemorrhoids.
Reproduced with kind permission © Burdett Institute 2008.

Haemorrhoids are usually classified as degree 1–4, as follows:
- First degree—internal, might prolapse into the lumen, but are only seen on proctoscopy. Might look like normal cushions, but bleed.
- Second degree—prolapse out of anus on straining or defaecation, return spontaneously or with minimal manual assistance to push back.
- Third degree—prolapse outside the anus continuously or often, not just with straining or defaecation. Often haemorrhoid needs manual replacement and might have associated external skin tags if long-standing.
- Fourth degree—thrombosed or strangulated external haemorrhoids. Venous return impaired; haemorrhoid becomes engorged and gangrenous. There may also be haemorrhoidal skin tags.

Symptoms

Symptoms can depend on the extent of the problem, although some people may be asymptomatic. Symptoms include:

- Dilated blood vessels
- Bleeding when defaecating, usually bright red arterial blood on stools, toilet paper, or in the toilet bowl
- Pain or discomfort, especially when sitting
- Pain during bowel movements
- Pruritus or irritation around the anal region
- Swelling around the anus
- Possible soiling of stool or mucus (if external)

Cause

Factors that may contribute to the development of haemorrhoids include:

- Constipation
- Straining during defaecation
- Ageing
- Heavy lifting
- Chronic cough
- Conditions that raise intra-abdominal pressure (such as pregnancy and childbirth).

Investigation

- Investigation should include digital examination and visual inspection
- Digital rectal examination—should be undertaken but internal haemorrhoids are often too soft to be felt during this examination
- Visual inspection—using a sigmoidoscope and/or proctoscope
- Note that not all rectal bleeding is the result of haemorrhoids. Consider bowel cancer and further investigation, regardless of age.

Treatment

Most cases of haemorrhoids can be self-treated using conservative methods. More serious or repeat cases may require medication or a surgical procedure. Haemorrhoids can recur after treatment; hence, they are controlled rather than cured.

Conservative treatment

Conservative treatment is generally for first and second degree haemorrhoids the following can be advised to control or provide symptomatic relief:

- Adequate dietary fibre intake by eating a balanced diet containing whole grains, fruit, and vegetables. Increasing dietary fibre should be done gradually to minimize flatulence and bloating.
- Adequate fluid intake is particularly important with an increased fibre diet to maintain soft, well-lubricated stools, and to prevent intestinal obstruction.
- Medication can be used for pain relief and to soothe symptoms.
- Simple analgesia (such as paracetamol) for pain relief.
- Over the counter topical haemorrhoidal preparations can soothe, contain local anaesthetic, mild astringent, and/or low-dose steroid (➔ p. 428) to provide symptomatic relief (avoid prolonged use of steroids).

  Pregnancy-related haemorrhoids usually resolve within a few months.

Surgery

Patients who do not respond to conservative treatment and/or have recurrent problems may require further treatment. However, depending on the severity of the symptoms and the degree of the haemorrhoid this could be non-surgical or surgical.

Non-surgical treatments include:
• Rubber band ligation
• Injection sclerotherapy
• Infrared coagulation/photocoagulation
• Bipolar diathermy
• Direct-current electrotherapy.

Surgical treatments include:
• Haemorrhoidectomy
• Stapled haemorrhoidectomy
• Haemorrhoidal artery ligation.

Further reading

NICE (2016). Haemorrhoids. https://cks.nice.org.uk/haemorrhoids (Accessed 20/7/2020).

Imperforate anus

An imperforate anus is a birth defect in which the rectum is malformed and/or the anus is missing. It is usually detected quickly and at birth, as the defect is obvious. Because of the defect, stool cannot be passed normally.

Symptoms

- No anal opening
- An anal opening in the wrong place, such as too close to the vagina
- No stool in the first 24 to 48 h of life
- Stool passing through the wrong place, such as the urethra, vagina, scrotum or the base of the penis
- A swollen abdomen
- An abnormal connection or fistula, between the baby's rectum and their reproductive system or urinary tract.

Causes

Imperforate anus is caused by abnormal development of the foetus.

Investigations

Usually seen on physical examination, may require an X-ray (➋ p. 230) or ultrasound (➋ p. 227) of the abdomen to reveal the extent of the abnormality. Other examinations may also be required, such as X-ray/ultrasound of the spine, echocardiogram, or MRI (➋ p. 222). This is because imperforate anus is associated with other anomalies.

Treatment

Imperforate anus usually requires immediate surgery to open a passage for faeces. The type of corrective surgery needed will depend on the severity of the defect, for example, how far the rectum has developed, whether there is sphincter involvement, and if any fistulae have developed. Taking these into consideration, imperforate anus can be treated surgically with a perineal anoplasty, pull through, and/or a colostomy formation.

Further reading

Yang G, Wang Y, and Jiang X (2016). Imperforate anus with rectopenile fistulas: a case report and systematic review of the literature. *BMC Paediatrics*, 16(65): 1–6.

Megarectum

Megarectum is the dilatation of the rectum and may occur as a result of underlying nerve supply abnormalities or muscle dysfunction, which remain after disimpaction of the rectum. Impaction occurs because of excessive laxity and hypomotility of the rectum, the threshold of sensation in the rectum is increased, which leads to accumulation of stool in the rectum.

Symptoms
- Faecal impaction
- Decreased defaecation
- Large/massive stools
- Abdominal pain
- Abdominal distension
- Slow transit constipation
- Overflow incontinence.

Causes
- Idiopathic
- Chronic constipation
- Hirschsprung's disease
- Evacuatory dysfunction.

Investigations
- Abdominal X-ray
- Anorectal manometry
- Transit study.

Treatment
The aim of treatment is to empty the rectum and produce a porridge-like stool to avoid faecal impaction:
- Enemas
- Daily use of laxatives, stimulant/osmotic (➜ p. 422–3)
- Behavioural training with evacuation techniques/habit training
- Transanal irrigation.

Surgery
Should only be considered when all other treatments have failed to adequately improve symptoms and as part of a multidisciplinary team decision.

Pilonidal sinus

Pilonidal sinus is also known as 'a nest of hairs', sacral fistula, hair cyst, or sacral dermoid (Fig. 5.4). A pilonidal sinus has a cystic structure and is often several centimetres in diameter. A pilonidal sinus can lead to abscess formation and may extend into the subcutaneous fat if other hairs become incorporated and promote a foreign-body reaction. Not all sinuses contain hairs. Subcutaneous sinuses are lined with granulation tissue and filled with debris, e.g. skin, scales, hair, and keratinocytes. The sinus usually discharges in the midline, often at the top end of the natal cleft.

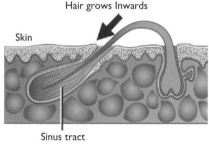

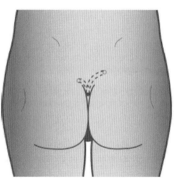

Fig. 5.4 Pilonidal sinus.
Reproduced with kind permission © Burdett Institute 2008.

Symptoms

Some patients with a pilonidal cyst will be asymptomatic. However, the following symptoms can occur:

- Pain/discomfort above the anus.
- Swelling above the anus, that may be intermittent
- Hairs may protrude
- Opaque yellow (purulent) or bloody discharge
- Unexpected moisture
- Discomfort when sitting or doing any activities that involve pressure in this area.

Causes

- Most commonly occurs in hirsute men <40 years.
- There might be a congenital predisposition (a family history is common).
- Obesity can predispose to the condition.
- Excessive sitting or inactivity is thought to predispose people to the condition, as sitting increases pressure on the coccygeal region. There are some cases where a pilonidal sinus can occur months after a localized injury or friction to the area.
- Excessive sweating. Moisture can fill a stretched hair follicle, which helps create a low-oxygen environment that promotes the growth of anaerobic bacteria, often found in pilonidal cysts. The presence of bacteria and low oxygen levels hamper wound healing and exacerbate a forming pilonidal cyst.

Investigations

A pilonidal sinus is usually seen on observation.

Treatment

- Asymptomatic/mild symptoms—shaving the area and good hygiene Acute symptoms—painkillers and surgical drainage, often under local anaesthetic. Post-operative shaving and hygiene is needed to promote healing
- Can be excised and sutured but could recur if infection and granulation tissue is not excised adequately
- Tendency to recur, especially if the tract is not drained adequately
- Might need wide surgical excision and healing by secondary intention if the pilonidal sinus becomes chronic
- Occasional need for plastic surgery
- Antibiotics may help.

Proctalgia fugax

Proctalgia fugax refers to the sudden onset of severe pain in the rectum. Sometimes known as recurrent anal pain.

Symptoms

- Smooth muscles in the anal canal and the sphincters suddenly tighten and go into spasm; often without warning, lasting from seconds to minutes
- Often occur at night
- Can be triggered by sexual activity, defaecation, constipation, or stress/anxiety.

Causes

The exact cause of the condition is unclear.

Investigations

Proctalgia fugax is usually a diagnosis of exclusion, requiring the exclusion of other causes such as haemorrhoids, abscesses, fissure or cancer.

Treatments

There is no known cure for proctalgia fugax. Most treatments may include topical GTN or nerve blocks, although there is no real evidence of their effectiveness. Many remedies include warm baths and/or relaxation techniques.

Further reading

Jevaraiah S and Purkayastha P (2013). Proctalgia fugax. *Canadian Medical Association Journal* 185(5): 417.

Pruritus ani

Pruritus ani is defined as intense, chronic itching affecting the perianal skin. The symptoms range from mild to intense and depression may result when symptoms are severe and persistent. Pruritus ani is classified as idiopathic when no cause can be found. However, 75% of cases have co-existing pathology.

Symptoms

- Perianal itching
- Perianal burning
- Perianal irritation
- Perianal pain.

Causes

The most common cause of pruritus ani is ineffective anal cleaning after defaecation, faecal incontinence, or minor faecal soiling due to faecal residue on the skin setting up a chemical reaction. Other causes are listed in Table 5.1 and Box 5.1. Once established, a vicious circle of irritation, scratching, and further skin damage results.

Table 5.1 Causes of pruritus ani

Anorectal conditions	• Haemorrhoids (⊃ p. 126–8) • Fissure (⊃ p. 120–1) • Fistula • Prolapse (⊃ p. 138–9) • Proctitis
Dermatological	• Psoriasis • Eczema • Contact dermatitis (e.g. faeces)
Infection	• Anal warts (⊃ p. 124) • *Candida albicans*
Malignant	• Anal cancer (⊃ p. 118–19) • Villous adenoma • Bowen's disease (perianal carcinoma in situ)

Box 5.1 Foods associated with pruritus ani

Most common
Coffee
Tea
Cola
Other caffeinated drinks
Alcohol, especially beer and wine
Chocolate
Tomato ketchup

Others
Milk products
Peanuts
Spices
Citrus fruits
Grapes
Spicy foods
Prunes

Treatment

Perianal skin cleansing is of utmost importance, plus avoiding soap, bubble bath, and strong chemicals used for washing and laundry. Some barrier creams may help, although occasionally they can exacerbate the problem. Advice should be given to resist scratching and avoiding some foods (see Box 5.1) may also help.

The nurse can also advise that dry anal wiping with paper does not always completely remove faecal residue from the perianal area. Small amounts of stool can also inadvertently be passed with flatus and any stool remaining can quickly result in skin sore. Advice needs to be given compassionately as some people may be offended by the suggestion that they might need to improve their perianal hygiene.

Rectal prolapse

A rectal prolapse is where the rectal mucosa has prolapsed to a degree that it can protrude beyond the anal verge. Essentially rectal prolapses can be classified as:

- Internal—the rectum folds in on itself but does not protrude out through the anus
- Mucosal prolapse or partial rectal mucosal prolapse—refers to loosening of the submucosal attachments to the muscularis propria of the distal rectal mucosal layer, meaning only the inner lining of the rectum protrudes from the anus
- Full thickness prolapse—where all the layers of the rectal wall prolapse.

Typically, a prolapse can occur during straining or defaecation and return to normal position after defaecation. In severe cases a prolapse can occur with minimal effort, such as walking and remain permanently or need manual replacement.

Symptoms

A rectal prolapse is often associated with discomfort, bleeding, copious mucus discharge, faecal incontinence (❷ p. 448–9), and/or difficulty in evacuation. Occasionally a prolapse presents as acute strangulation.

Cause

Most patients with a rectal prolapse have a long history of constipation, thus it is thought that prolonged, excessive, and repetitive straining during defaecation may progress to a rectal prolapse. Since a rectal prolapse itself causes functional obstruction, more straining may result from a small prolapse, with increasing damage to the anatomy. This excessive straining may be due to predisposing pelvic floor dysfunction such as obstructed defaecation and/or anatomical factors.

Investigation

A rectal prolapse might not be apparent during an examination in the left-lateral position, even with straining. If suspected, allow the patient to strain for 1–2 mins in the privacy on the toilet and then observe for a prolapse from behind. Look for:

- Partial or circumferential prolapse
- The protrusion beyond the anal verge in centimetres.

Anal ultrasound might show thickened internal anal sphincter resulting from repeated trauma.

Treatment

Treatment can be conservative or surgical.

Conservative

Some patients with a very minor, early prolapse can commence teaching to avoid straining. Education includes pelvic floor exercises, possibly with biofeedback (❷ p. 453) and manual replacement of the prolapse, as needed.

Surgery

Surgical methods in rectal prolapse can be classified into either perineal or abdominal.

A perineal procedure includes a transanal approach and Delorme repair, where redundant mucosa is excised and the rectal wall muscle is plicated. Medically high-risk or elderly patients are usually treated by perineal procedures, as they can be performed under a regional/local anaesthetic.

Abdominal procedures may involve a rectopexy (◑ p. 500), resection, or both. The procedure can also be performed laparoscopically.

Rectocele

A rectocele is a herniation of the rectovaginal septum, resulting in a bulging of the rectum forwards into the vaginal lumen (Fig. 5.5). A rectocele can be defined as:

- First degree—small rectocele on straining
- Second degree—moderate rectocele on straining
- Third degree—rectocele reaches into introitus on straining
- Fourth degree—rectocele reaches beyond the introitus.

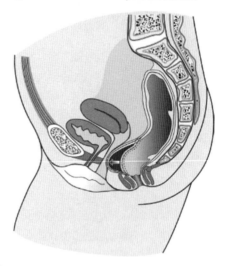

Fig. 5.5 Rectocele.
Reproduced with kind permission © Burdett Institute 2008.

Symptoms

Some women are asymptomatic however symptoms include:

- Sensation of a bulge or dragging
- Evacuation problems—incomplete evacuation, straining to evacuate, needing to digitate vaginally or perineally to complete evacuation
- Sexual discomfort
- Backache and discomfort on standing for long periods
- Soiling in some women when stools become 'trapped' in rectocele during attempted defaecation.

Causes

- Childbirth
- Straining and possibly congenital collagen weakness
- Exacerbated by obesity (possibly)
- Ageing; some degree of rectocele is probably normal in older women who have given birth
- Associated with anterior vaginal wall prolapse, vaginal vault prolapse, and an enterocele (small bowel herniation into the vaginal vault).

Investigations

- Vaginal examination—supine, at rest, and during straining
- Sims speculum enables the best visualization of the posterior vaginal wall—standing, at rest, and during straining
- Proctogram—barium paste can be seen in the bulge, at rest, during defaecation or trapped in the rectocele after defaecation (possible without the woman's knowledge).

Treatment

Treatment depends on the severity of the problem and includes:
- Digitation to support the posterior vaginal wall during defaecation
- Teach good defaecation dynamics and avoid excessive straining (➲ p. 446)
- Vaginal pessaries help some women
- Modification of stool consistency (firmer or looser, as indicated) to ease evacuation
- Manage any associated constipation using suppositories, enemas, or irrigation helps some patients.

Surgery

Surgery could be indicated for a 2–3 cm non-emptying/trapping rectocele or for cosmetic/comfort reasons. A gynaecologist will perform a posterior vaginal repair or sacrocolpopexy (if associated with vaginal vault prolapse). A colorectal surgeon will perform transrectal repair (usually with resection of excess tissue), with insertion of mesh to reinforce if necessary. The patient must avoid straining on defaecation after repair because it can cause recurrence of the rectocele. Complications can include new sexual dysfunction or faecal incontinence.

Rectovaginal fistula

A rectovaginal fistula is an abnormal epithelial lined connection between the anterior wall of the anal canal or rectum and the posterior wall of the vagina.

Symptoms

Depending on the size and location of the fistula, symptoms can be minor or major with significant problems of incontinence and hygiene, including:
- Passage of gas, stool, or pus from the vagina
- Foul-smelling vaginal discharge
- Recurrent vaginal infections
- Irritation or pain in the vulva, vagina, and the perineum (area between the vagina and anus)
- Pain during sexual intercourse
- Possible secondary dysuria
- Urinary tract infection.

Causes

Although a rectovaginal fistula can be idiopathic, the most common causes of a rectovaginal fistula include:
- Complications during childbirth, the perineum can tear during a long or difficult delivery
- Inflammatory bowel disease can cause inflammation and can increase the risk of developing a fistula
- Cancer in the vagina, cervix, rectum, uterus, or anus can cause a rectovaginal fistula
- Radiation to treat pelvic cancers can also create a fistula
- Surgical procedures on the vagina, rectum, perineum, or anus can cause an injury or infection that leads to an abnormal opening
- Perforated diverticula
- Congenital.

Investigations

- Contrast tests—a vaginogram or a barium enema can help identify a fistula located in the upper rectum.
- Blue dye test—a tampon is placed into the vagina and blue dye is inserted into the rectum. Blue staining on the tampon indicates a fistula.
- CT scan (➔ p. 220) of the abdomen and pelvis can locate a fistula and determine its cause.
- MRI (➔ p. 222) can show the location of a fistula and whether other pelvic organs are involved.
- Anorectal ultrasound can evaluate the structure of the anal sphincter.
- Anorectal manometry may be used when planning the fistula repair.

Treatments

Treating a rectovaginal fistula can be difficult. Successful treatment is dependent on the aetiology, size of the fistula, location, status of the sphincter, and any associated systemic disorders or possible infections.

Antibiotics

If a fistula has developed from an infection or the surrounding area is infected, a course of antibiotics will be prescribed prior to any other intervention.

Surgical

Many fistulas will simply heal on their own without the need for surgery. However, if the fistula persists, surgery may be necessary. Rectovaginal fistulas can be repaired through a multitude of approaches including transanal, vaginal, perineal, abdominal, and trans-sacral. The choice of operation is according to the patient's underlying pathology. Proper management of associated inflammatory diseases and systemic disorders is recommended for necessary complex cases.

Surgery may involve a gynaecologist and/or a colorectal surgeon with any of the following procedures:

- An anal fistula plug or biologic mesh to heal the fistula
- Repair the damaged anal sphincter muscles if damage occurred from a rectovaginal fistula
- A tissue graft or flap created from a nearby part of the body to cover the fistula
- In very complex cases, a colostomy may be created to allow healing to take place. In most instances, this is only a temporary measure and the colostomy will be reversed once the fistula is healed
- Seton stitch is possible.

Solitary rectal ulcer syndrome

Solitary rectal ulcer syndrome (SRUS) is an uncommon rectal disorder that does not necessarily end with an ulcer and may affect different parts of the rectum and other sites of the gastrointestinal tract. Ulcers are only found in 40% of the patients; 20% of the patients have a solitary ulcer. The rest of the lesions vary in shape and size, from hyperemic mucosa to broad-based polypoid.

Symptoms
- Rectal pain
- Rectal prolapse
- Bleeding
- Pain
- Tenesmus
- Mucus
- Chronic constipation
- Incomplete evacuation.

Causes
- Chronic constipation with straining
- Rectal prolapse/intussusception
- Digitation
- Paradoxical contraction.

Investigations
Investigations are usually combined with symptomatology and histology
- Flexible sigmoidoscopy/colonoscopy
- Defaecating proctogram
- Barium enema.

Treatments
- Prevention of constipation
- Behavioural changes
  - No digitation
  - No straining
  - Habit training.

Surgery—should only be considered when all conservative measures have failed to adequately improve symptoms and/or if SRUS is in the stages of prolapse.

Further reading
Forootan M and Darvishi M (2018). Solitary rectal ulcer syndrome: A systematic review. *Medicine*, 97(18), e0565.

Chapter 6

Liver

Alcoholic hepatitis

Inflammation of the liver as a result of excessive, long-term alcohol consumption.

Symptoms

Often alcoholic liver disease is symptom-free. Symptoms can include jaundice and liver failure. Continued drinking can result in cirrhosis, liver failure, and liver cancer.

Causes

High concentrations of alcohol damage the cells of the liver: the cells increase in size and retain water and protein. This results in accumulation of neutrophils, macrophages, and lymphocytes, followed by cell necrosis and deposits of collagen. Eventually, fatty liver develops, with 10% of people developing liver cirrhosis (➲ p. 152–4).

Prevention

To keep health risks from alcohol to a low level, it is safest not to drink more than 14 units a week on a regular basis.

Ascites

Ascites is the collection of fluid in the peritoneal cavity (between the layers of the peritoneum).

Symptoms

There are a number of symptoms associated with ascites:
- Abdominal distension
- Shifting dullness on percussion
- Abdominal pain
- Peripheral oedema.

Causes

Portal hypertension causes fluid to accumulate in the peritoneum as a result of cirrhosis. If the level of protein in the blood is ↓ the osmotic gradient is disturbed, leading to salt and water retention.

Lymphatic secondary tumours can block lymph drainage, with ascites being a response to secondary tumours in the peritoneum.

Investigations

- Mild ascites can be diagnosed using ultrasound.
- Moderate ascites causes some abdominal distension.
- Severe ascites causes marked abdominal distension.

Incidence

75% of patients with ascites have cirrhosis; 50% of patients with cirrhosis for at least 10 years will develop ascites. The mortality rate for ascites is 50% at 2 years.

Treatment

Initial treatment is diuretics (⊃ p. 419) and reduced salt intake but bedrest is not helpful.

If ascites is not controlled by non-invasive treatment, another option is paracentesis to drain the fluid. Up to 10 litres of fluid can be removed over several hours. It is necessary to monitor for hypotension, hypovolaemic shock, haematoma, leakage from drain site (might require a suture), and perforation (rare). Often an albumin infusion is required if a large volume is removed. A sample should be sent to the laboratory for analysis. Liver transplant may be considered.

Note that spontaneous bacterial peritonitis is common associated with a 20% mortality rate. Spontaneous bacterial peritonitis is treated with antibiotics (⊃ p. 408).

Autoimmune hepatitis

Autoimmune hepatitis is rare, but it is most common in young women, especially women with other autoimmune diseases. Diagnosis is made by exclusion of other causes of hepatitis.

Symptoms

Often autoimmune hepatitis is asymptomatic. Symptoms can include:
• Fatigue
• Jaundice.

Causes

The cause of autoimmune hepatitis is unknown.

Treatment

Response to treatment can be slow, possibly taking several years. Treatment is generally effective (90% of people). Medication for autoimmune hepatitis is steroids (➲ p. 428) and immunosuppressants (➲ p. 421), with possibly long-term treatment.

If treatment is ineffective after 4 years, a liver transplant may be necessary.

Cholangiocarcinoma

Cholangiocarcinoma is cancer of the bile duct—a rare and aggressive primary tumour.

Symptoms

Cholangiocarcinoma is generally symptom-free until the cancer blocks the bile ducts. When symptoms occur, the cancer has often spread and is incurable but symptoms include:
- Jaundice
- Itching
- Pale faeces
- Dark urine
- Anorexia
- Unexplained weight-loss
- Generally feeling unwell
- Abdominal pain
- Abdominal distention
- Pyrexia.

Causes

Although the exact cause is unknown cholangiocarcinoma is linked to:
- Primary sclerosing cholangitis (Ɔ p. 200)
- Bile duct cysts
- Bile duct stones
- Infection with a liver fluke parasite (uncommon in the UK)
- Exposure to certain chemicals
- Hepatitis B (Ɔ p. 164–5)
- Hepatitis C (Ɔ p. 166–7)
- Cirrhosis (Ɔ p. 152–4)
- Diabetes
- Obesity
- Smoking
- Excessive alcohol consumption.

Incidence

The prevalence in ♂ and ♀ is equal.

Investigations

Investigations include:
- Blood tests
- Ultrasound scan
- Computed tomography (CT) scan
- Magnetic resonance imaging (MRI) scan
- X-ray
- Biopsy.

Treatment

Cure is often not possible for cholangiocarcinoma. Treatment is usually used to control symptoms and includes:

- Surgery—providing a cure for a small number of people
- Stenting of the bile duct—to relieve jaundice
- Chemotherapy
- Radiotherapy.

Prognosis

Up to 50% will survive for at least 5 years: these are people with early cancer that had surgical removal of the cancer; 2% will live for at least 5 years if the cancer is at a later stage and surgery is not possible.

Cirrhosis

Definition

Cirrhosis is scarring of the liver, which negatively affects the liver function. Chronic (or occasionally severe acute) inflammation and scarring leads to diffuse damage/necrosis of hepatocytes (cells of the liver). Nodules may develop and fibrotic tissue will replace the normal cell architecture, harden tissues, and cause irreversible scarring of the liver (cirrhosis). Cirrhosis can result in derangement of the portal circulation, which impedes blood flow. It may eventually lead to:

• Functional failure
• Hepatocellular carcinoma.

Compensating cirrhosis is asymptomatic and can be followed by a decompensated phase. The decompensated cirrhosis is seen as obvious clinical symptoms: commonly ascites, bleeding, encephalopathy, and jaundice.

Symptoms

Cirrhosis may be asymptomatic until advanced. Symptoms can include:

• Fatigue
• Itching
• Right upper quadrant discomfort
• Fever
• Anorexia
• Nausea
• Arthritis
• Palmar erythema
• Dry eyes
• Diarrhoea
• Dark urine
• Loss of libido.

More severe symptoms include:

• Jaundice
• Haematemesis (→ p. 436–7)
• Melaena
• Ascites
• Encephalopathy
• Portal hypertension and collateral circulation
• Varices—oesophageal and gastric
• Changes in nitrogen metabolism
• Coagulation disorders of the blood
• Fetor hepaticus
• Skin changes, such as spider naevi
• Hepatic encephalopathy
• Osteoporosis
• Endocrine changes, such as gynaecomastia.

Cirrhosis may lead to:

• Liver failure.

Causes

There are three main causes of cirrhosis:
* Alcohol—50% of cases
* Chronic hepatitis, particularly hepatitis C
* Non-alcoholic steatohepatitis, a more severe form of non-alcoholic fatty liver disease.

Other causes include:
* Any form of chronic hepatitis
* Primary sclerosing cholangitis
* Haemochromatosis
* Wilson's disease—a congenital failure to excrete copper, leading to deposition of copper in the liver and brain.

Alcoholic cirrhosis

Alcoholic cirrhosis results from high consumption of alcohol. Alcoholic cirrhosis can be a chronic condition or related to binge-drinking. Susceptible individuals develop progressive liver disease from alcoholic hepatitis (➔ p. 146) and eventual cirrhosis. The disease can progress from a large fatty liver to a small shrunken liver with fibrous nodules and an impeded blood flow. Cirrhosis is more probable if the patient also has hepatitis C (➔ p. 166–7) or any other liver condition. Hepatocellular carcinoma can subsequently develop in 15–20% of patients with cirrhosis.

Incidence

In the UK, and other countries, the number of liver disease deaths is increasing. Liver cirrhosis is currently (2020) the fifth biggest killer in England and Wales.

Investigations

A series of biochemical tests (liver function tests) on blood samples are used to investigate hepatic disease:
* ↑ aminotransferase suggests hepatocellular disease
* A predominant ↑ in alkaline phosphatase indicates cholestatic or biliary tract problems.

Additionally, scans such as:
* Ultrasound
* CT
* MRI.

Liver biopsy is used as a diagnostic tool or to assess the extent of liver damage. Endoscopy can be useful to look for varices.

Further information

The European Association for the Study of the Liver (2018) EASL Clinical Practice Guidelines for the management of patients with decompensated cirrhosis. *Journal of Hepatology*, https://doi.org/10.1016/j.jhep.2018.03.024

Treatment

There is currently no cure for cirrhosis but symptoms and complications can be managed. Treating the underlying cause is needed such as viral hepatitis. Additionally, primary biliary cholangitis can be treated. In general treatment includes the management of the complications associated with cirrhosis. Nurses can advise on a number of measures to help, such as:

• Avoid alcohol
• Dry skin—moisturize
• Steatorrhoea—reduce fat intake
• Oedema—avoid dietary salt
• A balanced diet to prevent malnutrition
• Weight-loss if overweight
• Regular exercise
• Good hygiene and vaccinations are needed to reduce the risk of infections.

Primary biliary cholangitis is treated with ursodeoxycholic acid (❺ p. 428) and immunosuppressants. Complications associated with cirrhosis can be treated as follows:

• Treat alcohol dependence—consider naltrexone
• Colestyramine—itching
• Tear replacement—dry eyes
• Diuretics (❺ p. 419)—↓ fluid accumulation
• Vitamin supplements—malabsorption.

Nurses should also advise people:

• To monitor for osteoporosis
• With clotting disorders to take care with minor procedures that might cause bleeding, such as dental treatment.

Portal hypertension with bleeding varices is a serious complication of cirrhosis that can be treated by primary or secondary prophylaxis:

• Primary—banding to eradicate varices
• Secondary—beta-blockers.

People with complications, such as resistant ascites, may require a shunt procedure or liver transplantation.

Gilbert's syndrome

An inherited (recessive) condition in which an ↑ level of bilirubin is present within the blood system. Bilirubin is a natural yellow substance, the by-product of the breakdown of red blood cells.

Symptoms

Symptoms are often linked to certain scenarios:
• Dehydration
• Infection
• Physical exertion
• Surgery
• Menstruation.

Symptoms include mild jaundice (intermittent, short-duration) with:
• Abdominal pain
• Fatigue
• Anorexia
• Nausea
• Dizziness
• Irritable bowel syndrome (IBS)-type symptoms (➋ p. 96–8)
• Generally feeling unwell.

However, a third of people with Gilbert's syndrome are symptomless.

Cause

The liver has a faulty gene, resulting in difficulties in removing bilirubin from the bloodstream. The bilirubin is not passed into the bile at the normal rate.

Incidence

It is estimated that 5% of the UK population has Gilbert's syndrome. More men than women are affected. Diagnosis is usually made in the late teens or early twenties.

Investigations

Gilbert's syndrome is usually made using a blood test.

Treatment

Treatment is usually not necessary as there are limited symptoms, but avoidance of any stressors that bring on the jaundice can be useful.

Further information

Patients support group at http://www.gilbertssyndrome.org.uk

Haemochromatosis

Haemochromatosis is an inherited (recessive) condition, also called iron-overload disorder. The disease is characterized by the body absorbing too much iron from food, which is deposited in the liver, pancreas, heart, endocrine glands, and other organs, where iron levels in the body slowly build up over many years. Iron levels can be 20-fold greater than normal. A normal healthy adult absorbs 1–2 mg iron/day, which can ↑ to 3–6 mg/day in haemochromatosis.

Symptoms

Haemochromatosis is often asymptomatic. Symptoms can include:
• Fatigue, mood swings, and depression
• Weight loss
• Weakness
• Abdominal and joint pain
• Bronze skin pigmentation ('bronze diabetes')
• Diabetes mellitus—in two-thirds of patients—non-reversible
• Arthritis (especially in the first two finger joints)
• Heart arrhythmias
• ♀ might be asymptomatic because they lose iron during menstrual bleeding—irregular periods, absent periods, and early menopause are common
• In ♂ the genitals shrink, erectile dysfunction occurs and there is a loss of libido (pituitary effect)
• Liver enlargement
• Cirrhosis—non-reversible.

Symptoms can progress to:
• Liver damage
• Primary liver carcinoma.

Causes

Occasionally, haemochromatosis results from repeated blood transfusions, thalassaemia, or chronic liver disease. The latter may be due to cirrhosis (resulting in uncontrolled iron uptake) or excessive dietary iron intake (uptake increased by alcohol and vitamin C).

Incidence

Haemochromatosis is usually diagnosed in adults >40 years. Haemochromatosis is the most common genetic disorder in white people, affecting 1 out of 400 individuals in the UK. In addition, 10% of the population are carriers.

Investigations

Diagnosis of haemochromatosis is usually made as a result of investigations into abnormal liver function tests, investigation for other conditions (e.g. joint pain in diabetes), on routine blood test, or when screening affected family members.

Specific investigations for haemochromatosis include:
- ↑ blood ferritin levels (consider transferritin saturation levels)
- The presence of the *HFE* gene (blood test)
- Enlarged liver
- Liver biopsy—if liver damage is suspected.

Treatment

There is no cure currently known. Venesection may be necessary, initially weekly until iron levels are normalized. Venesection is contraindicated in patients with anaemia or cardiac disease and medication can be used.

For people who cannot use venesection to treat their haemochromatosis, a possible medication is deferasirox but it is not licensed for this indication as chelation therapy.

Occasionally, for severe liver damage, a liver transplant is required.

Nurses should provide support and counselling on the genetic implications, as siblings and children require testing. Advice can include avoidance of:
- Iron supplements
- Too much alcohol (promotes iron absorption and affects the liver)
- Vitamin C (encourages iron deposition)
- Cereals with added iron.

Prognosis

If identified before cirrhosis and diabetes develop, life expectancy remains normal.

Further information

The Haemochromatosis Society at https://www.haemochromatosis.org.uk

Hepatic encephalopathy

Hepatic encephalopathy is damage to the brain as a result of a build-up of toxins.

Symptoms

Symptoms of hepatic encephalopathy can include:
- Agitation
- Confusion
- Drowsiness
- Problems concentrating.

Potentially progresses to coma and death.

Cause

Hepatic encephalopathy may the inadequate management of toxins by the failing liver, as a result of hepatitis or cirrhosis.

Treatment

The main treatment is a laxative (➲ p. 422–3) to clear the build-up of toxins. In some cases, an antibiotic may be necessary or possibly Rifaximin. The nurse should also provide advice on a balanced diet, with a restriction in proteins.

Hepatitis

Hepatitis is characterized by inflammation of liver. Chronic hepatitis can lead to fibrosis, loss of liver function, and eventually cirrhosis (usually over the course of many years) and possibly liver cancer. There are several types of viral hepatitis:

- Hepatitis A (➲ p. 162)
- Hepatitis B (➲ p. 164–5)
- Hepatitis C (➲ p. 166–7)
- Hepatitis D (➲ p. 168)
- Hepatitis E (➲ p. 169).

Additionally:

- Alcoholic hepatitis (➲ p. 146)
- Autoimmune hepatitis (➲ p. 148).

Symptoms

There can be no symptoms, in the acute phase. Symptoms can include:

- Joint and muscle pain
- Pyrexia
- Nausea and vomiting
- Fatigue
- Generally feeling unwell
- Abdominal pain
- Dark urine
- Loss of appetite
- Pruritus
- Pale, grey-colour faeces
- Jaundice.

Chronic hepatitis may also be symptomless, until the liver begins to fail and it is identified by blood tests. Although the symptoms in the later stages can be:

- Jaundice
- Oedema in feet, ankles, and feet
- Confusion
- Hematemesis
- Melaena.

Causes

Hepatitis is usually the result of a viral infection or alternatively as a result of excessive alcohol intake.

Hepatitis A

Hepatitis A is categorized as viral hepatitis.

Symptoms

Incubation period is 2–6 weeks. Symptoms then include:
- Symptoms of hepatitis (➲ p. 161)
- Flu-like symptoms
- Nausea
- Diarrhoea.

Subsequently jaundice may develop a week later.

Hepatitis A can be severe in some patient groups, such as those with a weakened immune system.

A person with hepatitis is infectious to others for about two weeks before symptoms occur to a week after the first symptoms.

Causes

Hepatitis A is transmitted by contaminated water and food, passed on by the faecal–oral route. It can also be caught from close contact with someone who has hepatitis A.

Investigations

Blood tests can indicate the presence of the virus.

Treatment

There is no specific treatment for hepatitis A. Patients usually make a complete recovery after a few weeks/months, although it can be severe or even life-threatening. Alcohol consumption must be avoided.

Prevention

Vaccinations are recommended for travel to certain areas in the world.

Prognosis

No long-term damage resulting from hepatitis A is usually suffered. The immune system will also recover.

Hepatitis B

Hepatitis B is a viral hepatitis.

Symptoms

The incubation period is 1–6 months and can be acute or chronic. Symptoms include:
- Flu-like symptoms
- Tiredness
- Aches and pains
- Pyrexia
- Generally feeling unwell
- Nausea and vomiting
- Abdominal pain
- Pale, grey faeces
- Jaundice.

Symptoms will usually pass within 3 months (acute hepatitis B) but can last longer than this (chronic hepatitis B). If acute disease is severe, a liver transplant may be required.

Symptoms can progress to liver cirrhosis (➔ p. 152–4) or liver cancer (➔ p. 172–3). Rarely (less than 1% of cases) hepatitis B can progress to fulminant hepatitis B; the liver is damaged and can be fatal if not treated.

Causes

Hepatitis B is spread through contract with bodily fluids, most commonly blood but also semen, vaginal secretions, and additionally breast milk. Thus, hepatitis B can be spread from parents to children, among intravenous (IV) drug abusers, and be sexually transmitted. Patients can be carriers of hepatitis B and have additional risks of liver cirrhosis and primary liver cancer.

Incidence

About 1:1000 people are carriers in the UK.

Investigation

Blood test is used for viral antibodies. It can be important to test the whole family and vaccinate them all.

Treatment

Treatment varies on factors such as how long the person has been infected with hepatitis B. Emergency treatment can be used if the person was infected with the virus in the last few days. Acute hepatitis B (infected for up to a few months) is usually treated by symptom control. After six months with hepatitis B (chronic hepatitis B) long-term or possibly lifelong treatment is needed to keep the virus under control and reduce the risk of liver damage.

Nursing advice can include cautions in spreading the infection to others, such as avoiding unprotected sex, not sharing needles to inject drugs, and avoiding alcohol. Hepatitis during pregnancy risks transfer to the baby; vaccination of the baby is recommended soon after birth.

Medications can include:
- Peginterferon alfa-2a
- Antivirals.

Prevention

Vaccination against hepatitis B for travel in certain countries. A vaccine against hepatitis B is currently available for babies born in the UK.

Prognosis

If a baby contracts hepatitis B, there is a high chance (90%) of it becoming chronic. Most adults recover fully from hepatitis B within 3 months and are then immune to hepatitis B for life.

Further reading

European Association for the Study of the Liver (2017). EASL 2017 Clinical Practice Guidelines on the management of hepatitis B virus infection. *Journal of Hepatology* 67, 370–98.

Hepatitis C

Hepatitis C is a viral infection.

Symptoms

Often hepatitis C is symptomless until there is significant liver damage. Symptoms can be like chronic fatigue syndrome and include:
• Vague flu-like symptoms
• Tiredness
• Nausea and vomiting
• Anorexia
• Abdominal pain.

Hepatitis C can cause potentially life-threatening damage to the liver (cirrhosis), liver failure, or liver cancer over the years if untreated.

Causes

Hepatitis C is generally blood borne. It is usually spread through the use of IV drugs (at least half of cases), from mother to her baby, and rarely sexually transmitted. Historically prior to careful screening of blood used in blood transfusions, this was a further route of transmission.

Incidence

Up to 0.04% of the UK population are infected with hepatitis C, about 215,000 people.

Investigations

A blood test is required to detect antibodies, but may not be present in the initial incubation period.

Liver ultrasound can be necessary to look for liver damage.

Treatment

Nurses can advise on a balanced diet and exercise with minimal alcohol intake and smoking. People require advice about transmission, to avoid blood donation, not to share needles, razors, or toothbrushes, and additionally the small risk of sexual transmission. Medication may not be necessary in the acute phase but may be needed in the chronic phase (6 months or more after infection), although some people can become symptom-free without treatment.

Medication can include single or combinations of the following depending on the type of hepatitis C:
• Simeprevir
• Sofosbuvir
• Ledipasvir
• Dacatasvir
• Ombitasvir
• Paritaprevir
• Ritonavir
• Velpatavir

- Voxilaprevir
- Glecaprevir
- Pibrentasvir
- Ribavirin.

Most people are cured with treatment but it is possible to be re-infected with hepatitis C.

Prevention

Unlike some other types of hepatitis, there is no vaccine for hepatitis C currently available.

Prognosis

1 in 5 people infected with hepatitis C will recover, the rest become chronic carriers, and 60% will have chronic hepatitis C. The risk of cirrhosis is 20% but takes many years to develop; there is a small risk of liver carcinoma (2–3%) or non-Hodgkin lymphoma. Cirrhosis can develop within 10 years if the person takes regular or excessive alcohol, especially if they are female. Hepatitis C can slowly progress, with 90% of people being alive at 5 years and 80% at 10 years.

Further reading

European Association for the Study of the Liver. (2018). EASL Recommendations on Treatment of Hepatitis C 2018. *Journal of Hepatology* https://www.journal-of-hepatology.eu/article/S0168-8278(18)31968-8/fulltext

Hepatitis D

Hepatitis D is a viral infection and occurs only in conjunction with hepatitis B. It is most common in developing countries; but in the UK, hepatitis D is most common in IV drug users (75% of cases) and people who received a blood transfusion prior to careful testing prior to infusion.

Symptoms

There is an incubation period of 3–12 weeks. Symptoms can develop into cirrhosis or liver cancer.

Causes

Hepatitis D is usually spread through blood-to-blood contact, commonly through IV drug abuse.

Investigations

A blood test is required to detect antibodies.

Treatment

In general hepatitis D is self-limiting. Treatment with interferon (➔ p. 415) may be necessary.

Prevention

Vaccination against hepatitis B will prevent hepatitis D infection, as these are concurrent diseases.

Prognosis

People with concurrent hepatitis B and hepatitis D have a greater risk of cirrhosis, than people with hepatitis B alone.

Hepatitis E

Hepatitis E is a viral infection. Most cases are reported in developing countries, where epidemics can occur.

Symptoms

The incubation period is 2–12 weeks.

Causes

Transmission is via the faecal–oral route. Associated with eating raw or undercooked meats and shellfish.

Incidence

Hepatitis E is now the most common cause of acute hepatitis in the UK.

Treatment

Hepatitis E is usually self-limiting; there is no risk of long-term damage or chronic infection, except in the last trimester of pregnancy. In pregnancy, there is a risk of fatality (20%) and a high risk of miscarriage.

Prevention

There is no vaccination available to prevent hepatitis E.

Further reading:

European Association for the Study of the Liver (2018) EASL Clinical Practice Guidelines on hepatitis E virus infection. *Journal of Hepatology.* 68: 1256–71.

Hepatorenal syndrome

Hepatorenal syndrome is characterized by renal failure on the background of advanced cirrhosis and is usually fatal.

Symptoms

Symptoms of hepatorenal syndrome include:
- ↓ renal blood flow
- ↓ glomerular filtration rate
- ↓ urine output
- Sodium retention
- Disorders of the renin–angiotensin pathway
- Affects levels of aldosterone, norepinephrine, and vasopressin.

Cause

Hepatorenal syndrome is the outcome of advanced cirrhosis and additionally renal failure. The latter often results from:
- Gastrointestinal (GI) bleed
- Bacterial infection
- Hypovolemia (from the overuse of diuretics).

It can also be caused by hepatitis B or hepatitis C.

Treatment

To treat a GI bleed, bacterial infection, or hypovolemia, fluid replacement may assist if there is prerenal failure. Medication can be used to increase renal blood flow and filtration. Alternatively, dialysis may be necessary, either haemodialysis or peritoneal dialysis.

Medication to treat hepatorenal syndrome is a vasoconstrictor, such as terlipressin, which also increases renal blood flow and filtration. Plasma volume expansion is produced with albumin infusion.

Liver cancer

Primary liver cancer (hepatocellular carcinoma or hepatoma) where the cancer begins in the liver is uncommon. The majority of cases of liver cancer in developed countries are secondary to a primary tumour else-where in the body. Often liver cancer presents late in both primary and secondary cancers. The liver cancer can be staged to give an indication of cancer and the liver function:

* Stage 0—the tumour <20 mm, the person is well and liver function is normal
* Stage A—a single tumour <50 mm or up to three tumours, each tumour of <30 mm; the person is well and the liver function is normal
* Stage B—multiple liver tumours; the person is well and the liver function is normal
* Stage C—any previous stage BUT the person is unwell or the liver function is deranged, or the cancer has spread to the blood vessels, the lymph nodes, or other parts of the body
* Stage D—the liver has lost most of its function and other symptoms are occurring, such as ascites.

Secondary liver tumours occur when primary cancers spread to the liver, such as the:

* Bowel
* Breast
* Stomach
* Lung
* Ovary
* Skin
* Pancreas.

The tumour spreads through the bloodstream. Occasionally, the primary site is undetected. Treatment depends on the primary site, extent of the tumour, and the patient's general health.

Symptoms

Symptoms are vague and may not appear until the cancer is at an advanced stage. Symptoms can include:

* Unexplained weight-loss
* Anorexia
* Nausea and vomiting
* Abdominal pain or distention
* Jaundice
* Itching
* Tiredness.

Incidence

There are about 2500 new cases per year in UK. The ratio of prevalence in ♂:♀ is 2:1. Incidence is higher for people with cirrhosis (➋ p. 152–4). Obesity and an unhealthy diet are linked to liver cancer. Rates have in-creased considerably in the last few decades within the UK.

Investigations

Blood tests, scans, and biopsies are needed for a diagnosis.

Treatment

Early stage cancers (stage A) may be curable by:
- Resecting the affected section of the liver
- Liver transplantation
- RFA—radiofrequency ablation.

Stage B and C cannot often be cured, but chemotherapy can slow the disease progression and relieve symptoms, whereas stage D treatment is focused on symptom relief.

Treatment can include chemotherapy or radiotherapy.

Liver transplant

A liver transplant is the replacement of a liver with a healthy liver from a donor, who may be recently deceased or alive.

Causes

There are a number of reasons that a liver may need to be replaced when it is no longer working properly (liver failure).

Investigations

It is essential to undergo an assessment that includes several tests, such as:
- Blood tests
- X-rays
- Scans
- Upper GI endoscopy (⯁ p. 250).

Treatment

Prior to the transplant it is important to:
- Eat healthily
- Undertake regular exercise
- Avoid smoking.

The operation requires a hospital stay of up to 2 weeks. Subsequently life-long immunosuppressants will need to be taken to prevent rejection of the liver. Alcohol consumption should be avoided.

Non-alcoholic fatty liver disease

Non-alcoholic fatty liver disease (NAFLD) is an umbrella term for conditions that are caused by fat building up in the liver. There are four main stages of NAFLD:
- Steatosis—simple fatty liver—largely harmless
- NASH—non-alcoholic steatohepatitis—inflamed liver
- Fibrosis—persistent inflammation causing scar tissue
- Cirrhosis—severe scarring and damage with a change to the liver function (⊃ p. 152–4).

Symptoms

NAFLD is usually asymptomatic in the early stages. Thus, diagnosis is often through undergoing other tests for another reason. NASH and fibrosis can present with symptoms:
- Right upper quadrant abdominal pain
- Tiredness
- Unexplained weight-loss
- Weakness.

Fat within the liver can lead to:
- Diabetes
- High blood pressure
- Renal disease
- Liver damage including cirrhosis.

Cause

NAFLD is associated with metabolic syndrome (obesity, hypertension, diabetes mellitus, high cholesterol) and some medications, particularly steroid use.

Incidence

The number of new cases is ↑ and it is estimated that about a third of people in the UK have some fat in their liver—there should be none or very little within the liver. NAFLD may present at any age (including children), but most often appears in middle age. 5% of the UK population have NASH. 10% of people with NAFLD progress to cirrhosis.

Investigation

A routine blood test commonly detects abnormal liver function.

Treatment

Treatment includes life-style changes such as:
- Weight loss (not too rapid)
- Regular exercise
- Control of diabetes
- Low-fat diet
- Cholesterol lowering medication
- Limiting alcohol intake
- Stop smoking.

There is no medical treatment specifically for NAFLD, but if there are symptoms these may be medically treated.

Portal hypertension

Portal hypertension is ↑ pressure in the portal vein (↑ resistance to blood flow) due to the scarring within the liver making blood flow more difficult. As it is difficult for the blood to travel back to the heart, the blood flow often travels via smaller vessels that become stretched and weakened (varices). Normal pressure 1–5 mmHg; 12 mmHg ≥ risk of oesophageal or gastric bleeding.

Symptoms

Portal hypertension can be asymptomatic; however, symptoms can include:
- An enlarged spleen
- Collateral vessels may develop
- Varices
- Ascites
- Haemorrhoids
- Caput medusae—dilated veins around the umbilicus.

Causes

Portal hypertension occurs as a result of:
- Cirrhosis
- Chronic hepatitis
- Congenital atresia
- Splenic vein thrombosis.

Rarely, it is the result of parasitic disease (common in developing countries) or pancreatic disease.

Investigation

Investigations can include:
- Blood tests
- Scans including:
  - Abdominal ultrasound (➲ p. 227)
  - Doppler ultrasound
  - CT scan (➲ p. 220)
  - MRI scan (➲ p. 222).

Treatment

Abstain from alcohol consumption. Treatment may be necessary for varices and ascites. Liver transplantation may be indicated.

Prevention

Medication, such as beta-blockers, may prevent the development of varices. Endoscopic screening for varices is used.

Wilson's disease

A rare inherited (recessive) disorder of copper metabolism.

Symptoms

These symptoms can include:
- Brown rings around the cornea of the eye (Kayser–Fleischer ring)
- Abdominal pain
- Haematemesis—from bleeding varices
- Confusion
- Psychiatric symptoms
  - Personality changes
  - Bizarre behaviour
  - Anxiety
  - Depression
  - Delusions.
- Effects on the nervous system
  - Clumsiness
  - Dyscoordination
  - Loss of muscle control
  - Tremors.

These symptoms can progress to:
- Jaundice
- Ascites
- Liver failure
- Progressive fatal neurological disorders.

If Wilson's disease is not treated, it can be fatal.

Incidence

Symptoms occur in the teenage years most commonly. Wilson's disease affects about 1 in 30,000 individuals.

Investigation

Diagnosis is made using a blood test and eye examination. Additional tests may include urine test, liver biopsy, and scans such as MRI or CT.

Treatment

Treatment is the removal of excess copper from the body: this is termed copper chelation. Copper chelation is achieved with medication.

Medication to remove excess levels of copper in the body includes:
- D-penicillamine—cuprimine or depen
- Trientine dihydrochloride—syprine
- Zinc acetate—galzin.

Dietary manipulation to limit dietary copper may be useful. Foods that should be avoided include:

- Nuts
- Mushrooms
- Chocolate
- Offal
- Shellfish.

Alcohol should be taken minimally or avoided.

Further information

Patients can look at the patient information site at www.britishlivertrust.org.uk or www.wilsonsdisease.org.uk

Pancreas

Acute pancreatitis

Acute pancreatitis is a condition where the pancreas becomes inflamed.

Symptoms

Common symptoms of acute pancreatitis include:
- Sudden, severe central abdominal pain
- Nausea and vomiting
- Diarrhoea
- Pyrexia.

Causes

The cause of acute pancreatitis is not always known, but it is linked to:
- Gallstones
- Excessive alcohol intake
- Leak of pancreatic enzymes can be serious or occasionally fatal.

Investigations

Investigations include:
- Blood tests
- Computed tomography (CT) scan
- Magnetic resonance imaging (MRI) scan
- Ultrasound scan.

Treatment

Treatment for acute pancreatitis is within the hospital setting to allow an algesia and monitoring for intravenous (IV) fluids. Treatment also include treating the causal condition. If acute pancreatitis is due to alcohol, thi should be avoided. Most people begin to improve within a week and hav no long-term problems, but some develop serious complications.

For people with severe pancreatitis, intensive care therapy could b required.

Chronic pancreatitis

Chronic pancreatitis is a progressive inflammatory disease of the pancreas where the pancreas is permanently damaged and function is impaired.

Symptoms

The most common symptom of chronic pancreatitis is severe burning or shooting abdominal pain. The pain can be central or left-sided and travel backwards. The pain is intermittent but can last for hours or even days. Pain can be associated with eating or for no apparent reason. Also, symptoms can include:
- Nausea
- Vomiting.

As the pancreatitis progresses, the pain becomes more severe and frequent, becoming a continual dull pain within severe episodes of pain.

As symptoms develop to advanced chronic pancreatitis, there can be an inability to produce pancreatic enzymes, resulting in steatorrhoea. This can lead to symptoms, including:
- Weight-loss
- Loss of appetite
- Jaundice
- Diabetes.

Causes

The most common cause is excessive alcohol consumption. It may occur, rarely, in children with cystic fibrosis (➲ p. 186). Less common causes include:
- Smoking
- Autoimmune pancreatitis
- Genetics
- Pancreatic injury
- Gallstones blocking the pancreatic ducts
- Abdominal radiotherapy.

Incidence

Chronic pancreatitis can affect people of any age, but it is more common in men, aged 30–40, who are heavy drinkers over time.

Investigations

Investigations include:
- Ultrasound scan
- CT scan
- MRI scan—specifically MRCP (magnetic resonance cholangiopancreatography)
- Biopsy.

Treatment

Treatment controls rather than cures chronic pancreatitis or manages symptoms.

Chronic pancreatitis can be improved if people cease alcohol consumption and smoking.

Dietary changes such as a low-fat, high-protein, and high-calorie diet can help, but dietetic support is ideal. Supplements of fat-soluble vitamins and pancreatic enzymes may be useful. Steroids may be required by people with immune system problems that have resulted in chronic pancreatitis. Analgesia is needed. Surgery can be effective, including removal of the pancreas.

Cystic fibrosis

Cystic fibrosis is a hereditary disease affecting exocrine glands. A mutation in a specific gene controlling salt transport produces thick mucus. Cystic fibrosis predominantly affects the lungs and digestive system, including the pancreas and liver.

Symptoms

There are a number of symptoms associated with cystic fibrosis that include:
- Recurring chest infections
- Bronchiectasis
- Difficulty growing and increasing weight
- Jaundice
- Diarrhoea
- Constipation
- Malodourous faeces—fat not absorbed
- Meconium ileus in newborn babies.

There is also a risk of diabetes and liver problems and a greater risk of infections.

Causes

A genetic condition.

Incidence

In White people cystic fibrosis affects ~1 in every 2500 children and is usually diagnosed at birth. It is estimated that 1 in 25 people in the UK carries the gene for cystic fibrosis. There is an increased risk if one parent has cystic fibrosis.

Investigations

Investigations include:
- Newborn blood spot (heel prick) test
- Genetic testing—blood or saliva.

Treatment

There is currently no cure for cystic fibrosis, but treatment can control symptoms and prevent complications. The focus will be on lung and gastro-intestinal (GI)-related symptoms.

Physical exercise keeps lungs clear and is good for strength and overall health.

The mucus can make digestion and absorption difficult; thus, extra calories and nutrients may be required to avoid malnutrition.

Pancreatic enzymes may be necessary to help with digestion, as the pancreas may not be effective, and thus, fat is not digested properly.

Prognosis

Cystic fibrosis is a progressive disease and can be fatal if there is a serious infection or the lungs fail. About half of people with cystic fibrosis will live past 40 years old.

Further information

A useful website for patients is www.cysticfibrosis.org.uk

Pancreatic cancer

Definition

Cancer of the pancreas occurs when the growth of the pancreas cells is abnormal and uncontrolled. Cancer of the pancreas can originate from either the exocrine cells or the endocrine cells. The most common form is pancreatic ductal adenocarcinoma (exocrine tumour); other types are rarer and may require different treatment. There are two ways to stage a pancreatic cancer: the TNM (tumour, node, metastasis) system and the number system.

The TNM system

Tumour:
- Tis—tumour in situ (rarely diagnosed this early)
- T1—tumour is inside the pancreas but 2 cm or less
- T2—tumour is over 2 cm up to 4 cm
- T3—tumour is over 4 cm
- T4—cancer has extended outside of the pancreas into the blood vessels.

Node:
- N0—no lymph nodes contain cancer
- N1—means one to three lymph nodes containing cancer
- N2—four or more lymph nodes.

Metastasis:
- M0—no spread to distant organs, such as the liver or lungs
- M1—cancer has spread to other organs.

Exocrine pancreatic cancers have an additional grading system:
- G1—low grade—cancer cells look similar to normal cells
- G4—high grade—very abnormal cells.

Pancreatic neuroendocrine tumours (NETs) are graded differently:
- Well-differentiated NETs—low-grade and intermediate-grade tumours
- Poorly differentiated NETs—high-grade tumours.

There is also the number system:
Stage 1—cancer is <4 cm with no lymph node involvement
Stage 2—cancer has spread into nearby tissues or nearby lymph
Stage 3—locally advanced cancer—spread into the large, nearby blood vessels ± lymph nodes
Stage 4—advanced cancer—the cancer has spread to other areas of the body, such as the liver or lungs.

Symptoms

Early pancreatic cancers are often symptomless and thus can be difficult to diagnose in the early stages. Symptoms include:
- Abdominal pain
- Back pain (poor prognosis)
- Unplanned weight-loss
- Jaundice
- Dark yellow/orange urine
- Pale faeces
- Pruritus

- Nausea and vomiting
- Changes in bowel habit
- Fever
- Indigestion.

Diabetes may also develop.

Causes

The cause of pancreatic cancer is not fully understood, but there are a number of risk factors including:
- Age
- Being obese
- Smoking (associated in one-third of cases)
- Being diabetic
- Chronic pancreatitis (➔ p. 184–5)
- Stomach ulcer
- H. pylori infection (➔ p. 42)
- Family history of pancreatic cancer (one in ten cases)
- Lynch syndrome (➔ p. 104)
- Peutz–Jeghers syndrome (➔ p. 108–9).

Incidence

Pancreatic cancer is uncommon in people under the age of 40; it most commonly affects people aged 50–80, with half of all new cases being diagnosed in people aged 75 years or more. In the UK about 10,000 people a year are diagnosed with pancreatic cancer.

Investigations

Investigations may include:
- Blood tests
- CT scan (➔ p. 220)
- Abdominal ultrasound (➔ p. 227)
- Biopsy
- MRI scan specifically MRCP
- Endoscopic retrograde cholangiopancreatography (ERCP) (➔ p. 254–5)
- Positron emission tomography (PET) scan.

Treatment

If the cancer is Stage 1 or 2, it might be surgically resectable ± chemotherapy. Another surgical option is a bypass, to avoid obstruction ± chemotherapy. When the cancer is locally advanced, it is unresectable and chemotherapy might be offered. A person with an advanced or metastatic cancer might be offered chemotherapy or treatment for symptom control.

Surgery might include:
- Total pancreatectomy (➔ p. 496)—rarely performed in the UK
- Distal pancreatectomy (➔ p. 496)—for cancer in the pancreas body or tail
- Pylorus preserving pancreaticoduodenectomy (PPPD) (➔ p. 499)—for cancer in the pancreas head
- Whipple procedure (➔ p. 506)—for cancer in the pancreas head.

Alternatively stenting of the bile duct can reduce symptoms such as jaundice.

Chemotherapy can be given before surgery, after surgery, or if surgery is not possible.

Prognosis

In England and Wales, the prognosis for pancreatic cancer is poor, as often it is diagnosed late. About 20% of people will survive for 1 year after diagnosis. Less than 5% will survive for 5 years and 1% will survive for 10 years from diagnosis.

Chapter 8

Gall bladder

Acute cholecystitis

Acute cholecystitis is inflammation of the gall bladder (➲ p. 14). Usually associated with gallstones (➲ p. 198–9) in over 90% of patients when they block the cystic duct.

Symptoms

The main symptom of acute cholecystitis is a sudden sharp pain in the right upper quadrant of the abdomen that spreads towards the right shoulder or back. The area is very tender and deep breaths worsen pain, which is commonly persistent and lasts for several hours. Other symptoms include:
- Pyrexia
- Nausea
- Vomiting—stone in the bile duct
- Sweating
- Anorexia
- Jaundice—stone in the bile duct
- Distended abdomen.

An acute attack can occur after a large and/or fatty meal.

If the gall bladder is distended, its wall can perforate. The leak can form a chronic abscess.

Causes

Continued secretion by the gall bladder leads to a rise in pressure. Inflammation of the gall bladder wall results from the toxic effects of the retained bile and bacterial infection. The bile is usually turbid but may become frank pus (empyema of the gall bladder). There are two main categories of acute cholecystitis: calculous cholecystitis and acalculous cholecystitis. Calculous cholecystitis is the most common type and is and caused by biliary sludge, with about 20% of cases having a bacterial infection. Acalculous cholecystitis can be more serious, and is possibly caused by major surgery or sepsis.

Incidence

The typical person with acute cholecystitis is an obese, middle-aged woman.

Investigations

On examination there are a number of common signs:
- Right hypochondrial tenderness is present and is exacerbated by inspiration (Murphy's sign).
- Muscle guarding and rebound tenderness are common.
- The gall bladder is usually impalpable but occasionally a tender mass of omentum and gall bladder may be felt under the liver.
- Blood tests—elevated white cell count, elevated serum bilirubin concentrations
- Ultrasound scan.

Other investigations can include X-ray, computed tomography (CT) scan (➲ p. 220), or magnetic resonance imaging (MRI) (➲ p. 222).

Treatment

Acute cholecystitis can be potentially serious and usually requires a hospital admission for intravenous (IV) fluids, analgesia (→ p. 406), and antibiotics (→ p. 408). Cholecystectomy (→ p. 486) may be advocated after the acute inflammatory phase. The nurse can advise that to prevent further symptoms, it is advisable to have a healthy, balanced diet that includes reduction of high-cholesterol food. It is important to gradually lose weight, especially if obese and to take regular exercise.

Biliary malignancies

Cancer of the gall bladder can be adenocarcinoma or a squamous cell carcinoma. Adenocarcinoma affects the gland cells of the gall bladder lining and is the most common type of cancer in the organ. Squamous cell cancer affects the squamous lining of the gall bladder.

Symptoms

Initially gall bladder cancer is symptomless; thus, diagnosis is often made late. Symptoms can include:
- Abdominal pain
- Nausea or vomiting
- Jaundice.

Other symptoms can include:
- Anorexia
- Abdominal distention
- Dark yellow urine
- Pale faeces
- Pruritus.

Causes

The cause of gall bladder cancer is unknown. Risks are increased with:
- Age—most cases are in people over 70 years of age
- Family history—parent, sibling, or child
- A previous gall bladder condition—such as gallstones, cholecystitis
- Obesity
- Smoking.

Investigations

Investigations include:
- Blood tests
- Abdominal ultrasound
- CT scan—abdomen
- Biopsy
- Endoscopy—endoscopic retrograde cholangiopancreatography (ERCP).

Treatment

Treatment will depend upon factors including the type of cancer, the staging of the cancer, and any comorbidities. Treatment might include chemoradiation with or without surgery.

Surgery can be:
- Cholecystectomy (➲ p. 486) +/− resection of the associated liver +/− lymph nodes
- Whipple's procedure (➲ p. 506).

Prognosis

Prognosis is poor, often due to late diagnosis. Fewer than half of people with this cancer survive for 1 year after diagnosis.

Choledocholithiasis

Choledocholithiasis is the presence of gallstones within the common bile duct, commonly termed bile duct stones. In the main, the stones originate in the gall bladder.

Symptoms

The three common symptoms of choledocholithiasis are right upper abdominal pain (persistent, severe, and colicky), jaundice, and pyrexia. There may also be vomiting and dark urine due to the staining from the bilirubin and pale faeces. Additional symptoms include pruritus. In older people, there may be no symptoms. If there is prolonged biliary obstruction that last months or years, this can result in liver damage.

Investigations

A number of investigations are usually required:
- Blood tests
- Plain X-ray—rarely performed but can identify calcified gallstones
- Ultrasound—can show dilated bile ducts and gallstones, but may fail to detect stones
- ERCP (➜ p. 254–5).

Treatment

Common bile duct gallstones can be removed by endoscopic sphincterotomy or cholecystectomy.

Chronic cholecystitis

Chronic cholecystitis is inflammation of the gall bladder (⭗ p. 14) that persists over many months, as a result of gallstones.

Symptoms

Chronic cholecystitis often develops insidiously but symptoms may occur following an attack of acute cholecystitis. Some people report bouts of constant right hypochondrial or epigastric pain. The pain may last up to several hours and can radiate to the right shoulder or the back. Commonly symptoms of chronic cholecystitis are vague but include abdominal discomfort and distension, nausea, flatulence, and intolerance of fatty foods.

The complications of chronic cholecystitis include:
- Acute exacerbations (acute cholecystitis)
- Passage of stones into the bile duct (choledocholithiasis)
- Pancreatitis
- Cholecystenteric fistula formation
- Rarely carcinoma of the gall bladder.

Causes

Pathologically chronic cholecystitis is characterized by chronic inflammation and thickening of the gall bladder wall. In addition to stones, the gall bladder may contain brown sediment ('biliary mud').

Investigation

Examination of the abdomen may reveal tenderness over the gall bladder and a positive Murphy's sign (⭗ p. 199). Blood tests are usually not used for diagnosis. Imaging to diagnose chronic cholecystitis include:
- Ultrasound (⭗ p. 227)—looking for gallstones
- Plain X-ray—looking for calcified stones—is rarely used
- ERCP (⭗ p. 254–5).

Treatment

When chronic cholecystitis is established the treatment of choice is a cholecystectomy. When the diagnosis is less certain and symptoms are vague but the gall bladder is functioning well, a conservative approach is considered. Treatment in this scenario includes weight reduction and a low-fat diet, especially if fatty food is associated with the symptoms. Oral bile acid therapy may also be considered.

Gallstones

Gallstones are usually small (pea-sized) but can fill the whole gall bladder as multiple stones may be present. Most gallstones (75%) are yellow-green and made primarily of hardened cholesterol. The remainder are black or brown and formed from calcium, salts, and pigment (pigment stones).

Cholelithiasis is the formation of gallstones in the gall bladder, but about 15% of patients will also have stones in the common bile duct.

Symptoms

More than 80% of patients with gallstones are asymptomatic. Gallstones can be diagnosed by a chance finding on imaging for another problem. However, the following symptoms can occur if the gallstone blocks the bile duct:
- Pale stools
- Jaundice
- Colicky 'biliary colic' shooting abdominal pain, usually with or after eating (especially high-fat meals)
- Pain below the ribs on the right-hand side, possibly referred to the back or shoulder
- If symptoms are severe, 'biliary colic' may also present with fever, nausea, and vomiting. Severe pain can be caused by the stone passing along the bile duct or secondary to inflammation (cholecystitis)
- Pyrexia.

Cause

The cause is not fully understood but might be a chemical imbalance resulting in crystallization within the bile within the gall bladder. This can cause an increase in the size of the stones over many years, often with several stones forming.

Incidence

Gallstones are common: they occur in 10% of adults. The incidence ↑ with age (over 40 years of age), occurring in 30% of ♀ >50 years, and has a ratio of ♀:♂ of 2:1. There is a familial link, and the condition is more prevalent in White people.

Other risk factors include:
- Females who are on hormones, including some contraceptive pills
- Overweight or obesity
- Cirrhosis
- Primary sclerosing cholangitis (♦ p. 393)
- Irritable bowel syndrome (IBS) (♦ p. 96–8)
- Family history
- Recent weight-loss
- Taking ceftriaxone (antibiotic)
- Having been pregnant.

Investigations

- Blood tests
- Ultrasound scan—diagnoses 95%
- MRI scan
- Cholangiography
- ERCP (➲ p. 254–5)
- CT scan.

Murphy's sign can be used to determine an inflamed gall bladder. Use the hand/fingers on the right upper quadrant of the abdomen and ask the patient to breathe in: pain indicates inflammation.

Treatment

If there are no symptoms, it is possible to leave the gallstones. Treatment can include control of symptoms by using:

- A low-fat diet—to prevent worsening symptoms
- Analgesia (➲ p. 406)

Removal of the gallstones can include:

- Surgical removal of the gall bladder—cholecystectomy
- Endoscopic removal of the gallstones (ERCP)
- Lithotripsy—ultrasonic shock waves to breakdown the stones.

Primary sclerosing cholangitis

Primary sclerosing cholangitis is diffuse inflammation and fibrosis of the biliary system. Primary sclerosing cholangitis can often result in strictures of the bile ducts, which leads to occlusion of the bile ducts, biliary cirrhosis, and eventually cirrhosis.

Symptoms

There are a number of symptoms associated with primary sclerosing cholangitis including:
- Jaundice
- Pruritus (skin itching)
- Abdominal pain
- Possibly weight loss and fatigue
- Fat malabsorption leading to steatorrhoea
- Deficiency of fat-soluble vitamins.

In inflammatory bowel disease (IBD), the condition could progress to cholangiocarcinoma.

Cause

The cause of primary sclerosing cholangitis is uncertain. Primary sclerosing cholangitis can be associated with IBD (➔ p. 368–9) or other autoimmune diseases, such as systemic lupus erythematosus, systemic sclerosis, or type 1 diabetes mellitus. Primary sclerosing cholangitis is most common in young adult males with IBD.

Investigations

The investigations used to diagnose primary sclerosing cholangitis include:
- Blood tests—looking for ↑ alkaline phosphatase
- Imaging by ERCP
- Liver biopsy.

Treatment

Treatment is mostly targeted at avoiding complications:
- Correct nutritional deficiencies
- Treat pruritus
- Avoid infection.

Dilatation or stenting of the ducts might be possible. Antibiotics should be given if bacterial infection is present. The patient might need liver transplantation in end-stage liver failure.

Chapter 9

Nursing assessment

History taking—general

History taking is the key component of patient assessment, which enables a nurse to acquire significant and comprehensive knowledge to gain a better understanding of the patient's problems, and therefore identify the most appropriate interventions. Patient assessment is the first part of the nursing process, which views the patient holistically, and gathers information about a patient's physiological, psychological, sociological, and spiritual status. Therefore, identifies their needs and forms the basis of delivering high standards and quality of care.

Key factors:

- Active, attentive listening—attention to the details of what the patient is saying, either in a verbal or non-verbal manner
- Empathy—demonstrates the nurse understands the patient, recognizes their current situation and perceived feelings
- Communicating—in a non-judgmental, unbiased way of acceptance
- Focusing—brings the focus of the conversation to an essential area of concern, eliminating vague or rambling dialogue, and centres the assessment on the source of discomfort and pertinent details in the history
- Asking relevant questions—questions are general at first becoming more specific; asked in a logical, consecutive order; open-ended, close-ended, and focused questions may be useful during an assessment
- Responding appropriately to the information provided
- Providing information—to inform the patient what is about to happen, explain findings, and the need for further tests or observation to promote trust and decrease anxiety
- Taking time
- Not assuming a diagnosis.

The nurse needs to be able to appropriately process the information obtained from a comprehensive history. This, in conjunction with a physical assessment, will enable the nurse to plan care as required. This may include health promotion, treatment, follow-up, referral, or discharge.

SOAPIER

One assessment method to structure the history-taking process is the use of SOAPIER (subjective, objective, assessment, plan, implementation, evaluation, and review). The first four will be explored:

Subjective:
- A short statement in the patient's own words of their present illness or complaint
- History of present complaint—to include details of each problem, letting the patient tell their story, and asking questions if needed to clarify or elicit further information
- Past medical history—note all illnesses (non-trivial), operations, and hospital admissions
- Drugs and allergies—note all prescribed and over-the-counter drugs that the patient is taking
- Social and personal history—include alcohol and smoking history, use of recreational drugs, occupation, family history (particularly history of cancer, diabetes, or inflammatory bowel disease (➔ p. 368–9), recent exotic travel, whether they live alone, any use of social services).

Objective:
- Review of systems
- Physical examination
- Investigations.

Assessment:
- Formulation of diagnosis.

Plan:
- Development of a plan of care.

History taking—gastrointestinal

In addition to the SOAPIER method of history taking, there are gastrointestinal (GI)-specific considerations:
- Nutrition—appetite, change in eating pattern, recent weight loss or gain (planned or unplanned), food preferences, food intolerances, special diet, influences on diet (lifestyle, cultural)
- Difficulty in swallowing
- Jaundice, colour of urine, colour of stools
- Assessment of drugs—use of laxatives (➔ p. 422–3), stool softeners, antidiarrhoeal agents (➔ p. 411), non-steroidal anti-inflammatory agents (NSAIDS) (➔ p. 406), steroids (➔ p. 428), anticoagulants, prokinetics, iron supplements, antidepressants (➔ p. 410), diuretics (➔ p. 419), opiates (➔ p. 406), calcium channel blockers (➔ p. 416), antacids (➔ p. 407), anticholingerics (➔ p. 409), antibiotics (➔ p. 408), biguanides, and proton pump inhibitors (PPIs) (➔ p. 427)
- Stools—frequency, consistency, colour, odour (clarify the patients meaning of diarrhoea and constipation). Use bowel chart if an in-patient
- Bowel habit and any change in this habit. Consider use of Bristol Stool Form Scale chart
- Continence—post-defaecation soiling, urge incontinence, passive incontinence. Consider use of a continence scale, such as International Consultation on Incontinence Questionnaire-Bowels (ICIQ-B), St Marks Score
- Obstetric history (if applicable).

More in-depth questioning about topics reported:

Diarrhoea

- Onset and duration—gradual or sudden, frequency of stools, number per day, change in usual bowel habit
- Characteristics—watery, explosive, colour, mucous, blood, undigested food, fatty, odour
- Course—improving or worsening
- Associated symptoms—fever, chills, weight loss, abdominal pain, thirst, recent antibiotics
- Alleviating or precipitating factors.

Constipation

Consider use of constipation scale such as patient assessment of constipation quality of life (PAC-QOL), patient assessment of constipation symptoms (PAC-SYM).
- Onset and duration—recent occurrence or long-standing problem, sudden or gradual, last bowel movement
- Characteristics—dry hard stool, number of bowel movements per week, change in stool size, black stool, tarry stool, bright red blood, accompanied with abdominal or rectal pain, alternating with diarrhoea
- Feeling of incomplete evacuation
- Bulging towards vagina
- Post-defaecation soiling

- Course—continuous or intermittent
- Associated symptoms—feeling of incomplete evacuation, dragging sensation, prolapse, bloating
- Alleviating or precipitating factors—diet, fluid intake, use of drugs such as laxatives (➲ p. 422–3), manual evacuation.

Further reading

Black CJ and Ford AC (2018). Chronic idiopathic constipation in adults: epidemiology, pathophysiology, diagnosis and clinical management. *Medical Journal of Australia* 209(2): 86–9.

Cotterill N, Norton C, Avery K, et al. (2011). Psychometric evaluation of a new patient completed questionnaire for evaluating anal incontinence symptoms and impact on quality of life: The ICIQ-B. *Diseases of the Colon and Rectum* 54(10): 1235–50.

Maeda Y, Vaizey CJ, Norton C (2007) St Mark's Incontinence Score. *Diseases of the Colon and Rectum* 50(12): 2252.

Marquis P, De La Loge C, Dubois D, et al. (2005). Development and validation of the Patient Assessment of Constipation Quality of Life questionnaire. *Scandinavian Journal of Gastroenterology* 40(5): 540–51.

Yiannakou Y, Tack J, Piessevaux H, et al. (2017) The PAC-SYM questionnaire for chronic constipation: defining the minimal important difference. *Alimentary, Pharmacology and Therapeutics* 46(11–12): 1103–11.

History taking—liver

History

History taking is the same as for any general health history. Make a special note of drug/alcohol/substance use and misuse (important not to prejudge or stigmatize). Take a family history. Ask about diet and any symptoms of infection.

Physical examination

The liver may be enlarged or small in chronic alcoholic liver disease. In primary biliary cirrhosis, it may be enlarged. An enlarged spleen is common in chronic liver disease. Look for skin discoloration or sclera indicating jaundice.

Jaundice

- Diagnose on examination and blood tests
- Usually develops if bilirubin >45 µ mol/L of blood
- Pre-hepatic—haemolytic conditions
- Hepatic—liver damage
- Post-hepatic—obstruction of the flow of bile.

Stigmata of chronic liver disease—classic findings, usually associated with cirrhosis, are as follows:

- Palmar erythema—red discoloration of the palms of the hands
- Finger clubbing (rare)
- Spider naevi
- White nails (leuconychia)
- Skin pigmentation (jaundice or haemochromatosis).

History taking—nutritional

Nutritional assessment is a structured procedure that enables healthcare professionals to perform a systematic evaluation to identify the need for nutritional intervention in order to make a clinical decision using a person-centred approach.

This differs from nutritional screening with a tool such as malnutrition universal screening tool (MUST), which is a brief risk assessment which can be carried out by any healthcare professional and therefore may lead to a nutritional assessment by a dietitian.

There is no single measure for nutritional health. Several factors must be considered as part of the assessment, as outlined below.

History:
- Previous and current illness
- Surgery
- Sepsis/wound exudate, haemorrhage, fistula, healing
- Impaired digestion, vomiting, coeliac disease
- Weight history—including intentional or unintentional, recent changes in weight
- Drug therapy—which might affect dietary intake, nutrient absorption, and metabolism
- Socio-economic, psychological, cognition and physical ability.

Actual dietary and fluid intake:
- Appetite
- Meal pattern
- Food choice.

Body composition

Observation of physical appearance:
- Loss of fat
- Poor wound healing
- Pressure sores
- Poor mobility
- Oedema
- Dehydration
- Dyspnoea
- Lesion of lips and tongue
- Peripheral neuropathy
- Body mass index (BMI)
- Muscle mass, function.

Further reading

British Dietetics Association (BDA) (2016) Model and Process for Nutrition and Dietetic Practice. https://www.bda.uk.com/practice-and-education/nutrition-and-dietetic-practice/professional-guidance/model-and-process-for-dietetic-practice.html (Accessed 20/7/2020).

British Association of Parenteral and Enteral Nutrition (BAPEN) Malnutrition Universal Screening Tool (MUST) http://www.bapen.org.uk/pdfs/must/must_full.pdf (Accessed 04/02/2019).

Physical examination

Physical examination is used when disease is suspected or already identified. It may also be utilized as a screening examination when there is no suspicion/expectation of disease and used as part of the history taking.

The reasons pertaining to the procedure should be explained to the patient. The procedure itself should be explained and a chaperone should be offered. The environment for a physical examination needs to be private, warm, and well-lit.

Physical examination—rectal

A rectal examination includes visual inspection of the perianal area, and physical examination of the perianal area and the rectum. The nurse should inform the patient that the examination may be uncomfortable but not painful. There may be a feeling of rectal fullness and the desire to defaecate may be experienced. The patient should be positioned in the left lateral position, with hips flexed to 90 degrees, the knees flexed more than 90 degrees and the buttocks on the edge of the couch.

On inspection the nurse should examine for:
- Skin conditions—skin erosion, skin discolouration, skin disorders, such as eczema, fungal infections, or viral infections
- Scars from previous surgery or infection
- Anal fissures (⊃ p. 120–1)
- Anal fistula (⊃ p. 122–3)
- Haemorrhoids (⊃ p. 126–8)
- Pilonidal sinus (⊃ p. 132–3)
- Faecal soiling—poor hygiene, faecal incontinence
- Lumps or bumps—polyps, anal warts (⊃ p. 124), prolapsed piles, perianal haematoma, skin tags, sentinel pile, mucosal prolapse, rectal prolapse (⊃ p. 138–9), squamous cell carcinoma
- For prolapses or piles—ask the patient to bear down (strain) to observe for perineal descent, prolapse, or piles.

On perianal palpation, the nurse should feel the skin around the perineum for:
- Tracks that lead to external openings of fistulae
- Induration or fibrosis from sepsis.

Digital rectal examination or per rectum

Digital rectal examination (DRE) is also termed per rectum (PR) and is an examination of the anus and rectum to identify disease processes. The procedure is as follows:
- Lubricate a gloved index finger.
- Part the buttocks and gently insert finger into the anus to avoid trauma to the anal mucosa.
- Work with the anal reflex by putting your finger on the anus gently and wait a few seconds—this will allow the anus to contract and then relax.
- Note resting tone (slight resistance indicates good internal sphincter control).
- Note any spasm or pain on insertion. If the patient feels any pain, ensure that they are happy to continue with the procedure. If spasm or difficulty inserting the finger, ask the patient to talk or breathe out.

- Sweep clockwise and then anticlockwise.
- Palpate for irregularities internally.
- Note the presence of any tenderness, presence, and consistency of faecal matter (using the Bristol Stool Form Chart).

It is also possible to assess for the following:
- Resting tone (people with an acute fissure may not be able to tolerate a PR)
- Squeeze pressure
- Any thickening or masses in the anal canal or lower rectum
- Prostate (in men)
- Cervix (in women)
- Abnormalities in the recto-vaginal septum, such as a rectocele or weak perineal body.

After examination look at the gloved finger for blood and/or faeces. Document all findings, observations, and actions, including negative ones.

Further reading

RCN (2012). Management of lower bowel dysfunction, including DRE and DRF. RCN Guidance for Nurses. RCN, London.
RCN (2019). Bowel care: Management of lower bowel dysfunction including digital rectal examination and digital removal of faeces. RCN, London.

Abdominal examination

An abdominal examination is performed as part of the comprehensive physical examination that evaluates complaints such as pain, distension, enlarged organs, or masses. It consists of a predetermined sequence: inspection, auscultation, percussion, and palpation of all the quadrants. The examination begins with the patient in the supine position with the abdomen exposed.

Chapter 10

Investigating the gut

24-hour pH monitoring

A 24-h pH monitoring measures the amount of reflux into the oesophagus from the stomach over a 24-h period.

Indications for pH monitoring are:

- Patients with symptoms clinically suggestive of acid gastro-oesophageal reflux, who fail to respond during a high-dose therapeutic trial of a proton pump inhibitor (PPI)
- Patients with symptoms clinically suggestive of acid gastro-oesophageal reflux without oesophagitis or with an unsatisfactory response to a high-dose PPI in whom anti-reflux surgery is contemplated
- Patients with persistent acid gastro-oesophageal reflux symptoms despite anti-reflux surgery.

Contraindications:

- Suspected or confirmed pharyngeal or upper oesophageal obstruction
- Severe coagulopathy (but not anticoagulation within the therapeutic range)
- Bullous disorders of the oesophageal mucosa
- Cardiac conditions in which vagal stimulation is poorly tolerated.

Relative contraindications

There is an increased risk of complications from blind oesophageal intubation; if 24-h pH monitoring is required, risks can be reduced using endoscopic or radiological guidance.

- Peptic strictures
- Oesophageal ulcers
- Oesophageal or junctional tumours
- Varices
- Large diverticula.

Preparation

- Fast for a minimum of 4 h for solids and 2 h for liquids—a longer period of fasting may be appropriate for patients with evidence of fluid or food residues at endoscopy/radiology, such as those with achalasia.

Some prescription medications can affect the results of testing and should be stopped 7–14 days before the procedure, according to the unit where the test is carried out. Drugs that can affect the test results include:

- Adrenergic blockers
- Anticholinergics
- Some antacids
- Alcohol
- Cholinergics (drugs that produce the same effects as the parasympathetic nervous system)
- Corticosteroids
- H2 blockers
- PPIs.

Procedure

- A small probe is inserted through nostril and positioned near the lower oesophagus. The probe is plugged into a small unit (or monitor) worn on a belt or over the shoulder.

The small unit has several buttons that, when pressed, record:
- The occurrence of symptoms
- When patients eat
- When patients lie down.

The patient must return to the hospital to have the probe removed and return the equipment.

Further reading

Bodger K and Trudgill N (2006). Guidelines for oesophageal manometry and PH monitoring. *BSG Guidelines in Gastroenterology*.

Barium enema

A barium enema is introduced into the rectum via the anus, and a series of X-rays are taken to visualize the colon for anomalies—this gives a clearer image than with X-ray alone. Barium coats the bowel wall following changes in the patient's position after insertion of the enema and with insufflation of carbon dioxide or air.

Indications

A barium enema is rarely used now as it has been superseded by colonoscopy (⊃ p. 246–7) or computed tomography (CT) (⊃ p. 220).
- Altered bowel habit
- Suspected stricture
- Tumour or polyps
- Rectal bleeding
- Pain
- Ongoing diarrhoea/constipation
- Volvulus.

Contraindications

If barium escapes from the bowel into the mediastinum or peritoneum, it can cause irritation and, in some cases, severe inflammation. For this reason, in the immediate post-operative period or if perforation is suspected, an alternative iodine-based solution (gastrografin or another water-soluble agent) is given instead of barium.
- Suspected leak
- Known colonic stricture
- Severe dysphagia with an obvious oropharyngeal component: patient is unlikely to take sufficient contrast for a complete study
- Severe immobility and difficulty standing unaided.

Risk

Abdominal imaging that involves radiation (X-rays) is of potential harm to the patient in terms of a risk of inducing cancer. Furthermore, exposure during pregnancy, to even small amounts of radiation, has a risk of teratogenesis in the foetus. The use of X-rays should be kept to a minimum. If possible, good clinical history and examination findings, in addition to ultrasound, can help decrease the need for radiation-based investigations.

Preparation

- Low residue diet for 48 h
- Good oral fluid intake (about 2 litres)
- Two sachets of sodium picosulphate (Picolax), before the procedure, to help the bowel clear.

Procedure

- A barium enema is introduced per rectum with the patient in the left lateral position.
- The patient is turned prone, to encourage the barium to travel along the colon into the splenic flexure.
- The procedure takes 30–45 min.

Aftercare

The nurse should advise:

- A normal diet can be resumed unless otherwise indicated.
- An increase in fluids is needed to prevent constipation (2 litres daily).
- Stools may be chalky or light in colour when passed after the investigation, as the barium is not absorbed through the gastrointestinal tract.

Barium follow-through

Barium is ingested and a series of X-rays are taken to visualize the small bowel from the duodenum to the terminal ileum.

Indications

- Tumours
- Intermittent small-bowel obstruction
- Strictures
- Assessment of known small bowel disease and inflammation—Crohn's disease, coeliac disease, and polyposis syndromes
- Abnormal motility.

Contraindications

- As per barium enema (→ p. 214).

Risk

- As per barium enema (→ p. 214).

Preparation

- Fasting for 6 h prior to the examination.

Procedure

- Barium liquid is taken orally; alternatively, it may be given via a nasogastric tube.
- Images are taken at 20-min intervals, demonstrating a column of barium travelling along the small intestine.
- The procedure takes, on average, 2.5 h.

Aftercare

- As per barium enema (→ p. 215).

Barium meal

Barium is ingested and a series of X-rays are taken to visualize the upper gastrointestinal (GI) tract to the duodenum to observe for anomalies.

Indications

Since endoscopy has become more commonplace, the use of upper GI barium meal has continued to diminish. Nonetheless, a high-quality barium meal can provide excellent diagnostic information about the gastro-oesophageal junction and both gastric and duodenal mucosa.

* Dyspepsia
* Weight loss
* Upper abdominal mass
* Failure or contraindication to endoscopy oesophageal gastroduodenoscopy (OGD) (➲ p. 214–15)
* Hiatus hernia
* Polyps.

Contraindications

* As per barium enema (➲ p. 214).

Risk

* As per barium enema (➲ p. 214).

Preparation

* Nil by mouth for 4 h before examination.

Procedure

* The barium meal is ingested.
* The patient lies down and needs to turn into sideways, supine, and prone positions.
* Spasmolytic agents are given to decrease gastric motility. The procedure takes, on average, 15 min.

Aftercare

* As per barium enema (➲ p. 215).

Barium swallow

Barium is swallowed and then a series of X-rays are taken to visualize the oesophagus for anomalies.

Indication

- Dysphagia—difficulty swallowing solids or liquids
- Odynophagia—pain on swallowing
- Globus sensation—lump in throat
- As per barium enema (➲ p. 214).

Contraindications

- As per barium enema (➲ p. 214).

Risk

- As per barium enema (➲ p. 214).

Preparation

- Nil by mouth for 4 h before the procedure.

Procedure

- Patient should be in standing position.
- Barium is given orally and swallowed on instruction.
- A series of images are taken from the upper to the lower part of the oesophagus, at different angles.
- Procedure usually takes 15 min.

Aftercare

- As per barium enema (➲ p. 215).

Breath test

The hydrogen breath test uses the measurement of hydrogen in the breath to diagnose several conditions that cause GI symptoms. Anaerobic bacteria in the colon can produce hydrogen when exposed to unabsorbed food, particularly carbohydrates, such as sugars. In normal digestion, small amounts of hydrogen are produced. However, this can increase when there is a problem with digestion or absorption. Large amounts of hydrogen may also be produced when the colon bacteria move back into the small intestine (small bowel bacterial overgrowth). Some of the hydrogen produced by the bacteria, whether in the small intestine or the colon, is absorbed into the blood flow of the small/large intestine. The hydrogen-containing blood travels to the lungs where the hydrogen is exhaled in the breath and can be measured.

Indications
- Lactose malabsorption
- Bacterial overgrowth
- Abdominal pain
- Abdominal bloating
- Abdominal distension
- Increased amount of flatus
- Diarrhoea.

Preparation
Preparation can vary at different centres.
- Fasting 12 h before procedure.

Procedure
Devices and procedures used can vary from each centre.
- At the start of the test, the patient gives a base reading of hydrogen by blowing into a device.
- The patient then ingests a small amount of the test sugar.
- Additional samples of breath are collected and analysed for hydrogen every 15, 30, or 60 min for approximately 2–3 h.

Aftercare
- Patients with positive results should be seen by a dietitian.

Computed tomography

Computed tomography (CT) uses X-rays and high-powered computer reconstruction techniques to create a cross-sectional image or slices of anatomy through the body, showing all the different organs by their different water and fat contents, in addition to their vascularity. These slices are called tomographic images and contain more detailed information than conventional X-rays. A contrast agent may be used to improve the quality of images, to enhance the visibility of soft tissue, visceral organs, and blood vessels; the contrast can be drunk, given intravenously or as an enema into the rectum.

Indications

- CT is indicated if ultrasound is technically difficult or non-diagnostic.
- CT is used in conjunction with a colorectal cancer diagnosis to check for cancer spread—CT chest/abdomen and pelvis.

Contraindications

- No absolute contraindications
- Difficulty of transferring sick and unstable patients to the scanner
- A recent barium test can result in severe artefacts in CT scans.

Risk

- There is a risk of 1 in 1000 of inducing cancer due to a relatively high radiation dose.
- Exposure during pregnancy has a risk of teratogenesis in the foetus.
- Patients with kidney problems carry an increased risk of potential problems eliminating the contrast material from their system after the examination, risking renal failure.
- The risk of an anaphylactic reaction to the contrasts.

Procedure

Most commonly, an abdominal CT scan requires the use of a contrast agent.

- The patient lies on the examination table which advances through the CT scanner, while the X-ray tube rotates continuously around the examination table, emitting controlled beams of radiation. Each time the X-ray tube makes a 360° rotation, a digital image of a thin transverse section of the abdomen is acquired.
- The patient must lie still and hold their breath, usually for 6–10 s at a time.
- The average procedure time is 20 min.

Aftercare

Nurses should advise patients that occasionally there can be a laxative effect from the oral contrast.

Defaecating proctogram

A defecating proctogram is imaging (X-ray) of the mechanics of a patient's pelvic floor and defecation in real time. The anatomy and function of the anorectum and pelvic floor can be dynamically studied at various stages during defaecation (defaecation is not replicated only simulated).

Indications

- Intractable constipation—to exclude obstructed defecation
- Perineal herniation—to exclude anismus as a predisposing factor
- Suspected rectal intussusception or rectal prolapse.

Risk

Imaging that involves radiation (X-rays) is of potential harm to the patient in terms of a risk of inducing cancer. Furthermore, exposure during pregnancy, to even small amounts of radiation, has a risk of teratogenesis in the foetus.

Procedure

- The patient swallows oral diluted barium to delineate the small bowel so that any hernia (enterocele) can easily be demonstrated.
- Barium paste is inserted into the rectum.
- The patient sits in an upright position on a commode and tries to evacuate the barium from the rectum with real time imaging from the start of straining to the completion of evacuation.

Patient privacy and a relaxed reassuring environment are essential, and the test is usually only performed in centres at which this environment can be developed. Evacuation of the barium paste is recorded using fluoroscopy (an X-ray 'movie').

Aftercare

The nurse needs to advise patients that:

- Constipation can occur after the investigation; to prevent this drinking plenty of fluids (2 litres) is necessary after the test each day until 'normal' bowel function returns.
- Bowel motions may be pale in colour for a short period due to the barium.
- Some may experience faecal incontinence for a short period after the investigation.

Magnetic resonance imaging

Magnetic resonance imaging (MRI) produces cross-sectional images of the body and internal organs. MRI scans use a large bore high field strength magnet technique, not ionizing radiation (X-rays). An MRI scanner is a noisy, narrow, confining tube. A benefit of an MRI is that the computer software enables display of the information in any plane, which affords a better understanding of the relationships between different organs/structures and the abnormality; this is useful in surgical planning. The magnet aligns the protons within the atoms of the patient's body in one direction. High-energy audible-frequency sound is used to transfer energy to these protons, which deflects their alignment. When they return to a normal relaxed state, energy is emitted, which is detected by the scanner, and the information is used to map the internal structure of the body in terms of tissue structure and characteristics.

Indications

- Primarily used for assessment of rectal and perineal disease caused by inflammatory bowel disease (IBD) (➲ p. 368–9) or as part of staging of anorectal cancer.
- Increasingly used for exclusion of pancreatic and biliary pathology, if ultrasound is inconclusive.
- Specialist centres might use MRI to identify small and large bowel pathology.
- The contrast resolution between different tissue types enables characterizations of abnormal tissue.

Contraindications

- Metallic implants, e.g. cardiac pacemaker or other metallic mechanical/ electrical device in the heart or brain
- Metal in crucial or sensitive areas, e.g. shrapnel in the eyeball.

Relative contraindications

- Claustrophobia
- Ventilated or monitored patients
- The safety of MRI during the first trimester of pregnancy is uncertain.

Procedure

- The patient lies inside the tunnel.
- For some small bowel and pancreatic studies, injections of antispasmodic (➲ p. 409) or antisecretory agents (➲ p. 414) might be required.
- Some staging examinations might require an intravenous contrast agent.
- The patient must be able to lie still on the scanner table, inside the magnet bore.
- The procedure, on average, takes between 15–45 min.

Manometry—anorectal

Anorectal manometry is a functional test that assesses the tone and function of the anal sphincters. The test provides a measure of the effectiveness of anal muscles, the rectoanal inhibitory reflex, sensation, and the co-ordination of the anal sphincters, as well as volume compliance of the rectum. It is not a definitive test and is usually used in combination with endoanal ultrasound and X-rays.

Indications
- Faecal incontinence
- Hirschsprung's disease
- Prior to surgery.

Procedure
The procedure can vary from unit to unit.
- Usually anorectal manometry involves the insertion of a flexible probe into the rectum ± a small balloon filled with water, while the patient is lying in the left lateral position.
- The patient relaxes, squeezes, and pushes down, whilst the healthcare professional takes measurements.
- The test typically takes approximately 30 min to 1 h.

Manometry—oesophageal

High resolution oesophageal manometry is a test to measure the pressure activity within the oesophagus and the sphincter at the top of the stomach. The multi-pressure sensor catheter (tube) has sensors situated at 1 cm intervals, allowing for measurements along the entire length of the oesophagus.

Indications for oesophageal manometry:

- To diagnose suspected primary oesophageal motility disorders, including achalasia (➲ p. 18) and diffuse oesophageal spasm (➲ p. 54)
- To diagnose suspected secondary oesophageal motility disorders occurring in association with systemic diseases, such a systemic sclerosis
- As part of the pre-operative assessment of some patients undergoing antireflux procedures
- To reassess oesophageal function in patients who have been treated for a primary oesophageal disorder or undergone antireflux surgery, including dysphagia (➲ p. 24) following fundoplication.

Contraindications

- Suspected or confirmed pharyngeal or upper oesophageal obstruction
- Severe coagulopathy (but not anticoagulation within the therapeutic range)
- Bullous disorders of the oesophageal mucosa
- Cardiac conditions in which vagal stimulation is poorly tolerated.

Relative contraindications

There is an increased risk of complications from blind oesophageal intubation; if oesophageal manometry is required risks can be reduced using endoscopic or radiological guidance.

- Peptic strictures
- Oesophageal ulcers
- Oesophageal or junctional tumours
- Varices
- Large diverticula.

Preparation

- Fast for a minimum of 4 h for solids and 2 h for liquids—a longer period of fasting may be appropriate for patients with evidence of fluid or food residues at endoscopy/radiology, such as those with achalasia.

Some prescription medications can affect the results of testing and should be stopped 7–14 days before the procedure, according to the unit where the test is carried out. Drugs that can affect the test results include:

- Adrenergic blockers
- Anticholinergics
- Some antacids
- Alcohol
- Cholinergics (drugs that produce the same effects as the parasympathetic nervous system)
- Corticosteroids
- H2 blockers
- PPIs.

Procedure

- The nostril and throat are numbed with a topical anaesthetic while the patient is in a sitting position.
- A thin flexible catheter, about 4 mm in diameter, is passed through the nostril, into the oesophagus and the stomach, while the patient swallows water. The tube has holes in it that sense pressure along the oesophagus. It will be positioned so that the pressure sensors cover the entire length of the oesophagus.
- The patient lies in a comfortable position.
- Pressure recordings are made over a period at different timed intervals while the patient takes sips of water.
- The catheter is removed at the end of the investigation.
- The procedure takes about 45 min.

Further reading

Bodger K and Trudgill N (2006). Guidelines for oesophageal manometry and PH monitoring. *BSG Guidelines in Gastroenterology*.

Scintigraphy

Scintigraphy is also termed radionuclide imaging or nuclear medicine studies. A low-dose radioactive chemical is given orally or intravenously and a gamma camera is used to create two-dimensional images or the pick up of this chemical.

Indications

- White cell scan—to look for inflammation or abscesses.
- Hepatobiliary iminodiacetic acid (HIDA) scan—to examine hepatic excretory and gall bladder functions. Might be used to delineate bile leaks or congenital anomalies in infants with jaundice.
- Positron emission tomography (PET) (or PET/CT) scan—excludes the spread of tumours to distant sites if major surgery is being considered. Can identify small areas of recurrence, if these cannot be identified by other imaging techniques.

Risks

- Similar to X-rays (➲ p. 230).

Preparation

- It is usual to be nil by mouth but length of time varies in different units.
- Some medications need to be stopped prior to the test.

Procedure

- The test can involve putting a small amount of radiotracer into a meal, such as milk or porridge, or giving the radiotracer intravenously.
- Images are taken at intervals over a 1–4 h period, depending upon the test.

Aftercare

The nurse needs to explain the minimal risks of excretion of the radioactive material in the faeces and/or urine.

Ultrasound—abdominal

An abdominal ultrasound uses high-frequency sound waves, in a similar way to radar, to map out different tissue interfaces and display the information in a two-dimensional real-time image that represents the internal tissues of the body. Some detail can be lost because parts of the bowel containing gas obstruct the view of deeper structures. Ultrasound is best used to examine solid or fluid-containing organs of the abdomen, such as for detecting gallstones. Although loops of bowel can make examining the abdomen and pelvis difficult, good detail of the bowel wall makes it possible to identify bowel inflammation in colitis, thickened bowel loops suggestive of inflammatory bowel disease, diverticulitis, or inflammatory conditions of the small bowel.

Indications

- Abdominal pain
- Liver enzyme levels
- Jaundice
- Hepatomegaly
- Symptoms of biliary tract pathology
- Renal insufficiency
- Abdominal masses
- Suspected abdominal sepsis
- IBD.

Relative contraindications

- Multiple abdominal dressings/stoma bags make access to the abdominal wall difficult.
- Pancreatic imaging may be poor because of overlying bone and gas.

Preparation

- Patients should be nil by mouth for 4 h before the examination.

Procedure

- The test involves the use of a handheld probe on the abdominal wall with lubricating gel and a screen to see images.
- The procedure usually is less than 30 min.

Ultrasound—endoanal

An endoanal ultrasound uses high-frequency sound waves, in a similar way to radar, to map out different tissue interfaces and display the information in a two-dimensional real-time image that represents the internal tissues of the body.

Indications
- Faecal incontinence (also require anorectal manometry)
- Obstetric injury
- Anal sphincter defect.

Procedure
- A probe is placed into the anal canal.
- The patient is usually scanned in the left lateral position; although the prone position may also be used.
- The probe is inserted into the anal canal up to approximately 6 cm and then gently withdrawn down the anal canal, during which cross-sectional images of external anal sphincter and internal anal sphincter can be acquired.

Virtual colonoscopy

Virtual colonoscopy (VC), also known as CT colonography, is a CT scan
(➔ p. 220) of the lining of the large bowel.

Indications

Suspected colorectal cancer, such as when an obstructing cancer cannot
be traversed at colonoscopy (➔ p. 246–7) but a biopsy is not possible
Colonic polyps.

Contraindications

Previous surgery that has left an oversewn rectal stump or mucous
fistula
The presence of IBD is a relative contraindication owing to the
increased risk of perforation, particularly in active disease.

Risk

As per X-rays—abdominal (➔ p. 230).

Preparation

Varies between units but includes:
A special diet
Laxative to empty the bowel.

Procedure

The patient lies on the CT scanner table in the left lateral position.
A soft thin rectal catheter is inserted.
Carbon dioxide is introduced by a pressure-controlled pump to
insufflate the colon.
An antispasmodic may be given.
Two scans are acquired: supine and prone.
The average time for the procedure is approximately 20 min.

Complications

Perforation is a rare complication; the incidence is significantly less than
that reported in conventional colonoscopy.

X-ray—abdominal

A plain abdominal X-ray is non-invasive and helps shows an overview of the bony and soft tissue structures in the abdomen and can show gas within an obstructed or diseased bowel.

Indications

- Suspected bowel obstruction and abdominal distension accompanied by nausea and vomiting with decreased bowel output
- Assessment of the extent of disease in acute colitis.

Risk

- Imaging with X-rays involves exposing a part of the body to a small dose of ionizing radiation, giving a small risk of cancer.
- There are potential risks to the foetus of pregnant women.

Procedure

- The patient may be asked to stand or lie still for a few seconds.
- An average time for the procedure is approximately 15 min.

X-ray—transit

A transit X-ray is used to assess the whole gut transit time; it is simple to perform and cost-effective. The radio-opaque marker test, which usually uses plastic shapes enclosed in a capsule, is the most widely used. However, this technique produces radiation exposure and requires good compliance by the patient.

Indications
• Assess gut transit time.

Risks
• As per X-rays (⟶ p. 230).

Preparation
Laxatives and suppositories are to be stopped from day 1 of taking a capsule until after the X-ray has been taken. Normal diet can be continued.

Procedure
Methods may vary between units.
• The procedure can include ingestion of single/multiple capsules.
• Followed by several abdominal X-rays or a single abdominal X-ray several days or a week later.

Aftercare
The nurse can advise on resuming laxatives after the X-rays have been completed.

Chapter 11

Endoscopy

Pre-assessment/admission

Patients undergo an assessment prior to any endoscopy procedure which includes the following. A consensus document proposes that pre-procedural checklists should be used, and all aspects of care throughout the procedure, including any changes in health status, must be documented and reported to the endoscopist.

- A full, relevant history is taken, and any significant findings communicated to the endoscopist.
- Ensure that the preparation and fasting instructions are followed.
- If the patient has diabetes, check their blood sugar level at admission.
- History of cardiac problems, especially endocarditis or heart valve replacement.
- Medication usage—particularly oral anticoagulants, iron supplements, and any drugs that could affect/interact with the sedation used during the endoscopic procedure.
- Informed consent—obtained by the admitting nurse as per strict procedural guidelines.
- Insertion of a flexible intravenous (IV) cannula for access and administration of sedatives, pain relief, and antispasmodic agents.
- Check whether the patient has loose or broken teeth or dentures before upper gastrointestinal (GI) procedures.
- The patient should be wearing the correct identification bracelet.
- Informed consent must be obtained by the endoscopist.

Consent

Consent is a legal and ethical standard that must be obtained before starting any treatment or physical investigation. This principle reflects the right of patients to determine what happens to their bodies and is a fundamental part of good practice.

Consent should be obtained by the endoscopist or delegated to a suitably trained individual, such as a nurse. The formal consent process should be completed before entry into the procedure room. Final validation of that process should occur before the procedure starts.

Capacity for consent

The UK guidelines around law on mental capacity advise that every adult patient has the capacity to make decisions about their care and treatment and to agree or disagree to any planned investigation/intervention.

A person lacks capacity if there is an impairment or disturbance (e.g. a disability, condition, or trauma, or the effect of drugs or alcohol) that affects the way the mind or brain works. As a result, this means that the individual is unable to make a specific decision at the time it needs to be made.

Emergency endoscopy consent

In an emergency, full compliance with written consent may not be possible. In such circumstances, it is recommended that verbal consent is used but must be fully documented in the medical notes.

Where written or verbal consent cannot be obtained in an emergency, it is recommended that the investigation/intervention taken must be the least restricting of the patient's future options.

Further reading

https://www.bsg.org.uk/resource/obtaining-valid-consent-for-gastrointestinal-endoscopy-procedures.html (Accessed 09/04/2019).

Endoscopic procedures

- A minimum of two endoscopy assistants (one of whom must be a registered nurse) must be present during all endoscopic procedures:
  - One assistant to monitor the patient's condition
  - One assistant to aid the endoscopist with practical aspects.
- Correctly position the patient on the trolley (on their left-hand side) for insertion of the endoscope.

The following recommendations are for sedated or high-risk unsedated patients:

- Administration of oxygen through nasal cannula throughout the procedure
- Monitoring oxygen saturation and the pulse rate throughout the procedure
- Additional blood pressure and electrocardiogram measurements might be required.

Recovery/post-procedure care:

- Continuously monitor patient observations until fully alert.
- Record and manage any adverse events or complications.
- Provide the patient with specific discharge instructions and emergency contact details in case of complications.
- Consultations with sedated patients should take place in the presence of a relative because of possible amnesia from sedation.
- Check follow-up appointment or management has been arranged.
- Ensure a responsible adult is available to accompany the patient home, if they have undergone sedation.
- Provide the patient with relevant information regarding the procedure and instruct sedated patients not to drive or take any responsible action on that day.
- Remove the IV cannula and check for swelling or erythema—apply an appropriate dressing to the site.

The recovery process can apply to most procedures; however there may be additional factors required in specific procedures, which will be included under the individual heading.

Further reading

https://www.bsg.org.uk/clinical-resource/guideline-for-obtaining-valid-consent-for-gastrointestinal-endoscopy-procedures/ (Accessed 10/07/2020).

Sedation and anaesthesia in endoscopy

In the endoscopy setting, sedation and anaesthesia play an integral role in relieving anxiety, reducing pain, and providing amnesia. Sedation techniques have the potential to render uncomfortable diagnostic and therapeutic procedures more acceptable for patients. However, it is not without risk, and therefore should be discussed with the patient before obtaining informed consent for the procedure.

Conscious sedation

Most procedures in endoscopy are performed under 'conscious sedation', which is a drug-induced depression of consciousness during which patients can cooperate and participate by responding to verbal or tactile stimulation, and cardiorespiratory function remains intact. Generally, a benzodiazepine is titrated to the patient's response level, and is considered a safe target state because ventilation and cardiovascular function is maintained. The drug of choice is midazolam, mainly because of its rapid onset and short duration of action.

Often in colonoscopy, because of looping and stretching the bowel, an analgesic is also intravenously administered concomitantly with sedation. A small dose of an opioid, e.g. pethidine or fentanyl, is administered before sedation.

Contraindications

- Known benzodiazepine sensitivity
- Previous history of complications with sedation
- Patients with respiratory insufficiency or other multiple comorbidity.

Monitoring the sedated patient

Once the patient is sedated, the endoscopist undertakes the procedure and an assistant monitors the patient. The British Society of Gastroenterology (BSG) guidelines state that all patients requiring sedation must have an IV access cannula in place throughout the procedure. This enables rapid administration of further sedation or, indeed, reversal drugs. The patient should also have continual administration of oxygen and pulse oximetry monitoring. Because both benzodiazepines and opiates can cause respiratory depression, careful monitoring of the patient's respiration rate and oxygen saturation are required.

Local anaesthetic

Lidocaine is an effective local anaesthetic agent which can be used in the following three ways:

- A subcutaneous injection before surgical incision and insertion of a percutaneous endoscopic gastrostomy (PEG) tube into the stomach.
- It is most commonly used in endoscopy as an anaesthetic throat spray before gastroscopy: 10 mg/spray, maximum dose 20 sprays. The patients are given three to eight sprays at the back of the throat and then asked to swallow. This helps block the gag reflex and ease the passage of the scope. The risks are minimal, but the patient must be advised to refrain from taking hot drinks until the spray has worn off (about 30 min). The administration of local anaesthesia will depend on local policy.
- A topical agent, such as lidocaine gel, in painful perianal disease, e.g. an anal fissure (⊃ p. 120–1) can cause severe pain and anal sphincter spasm, possibly preventing the insertion of the colonoscope.

General anaesthetic

This option is rarely used, because it carries an increased risk of medical and mechanical complications. One example of this is the patient will not be able to move on request and therefore must be moved by staff throughout the procedure.

Further reading

https://www.asge.org/home/guidelines (Accessed 10/07/2020).
http://www.aomrc.org.uk/wp-content/uploads/2016/05/Safe_Sedation_Practice_1213.pdf (Accessed 19/03/2019).
https://www.ncbi.nlm.nih.gov/pmc/articles/PMC3558570/ (Accessed 19/03/2019).

Biopsies, aspiration, and handling specimens

The collection of mucosal specimens for examination in the pathology laboratory is an important part of differential diagnosis in the endoscopy department. An experienced assistant who can correctly use the equipment and handle specimens should have sole responsibility for the collection and transfer of the specimens from the clinical environment.

Communication

Important communication points:
- Anatomical location is of major importance for future treatment.
- Establish the equipment requirements, e.g. forceps, a snare (a loop of wire), or a sheathed cytology brush, CLOtest® (urease test strip for *Helicobacter pylori*).
- Appropriately labelled containers with the correct medium for transport must be available.
- Biopsies from different anatomical sites must be submitted in separately labelled containers and placed in a plastic bag with a pathology request form and adequate information regarding the patient's demographic details and presenting symptoms.
- Check that the patient's demographic details are correct on the container and request form before removing them from the clinical environment.

Procedure for taking specimens

Personal/universal protective equipment must be worn at all times.

Forceps
- Pass the forceps to the endoscopist, who will pass them down the biopsy channel of the endoscope or laparoscope under direct visualization.
- When the forceps are in contact with the mucosa, the assistant will open and close the forceps on the instruction of the clinician.
- The forceps are then removed from the biopsy channel in the closed position, while the assistant holds a gauze swab over the opening to prevent spillage of gastric contents.
- The specimen is extracted and handled as indicated below.

Polypectomy

Snare

As for the forceps procedure.
- On visualization, the endoscopist will ask for the snare to be opened, placed over the polypoid area and closed to the predetermined mark.
- The polyp can be removed, as described above (as per forceps removal), and the polyp retrieved using suction into a polyp trap attached to the suction port, appropriate retrieval forceps, or a snare (on removal of the scope).
- The specimen should be handled as indicated in the next section.

Specimen handling

• Biopsies should be extracted gently from the forceps, with a blunt needle, onto a piece of filter paper which is shaped at one end to differentiate the proximal and distal anatomical orientations—check with your local pathology laboratory for their preference.
• Multiple samples from similar anatomical areas can be placed on one sheet of paper but place them centrally to enable accurate orientation in the histology laboratory—check with your local pathology laboratory for their preference.
• All the patient's specimen samples should be placed in correctly labelled containers before commencing another patient's samples.
• Place the containers in an appropriate plastic bag, with the appropriate documentation, for transportation.

Cytology

Cytology specimens can be taken if a biopsy is contraindicated, e.g. anticoagulation therapy, or cannot be obtained.

Procedure

• Place a sleeved disposable brush down the biopsy channel.
• On direct visualization and instruction by the clinician, open the brush to enable the head to extend out of the plastic sheath.
• The clinician will brush the surface mucosa and then request that the brush be withdrawn back into the sheath.
• The sheath is then withdrawn from the scope.
• The brush is extended and brushed against two or three glass slides, which are fixed immediately with liquid fixer to prevent the cells drying, causing damage to the specimen.
• Each glass slide should be labelled with the patient's demographic details and placed in an appropriate slide box for transportation with the correct documentation.
• Alternatively, some clinical areas cut the brush off at the sheath using sterile scissors and place it straight into a specimen pot containing formalin solution.
• All the patient's specimen samples should be placed in correctly labelled containers (pots or slides) before commencing work on another patient's samples.
• Place the containers in an appropriate plastic bag, with the appropriate documentation, for transportation.

Disposal of single-use equipment

All the equipment used for collecting specimens should be single use if possible.

• Used blunt-ended needles and forceps should be treated as sharps and disposed of in the correct bins provided.
• Reusable forceps should be cleaned and sterilized according to the national guidelines—decontamination of all reusable equipment should be tracked. Single-use items also have tracking labels, and these should be placed in the patient's notes.

Management of cleaning and disinfection

The following procedures and protocols should be followed to ensure maximum safety is attained:

- Trained personnel only
- Appropriate immunization/assessment by the occupational health department
- Appropriate protective clothing—single-use nitrile gloves, long-sleeved waterproof gowns, and goggles/face visor
- Dedicated washing area
- Automated machine—compatible with HTM2030 guidance
- Extraction facilities
- Comprehensive documentation to track scope disinfection and validation available—ongoing review of the traceability of scope accessories that are not decontaminated with the scope.
- Disinfection exposure no more than 3 h before use—check the risk assessment guidance of your local trust
- Health and Safety Executive (HSE)-approved vapour mask and spillage kit for emergencies—check the guidance of your local trust
- Compliance with Health and Safety at Work Act 1974 and the Control of Substances Hazardous to Health (COSHH) Regulations 1994
- All the substances used in the decontamination of medical devices must have a risk assessment by COSHH.

Management of the process

The *MDA Device Bulletin* includes information regarding compatible processes recommended by the device manufacturers and can be used as a source of reference for all departments.

Ensure decontamination of the instrument before service or repair. All equipment should be decontaminated if possible, unless the insertion tube is leaking (socially clean manual cleaning is required before sending an endoscope for repair). A decontamination certificate must accompany the equipment (e.g. MHRA DB 2003).

Single-use items must clearly display the International Organization for Standardization (ISO) symbol (Fig. 11.1), with a diagonal line drawn through it.

Store the scopes in a room separate from the reprocessing area; hang the instruments vertically in a dry well-ventilated cupboard.

Fig. 11.1 ISO symbol for single-use items.
Reproduced with kind permission © Burdett Institute 2008.

Further reading

www.bsg.org.uk/resource/guidance-on-decontamination-of-equipment-for-gastrointestinal-endoscopy-2017-edition.html (Accessed online 09/04/2019).

Cleaning and disinfection of endoscopes

Transmission of infection

A guiding principle for decontamination is that of standard precautions—any patient must be considered a potential infection risk and each endoscope and device must be reprocessed with the same rigour following every endoscopic procedure. Few data exist as to the absolute risk of transmission of infection from patient to patient at endoscopy. Additionally, infections complicating endoscopy may commence only after the patient has been discharged home, following their procedure. Because of the complexity of these reusable instruments, decontamination must strictly adhere to local and national guidelines.

Limited data are available regarding the absolute risk of transmission. However, transmission of infection at endoscopy can be associated with the following:
- Onset following discharge
- Endoscopic retrograde cholangiopancreatography (ERCP) (➲ p. 254–5)—septicaemia could be due to endogenous infection, rather than endoscopically induced infection
- Endoscopically induced infection is usually caused by procedural errors in decontamination:
  - Use of old scopes—more likely to have associated channel and surface irregularities
  - Inadequately designed or poorly maintained automatic endoscope reprocessors
  - Substandard disinfection
  - Inadequate drying and storage.
  Transmission of viral infection occurs for the following reasons:
- Failure to brush the biopsy channel
- Failure to sterilize reusable biopsy forceps ultrasonically or with steam
- Inadequate chemical exposure

Types of micro-organism are associated with endoscopy:
- Mycobacteria
- Bacterial spores—*Bacillus* and *Clostridium*
- Multi drug resistant gram-negative bacilli
- Pathological prions, including Creutzfeldt–Jakob disease (CJD) and vCJD.

Further reading

www.bsg.org.uk/resource/guidance-on-decontamination-of-equipment-for-gastrointestinal-endoscopy-2017-edition.html (Accessed online 09/04/2019).

https://assets.publishing.service.gov.uk/government/uploads/system/uploads/attachment_data/file/372220/Endoscope_decontramination.pdf (Accessed online 09/04/2019).

https://www.gov.uk/government/collections/decontamination-and-infection-control (Accessed online 09/04/2019).

Decontamination

If the endoscope is correctly decontaminated and it is assumed that all patients are potentially infectious, there is no need to schedule patients with known infections at the end of an endoscopy list. However, a prevailing infection control policy should be in place and often includes scheduling patients who are known to have methicillin-resistant *Staphylococcus aureus* (MRSA) at the end of the endoscopy session list.

Endoscopes are routinely exposed to mucus and other gastrointestinal secretions, blood, saliva, faeces, bile, and sometimes pus. The process of decontamination comprises two key components with a number of stages:

• Manual cleaning—including a pre-cleaning routine in the procedure room before the endoscope is disconnected from its stacking system. This is followed by a manual cleaning process in a dedicated decontamination facility, which includes brushing of all accessible channels with a purpose-built single-use cleaning device and exposure of all external and accessible internal components to a low-foaming medical grade detergent known to be compatible with the endoscope.

• Automated disinfection, followed by rinsing of internal and external surfaces and drying of all exposed surfaces of the endoscope.

Table 11.1 Stages of reprocessing (BSG Guidelines 2016)

Stage	Why
Bedside procedure (pre-clean)	To remove readily detachable organic matter. This will help to reduce the possibility of drying and causing channel blockages, especially if there is a delay before manual cleaning takes place
Leak test	To ensure the integrity of the endoscope. Any damage to the outer surface could allow body fluids or chemicals into the internal workings of the endoscope
Manual clean	Brushing of accessible channels and flushing of all channels to remove organic matter. This stage will also allow the detection of channel blockages
Rinsing	To remove detergent residues that may affect the performance of the disinfectant
Drying	To expel excess fluid that may dilute the disinfectant
Disinfection	To eradicate potentially pathogenic microorganisms, i.e. bacteria, including mycobacteria and viruses
Rinsing	To remove disinfectant residues that could cause a harmful effect to the patient
Drying	To expel excess fluid before use on the patient or storage

Further reading

www.bsg.org.uk/resource/guidance-on-decontamination-of-equipment-for-gastrointestinal-endoscopy-2017-edition.html (Accessed 09/04/2019).

https://assets.publishing.service.gov.uk/government/uploads/system/uploads/attachment_data/file/372220/Endoscope_decontramination.pdf (Accessed 09/04/2019).

https://www.gov.uk/government/collections/decontamination-and-infection-control (Accessed 09/04/2019).

Capsule endoscopy

Capsule endoscopy is an endoscopic procedure used to record images of the GI tract for use in medical diagnosis. The capsule is similar in shape to a standard pharmaceutical capsule, although a little larger, and contains a tiny camera and an array of LEDs (light emitting diodes) powered by a battery.

Indication

The primary use of capsule endoscopy is to examine areas of the small intestine that cannot be seen by other types of endoscopy procedures:
- Bleeding—melaena/haematochezia/obscure GI bleeding
- Polyps
- Ulcers
- Tumours
- Crohn's disease/suspected active disease
- Refractory coeliac disease
- Suspected non-steroidal anti-inflammatory drug (NSAID) p. 406 induced enteropathy
- Small bowel transplantation.

Preparation

This can vary from hospital to hospital; the general consensus is as follows:
- Nil by mouth (NBM) for 12 h
- Bowel preparation to be taken the day before the procedure
- Some medications may need to be stopped.

Procedure

- The capsule is activated once it is removed from the sterile blister pack.
- Capsule is swallowed or it can also be delivered endoscopically.

Complications

- Retention of capsule is possible although the rates are low; on occasion removal may be required
- Perforation
- Aspiration or displacement of the capsule
- Fracture of the capsule (very rare).

Recovery

- Can drink 2 h after swallowing the capsule
- 4 h after swallowing capsule can eat a light diet
- Capsule is generally passed in stool, dependent on bowel frequency
- Connect the data recorder to the workstation to download the data.

Timings for the above may vary according to the individual hospital protocol.

Further reading

https://www.nice.org.uk/guidance/ipg101/chapter/2-The-procedure (Accessed 22/03/2019).

Colonoscopy

A colonoscopy is an endoscopic procedure used to examine the entire large bowel and rectum. The mucosa of the bowel can be visualized directly, and an assessment, biopsy, and diagnosis can be made. To further clarify the findings, a barium enema/CT scan can be performed.

Indications

- Rectal bleeding—which is darker and mixed with the stools
- Change in bowel habits—especially diarrhoea/looser stools
- Iron-deficiency anaemia
- Abdominal pain/mass
- Surveillance for inflammatory bowel disease
- Surveillance for cancer
- Surveillance for polyps
- The procedure can be both diagnostic and therapeutic.

Preparation

Preparation of the bowel is the most important factor in the success of a colonoscopy examination. The bowel lumen must be free of faecal matter to visualize the vascular pattern and mucosal lining.

- Low-residue diet for 2 days before the investigation
- Oral sodium picosulfate is taken in drink form 1 day before the investigation. This induces diarrhoea and facilitates cleaning of the bowel.
- The patient is advised to take only clear liquids during the preparation period
- Patients need to be NBM for 2 h before the procedure if they are to be sedated.
- Preparation may vary in each hospital protocol.

Procedure

The procedure takes 20–30 min and commences with a digital rectal examination. The lubricated colonoscope is then inserted into the rectum and insufflated. The instrument is slowly advanced, under direct visualization, along the colon. If the ileocaecal valve is visualized when the scope reaches the caecum, it can be entered. The appearance of the ileal mucosa differs from that of the large bowel because of the presence of villi, which increases the absorptive surface area of the ileum significantly. The instrument should be withdrawn carefully; note any polyps, lesions, mucosa, and vessels (e.g. angiodysplasia).

Biopsies can be taken of any pathology encountered or inflamed mucosa, which aids diagnosis—note the location and size (in mm).

Complications

- Perforation—1:5000 cases for diagnostic procedure; <1:500 for polypectomy
- Failure to complete the investigation—requiring retesting or further investigations
- Haemorrhage from therapeutic procedures.

Recovery

The patient must stay in recovery for up to 2 h, to be monitored following sedation and any therapeutic procedure. The follow-up plans will then be explained to the patient and their relative/carer; consideration should be given to the effect of the sedative on the patient.

Double balloon enteroscopy

Double balloon enteroscopy (DBE) is an endoscopic procedure used to examine the small bowel through the use of two balloons. One balloon is attached to the distal end of the scope and the other is attached to a transparent tube sliding over the endoscope.

Indications
- Small bowel bleeding
- Pathologies of the upper and lower GI system that doctors may suspect originate from the small bowel.

Preparation
- Colonoscopy preparation applies; can depend on local protocols.

Procedure

When inflated with air, the balloons can grip sections of the small bowel and 'shorten' the small bowel by pleating it over the endoscope. Sequential shortening of the small bowel over the endoscope and advancement of the endoscope enables a comprehensive examination of the entire small bowel. The procedure can be performed via the upper GI tract (antegrade) or through the lower GI tract (retrograde).

Complications
- Related to colonoscopy
- Rare instances of mild pancreatitis or ileus (less than 1%) have been reported.

Recovery
- As per general recovery/post-procedure care (➲ p. 236). Can depend on type of sedation given.

Flexible sigmoidoscopy

A flexible sigmoidoscopy is an endoscopic procedure to examine the left side of the colon from the rectum to the splenic flexure using a flexible endoscope. The lining of the bowel can be visualized directly. An assessment, biopsy, and diagnosis can be made and treatment can be performed as necessary.

Indications

- Outlet-type rectal bleeding—bright red and not mixed with the stool
- Localized lower-left quadrant pain
- To further examine/clarify the results, a barium enema/CT scan of the left side of the colon can be performed.

Preparation

If sedation is required, the patient should refrain from eating and drinking 2 h before the procedure. An enema is administered at least 1 h before the procedure, to clean the descending colon, sigmoid, and rectum.

Procedure

- The procedure takes 5–20 min and commences with a digital rectal examination.
- The lubricated sigmoidoscope/colonoscope is inserted into the anus under direct vision and the rectum is insufflated.
- The endoscopist slowly withdraws the scope, if required, so that the lumen of the rectum is in full view.
- The instrument is slowly advanced, under direct visualization, up to the splenic flexure. In the sigmoid colon the circular haustral folds will be visible. Careful examination is required to ensure that no polyps or lesions are missed.
- Once through, the triangular haustral folds of the transverse colon are visible and the insertion is complete.
- Careful withdrawal of the scope is required, while noting any abnormal mucosal polyps, lesions, or vessels, such as angiodysplasias.

Biopsies can be taken of any pathology encountered or inflamed mucosa, which aids diagnosis—note the location and size (in mm).

Complications

- Perforation—1:5000 cases for diagnostic procedure; <1:500 for polypectomy.
- Failure to complete the investigation—requiring retesting or further investigations.
- Haemorrhage from therapeutic procedures.

Recovery

If the patient is not sedated, they can be discharged as soon all relevant documentation and post-procedure assessment is completed. The follow-up plans should be explained to the patient before discharge.

Oesophageal gastroduodenoscopy

Oesophageal gastroduodenoscopy (OGD) is an endoscopic procedure where an endoscope is used to look inside the oesophagus, stomach, and duodenum.

Indications for an OGD

Diagnostic:

- Dyspepsia (➲ p. 22–3)—reflux or *H. pylori*
- Haematemesis (➲ p. 43)
- Dysphagia (➲ p. 24)
- Upper GI malignancy
- Peptic ulcer (➲ p. 30–1)
- Coeliac disease (➲ p. 64–5)
- Post gastrectomy
- Familial adenomatous polyposis (➲ p. 92–3)—will require long-term surveillance
- Barrett's oesophagus (➲ p. 19)—will require long-term surveillance
- Ingested foreign body (➲ p. 264–5)
- Vomiting.

Therapeutic indications

- Treatment of oesophageal varices (➲ p. 443)
- Placement of feeding tube—percutaneous endoscopic gastrostomy (PEG)
- Removal of foreign bodies
- Treatment of oesophageal malignancies—dilating/stenting, laser
- Dilatation of stricture.

Complications

- Significant bleeding is a very rare complication of diagnostic upper GI endoscopy
- Perforation is uncommon—about 0.03%
- Mortality is rare—about 0.001%.

Contraindications

- Known or suspected gastrointestinal perforation
- Lack of informed consent
- Unstable cardiac patient
- Uncorrected coagulopathy
- Airway protection—GI bleed if semi-conscious and not intubated
- Food taken with 4 h of procedure
- Known achalasia (➲ p. 18) and not fasted for 24 h
- Lack of trained personnel to perform and support the procedure
- High oesophageal obstruction.

Recovery

As per general recovery; may change depending on whether sedation has been used.

Further reading

British Society of Gastroenterology. Endoscopy Guidance https://www.bsg.org.uk/clinical-resources/endoscopy/endoscopy-guidance/ (Accessed 10/07/2020).

Colonic stents

Colonic stenting is a therapeutic endoscopic procedure and is a management option for acute large bowel obstruction. Colonic stents are associated with lower mortality and morbidity compared to emergency surgery in cases of acute suspected malignant large bowel obstruction. However, current evidence does not recommend use of colonic stent as a bridge until surgery in these cases, but it is a preferred treatment to relieve obstruction in palliative settings.

Types of stent

Originally, oesophageal stents were used, but now custom-designed colonic stents are available. Various types are available.

- Self-expanding metal stents—most commonly used
- Plastic—migrate easily and can occlude the colonic lumen.
- Rigid—more difficult to place through an obstruction than other types of stent.

Indications

- Acute large bowel obstruction.

Colonic stenting in the acute setting has some definitive advantages compared to emergency surgery. However, the long-term impact of colonic stent insertion requires consideration in relation to oncological outcomes, especially in cases of curable and resectable cancers at presentation.

Preparation

Preparation is not usually required.

Procedure

It is also unusual to sedate the patient; most need no analgesia during stent placement. Most stents are placed under fluoroscopic control; they are deployed over a guidewire. The stent expands during the 48 h following the procedure.

Complications

- The mortality rate is 2%—lower than that of emergency surgery (20%)
- The risk of perforation is 3%—potentially fatal and more common following balloon dilatation of a stricture
- Failure to deploy stent—rates of 0–30% have been reported
- Migration (up to 4 weeks later)—re-stenting is often required
- Bleeding—minor bleeding owing to mucosal pressure is common
- Faecal impaction
- Occlusion (all types but plastic most likely)
- Re-obstruction—tumour in-growth of 25% over time
- No evidence of the promotion of tumour growth or spread—local or metastases
- It is easier to place stents in a more distal (lower) position in the colon, but these are more likely to be dislodged and/or cause symptoms, e.g. discomfort, tenesmus, bleeding, or faecal incontinence (⊃ p. 448–9).

Recovery

- Monitor blood pressure, temperature, and pain—possible perforation or bleeding.
- Expect some abdominal discomfort—mild analgesics or antispasmodics.
- The patient could have repeated bowel actions as the colon decompresses—ensure toilet access for frail patients.
- Stool softeners are used to keep the stent patent—loose or liquid stool might be needed to prevent blockage (but watch for faecal incontinence).
- Give patient/carer education to watch for complications.

Further reading

www.ncbi.nlm.nih.gov/pmc/articles/PMC4766252/pdf/WJGE-8-198.pdf (Accessed 09/04/2019).
https://www.nice.org.uk/guidance/cg131/evidence/full-guideline-pdf-183509680 (Accessed 09/04/2019).

Endoscopic retrograde cholangiopancreatography

Endoscopic retrograde cholangiopancreatography (ERCP) is a technique that combines the use of endoscopy and fluoroscopy to diagnose and treat certain problems of the biliary or pancreatic ductal systems.

Indications

Diagnostic procedure

- Chronic pancreatitis (➔ p. 184–5)
- Obstructive jaundice—this may be due to several causes
- Gallstones (➔ p. 198–9) with dilated bile ducts on ultrasonography
- Indeterminate biliary strictures and suspected bile duct tumours
- Suspected injury to bile ducts either as a result of trauma or of iatrogenic origin
- Sphincter of Oddi dysfunction.

Therapeutic procedure

- Endoscopic sphincterotomy (of the biliary or the pancreatic duct sphincter)
- Removal of stones or other biliary debris
- Insertion of bile duct stent(s)
- Dilatation of strictures, e.g. primary sclerosing cholangitis (➔ p. 200), anastomotic strictures after liver transplantation.

Preparation

Preparation for an ERCP is NBM for 6 h.

Procedure

An endoscope is passed through the mouth to the oesophagus, stomach, and into the duodenum. The opening where the bile and pancreatic ducts empty into the duodenum is located.

A flexible catheter is passed through the endoscope and into the ducts where contrast is injected to make the ducts more visible on X-ray. The ducts are examined for narrowed areas and/or blockages. Biopsies may be taken, stones removed, and stents inserted if required.

Complications

- Pancreatitis (➔ p. 182)
- Infection of the bile ducts or gallbladder
- Haemorrhage
- Perforation in the bile/pancreatic ducts.

Recovery

As per general recovery/post-procedure care (→ p. 236) with the addition of the following:

- Stay in recovery depends on sedation
- Bloating and/or nausea may occur
- Sore throat may last for 1–2 days.

Further reading

https://www.niddk.nih.gov/health-information/diagnostic-tests/endoscopic-retrograde-cholangiopancreatography (Accessed online 22/03/2019).

Szary NM and Al-Kawas FH (2013). Complications of endoscopic retrograde cholangiopancreatography: how to avoid and manage them. *Gastroenterology and Hepatology* 9(8): 496–504.

Endoscopic retrograde cholangiopancreatography: biliary duct dilatation

ERCP (➲ p. 254–5) can be used as a therapeutic endoscopic procedure to dilate the biliary duct.

Indications

- Fibrosis after treatment for sclerosing cholangitis
- Malignant strictures.

Preparation

Preparation for an ERCP is NBM for 6 h.

Procedure

The equipment required for ERCP dilatation is:

- Rigid stepped dilators: 5 Fr, 7 Fr, or 9 Fr gauge stepped
- Standard guidewire
- Balloon catheters.

Balloon catheters need to be:

- 4–10 mm in diameter when inflated
- 2–5 cm in length
- 5 Fr or 7 Fr gauge
- Radio-opaque marks.

The procedure is as per ERCP and sphincterotomy (➲ p. 262–3) with the following additional procedures:

- Pass the guidewire into the common bile duct (CBD) (➲ p. 15).
- The balloon is inserted over the guidewire—flush the internal catheter with saline before handing it to the endoscopist.
- Inflate the balloon to the predetermined pressure.
- Monitor under fluoroscopy for 'waist' (dilatation of stricture) disappearance.
- The procedure is painful—limit the dilatation time to no more than 10–20 seconds.
- Rigid dilatation, as above.
- Gently insert the catheter up to the maximum gauge of the dilator, using imaging as a guide.

Recovery

During the procedure—observe the patient for pain and signs of perforation of the duct on imaging.

Post-procedure as per ERCP (➲ p. 255).

Further reading

http://www.spg.pt/wp-content/uploads/2015/07/2017-Updated-guideline-on-the-management-of-common-bile-duct-stones-CBDS.pdf (Accessed online 07/04/2019).

Endoscopic retrograde cholangiopancreatography: biliary stent placement

Biliary stenting is a therapeutic endoscopic procedure to place a stent into a biliary stricture.

Indications
- Gallstones—in the gall bladder or within the bile ducts
- Pancreatitis (➔ p. 182)
- Sclerosing cholangitis (➔ p. 200)
- Pancreatic cancer (➔ p. 188–90)
- Gallbladder cancer (➔ p. 194)
- Bile duct cancer
- Liver cancer (➔ p. 172–3)
- Enlarged lymph nodes in the region of the pancreas and liver due to various types of tumour
- Injury to bile ducts during surgery
- Infection
- The stent is placed after sphincterotomy, ± stone extraction to aid duct drainage.

Preparation
As per ERCP (➔ p. 254) using radiological identification of the stricture through cannulation of the duct and injection of radio-opaque contrast.

Procedure
Equipment
Types of stents may vary according to individual hospital protocols:
- A large-channel duodenoscope—4.2 mm for 10/12 Fr stent. (3.2/2.8 mm scope for 7 Fr stent only)
- Guidewire—a hydrophilic-coated wire is suggested, which is 400–480 cm in length, with an atraumatic tip
- A stent introducer set
- Various sized stents or a single-action set
- Prime the guidewire and stent catheter using saline.

The procedure is as per ERCP (➔ p. 254) plus:
- Introduce the wire down the accessory channel, maintaining fluoroscopic visualization to aid advancement of the wire and stent placement.
- The stent introduction set is mounted over the guidewire—the assistant maintains gentle traction.
- The equipment is held straight to aid process.
- Continue traction to prevent looping of the wire in the duodenum as the stent introducer enters the bile duct.
- Fluoroscopic checks are used to monitor the placement of the guidewire.
- The catheter is guided over the obstruction and the stent is positioned.
- Maintain gentle traction.

- The guidewire is removed at this point for injection of contrast medium and observation of bile drainage.
- Metal expanding stents are placed as outlined in the first two steps.
- Follow the individual manufacturer's guidance.

Change stent: if blocked or life expectancy expired
- Insert a standard catheter into the stent tip, inject the contrast medium, and check the position of the stent.
- Flush the catheter with saline.
- Introduce the guidewire down the catheter.
- Pass a Soehendra stent retriever over the wire.
- Screw the end into the stent—turning clockwise.
- Once secure, the endoscopist pulls the stent back into the duodenum, while the assistant pushes gently on the guidewire to maintain the position.
- The stent is either removed or left to pass through the gut.
- Normal stenting procedure for replacement.

Stent removal
- The stent is removed by a snare, Dormier basket, or grasping forceps used with a scope.

Complications
As per ERCP (➲ p. 254).

Recovery
As per ERCP (➲ p. 254).

Further reading
https://www.bsir.org/patients/biliary-drainage-and-stenting/ (Accessed 29/03/2019).
https://www.cochranelibrary.com/cdsr/doi/10.1002/14651858.CD004200.pub2/epdf/full (Accessed 29/03/2019).

Endoscopic retrograde cholangiopancreatography: biliary stone extraction

Removal of biliary stones from the CBD using ERCP (➔ p. 254–5) is a therapeutic endoscopic procedure. Biliary stones may pass spontaneously after a sphincterotomy if they are 10 mm or smaller. The procedure can be undertaken either using a balloon or a basket technique.

Indications
- Biliary stones.

Preparation
Patient preparation is as per ERCP (➔ p. 254).

Equipment
Balloons comprising the following:
- Catheter-tipped—5 Fr or 7 Fr in diameter
- Various balloon sizes—8.5–18 mm in diameter
- Wire-guided balloons are available.

Dormier basket comprising the following:
- A rectangular or spiral wire basket of six or eight wires
- A Luer port for injection of contrast medium
- Some baskets are wire-guided.

Sphincterotomy is often required before stones can be extracted. Check the basket or balloon and prime with contrast medium before insertion.

Procedure
Balloon procedure
- Fluoroscopic guidance should be used throughout the procedure.
- Advance the deflated balloon into the CBD above the stones.
- Inject the contrast medium to establish the position of the stones— prevent trapping air in the catheter, because this can mimic stones on imaging.
- Inflate the balloon while observing the imaging screen—inflate the balloon accordingly.
- The endoscopist will retract the balloon slowly, drawing the stones down the duct.
- Repeat the procedure until the duct is clear.
- A wire-guided balloon can also be used for impacted stones or extraction of multiple stones.
- Place the wire into the duct first and then advance the balloon over the wire.

Basket procedure

Advancement of the basket follows the first three steps above and then the following steps:

- Open the basket in the duct with care not to push the stone further up the duct.
- The endoscopist should pull down to engage the stones—a gentle movement forwards and backwards might be useful.
- The basket should be closed on communication from the endoscopist or before removal of the basket from the duct.

Mechanical lithotripter

Various types of device are available. Extraction of a large stone is performed using the basket method: check the manufacturer's guidelines for the use of particular accessory baskets.

The following procedure with relevant equipment should be followed:

- Use a large-channel scope.
- Use fluoroscopic imaging throughout the procedure.
- Sphincterotomy.
- The metal sheath of the lithotripter is passed over the plastic catheter of the basket according to the manufacturer's guidance.
- Attach a torque handle.
- Close the basket slowly using a mechanical torque to crush the stone.
- The basket could break if the stone is hard.
- The procedure should only be undertaken by an experienced team.

Complications

- Bleeding can occur.
- Pancreatitis (● p. 182) occurs in 5–10% of patients undergoing ERCP and is the most common complication. Studies are been done to determine drugs that can help prevent this occurring.
- Perforation can occur due to damage by instruments at the time of investigation.
- Cholangitis (● p. 200) can occur. Antibiotics are given to all patients with suspected bile duct obstruction to prevent infection.

Recovery

As per ERCP (● p. 255).

Further reading

https://www.bsg.org.uk/clinical-resource/updated-guideline-on-the-management-of-common-bile-duct-stones-cbds (Accessed 10/07/2020).

Endoscopic retrograde cholangiopancreatography: sphincterotomy

Sphincterotomy is a therapeutic endoscopic procedure to drain the bile duct or pancreatic duct of stones.

Indications
- Stones in the bile duct
- Stones in the pancreatic duct.

Preparation
As per ERCP (➲ p. 254) with the following additional checks:
- Check whether the patient has a pacemaker or internal metal fittings (e.g. hips or pins)—contact the local cardiology department regarding the suitability of using electrical diathermy with a pacemaker.
- Clotting screening.
- Gain consent for therapeutic intervention.
- Apply the diathermy plate to the patient's thigh.
- Place the patient's hands and arms on the X-ray mattress.

Equipment
- A selection of sphincter tomes
- A selection of guidewires
- Saline flushes—20 ml
- Diathermy.

Procedure
To gain better access to the ampulla and use a therapeutic accessory, a small cut is made in the papilla of Vater to enlarge the opening of the bile duct and/or pancreatic duct. This is done to improve the drainage or to remove stones in the ducts. Removed stones are usually dropped in the intestine and pass through quickly.
- Prime the sphincter tome with saline. Check the bowing of the wire at the tip of the sphincter tome.
- Check the diathermy connections are correct and in working order.
- Visual fluoroscopy is required throughout the procedure.
- The endoscopist cannulates the ampulla or passes over the wire *in situ*.
- The assistant bows the sphincter tome slowly according to the endoscopist's instructions.
- The endoscopist cuts through the ampulla with the wire intermittently and the assistant releases and tightens the handle to bow the wire accordingly.
- If the wire cannot be cut, check that the accessory wire is far enough away from the scope—check on screen that the wire is visible at the ampulla opening (prevents internal injury to the duct on cutting blind).
- Observe for excessive bleeding during the procedure.

Recovery

The post-procedure care required is similar to that for diagnostic ERCP (⊃ p. 255); however, special precautions regarding bleeding must be noted.

Further reading

https://emedicine.medscape.com/article/1829797-overview (Accessed 05/04/2019).

Foreign-body removal from the upper gastrointestinal tract

Removal of a foreign body from the upper GI tract is a therapeutic endoscopic procedure.

Indications

- Ingested foreign body (non-food) from a child, an elderly person, patients with psychiatric disorders, or prisoners (ingested accidentally or to self-harm)
- Patients with oesophageal narrowing may experience food bolus impaction.

Investigation

The European Society of Gastrointestinal Endoscopy (ESGE) does not recommend radiological evaluation for patients with non-bony food bolus impaction without complications.

- Plain X-ray is advocated to assess the presence, location, size, configuration, and number of ingested foreign bodies if ingestion of radiopaque objects is suspected or type of object is unknown.
- CT scan (→ p. 220) in all patients with suspected perforation or other complication that may require surgery.
- Barium swallow (→ p. 218) is not recommended because of the risk of aspiration and worsening of the endoscopic visualization.

Procedure

- The patient should be placed in a left-lateral position—sedation might be required if the patient is agitated.
- During the procedure and recovery phase, monitor vital signs for respiratory distress, perforation, haemorrhage, and pain.
- There is a danger of dropping the object into the pharynx during removal and inhaling.
- Use an overtube (well lubricated) for sharp objects, or if repeated intubation is needed for multiple objects, to protect the oesophagus and prevent dropping objects into the airway. If the object is too large for an overtube, use a hood (e.g. condom).
- The method used depends on the size, shape, location, and material of the foreign body.
- Upper oesophagus—if there are problems with excessive saliva, suction from the mouth and keep the airway clear (antisecretory agents might be needed for good vision). Use a laryngoscope and McGill forceps if they can reach the object. Use a rigid oesophagoscope for sharp objects (e.g. open safety pins) in the upper oesophagus.
- Solid object—Dormier basket or snare.
- Food bolus—break up or use forceps or suction to grasp the bolus. Take care if bones are involved.
- If present at the same time, the stricture can be dilated to prevent recurrence.
- Soft object—break up with the end of the endoscope, biopsy, or use grasping forceps.
- Use magnetic or rubber forceps for sharp metal objects, e.g. needles or nails.

Recovery

- If the foreign body cannot be retrieved endoscopically, in-patient treatment and close clinical observation is mandatory for sharp pointed objects and batteries.
- Radiographic follow-up examinations should be performed to assess the object's passage through the gastrointestinal tract.
- Daily radiographs are recommended for sharp-pointed objects.
- For batteries beyond the duodenum, plain radiography every 3–4 days is adequate.
- Surgery must be considered for removal of dangerous foreign bodies that have passed the ligament of Treitz and fail to progress within 3 days after ingestion

Further reading

https://www.esge.com/assets/downloads/pdfs/guidelines/2016_s_0042_100456.pdf   (Accessed 05/04/2019).

Oesophageal dilatation

Oesophageal dilatation is a therapeutic endoscopic procedure to dilate a stricture in the oesophagus. The first aim of oesophageal dilatation is to alleviate symptoms and improve nutritional intake, in addition to preventing complications, e.g. aspirate pneumonia. Oesophageal dilatation has evolved considerably over the years, in addition to development of a large range of purpose-built dilators.

Indications

- Treatment of symptomatic obstruction—functional or anatomical oesophageal disorders
- Acid reflux (● p. 36)
- Malignancy
- Achalasia (● p. 18)
- Anastomotic stricture
- Corrosive induced stricture
- Sclerotherapy
- Radiation.

Contraindications

- Active perforation
- Recent perforation or upper GI tract surgery
- Pharyngeal or cervical deformity, increased risk
- Thoracic aneurysm (large)
- Severe cardiac disease
- Severe coagulopathy.

Preparation

The procedure is performed by an endoscopist, with two trained endoscopy assistants.

- Fasting for 6 h before the procedure; patients who have known achalasia could require a longer period of fasting.
- Informed consent—identify patients at high risk of perforation ± surgical intervention. Risk of perforation during dilatation 1:260. Risk of death 1%.
- Review oral anticoagulation and antiplatelet agents—document the prothrombin time in the medical/nursing notes.
- Administer antibiotic prophylaxis, according to BSG guidelines, to all at-risk patients.
- Use IV sedation, according to local guidance and the BSG guidelines. It is usual to use opiates + benzodiazapines for dilatation. All patients should be classified according to the American Society of Anesthesiologists (ASA) grade I–V scale of physical status.
- Ensure IV access at all times.
- A qualified nurse should administer supplementary oxygen and monitor pulse oximetry.
- Ensure that relevant X-rays are available with patient.

Procedure

- The initial dilator choice should be based on the known or estimated stricture diameter, length, and the underlying pathology.
- Consider limiting the initial dilatation to 10–12 mm in diameter (corresponding to 30–36F) in cases of very narrow strictures not passable by the adult gastroscope.
- Consider using no more than three successively larger diameter increments in a single session for both bougie and balloon dilators.
- Patients usually need several sessions to achieve resolution of dysphagia and they should be informed of this possibility before the first procedure.
- Use wire-guided (bougie or balloon) or endoscopically controlled (balloon) techniques for all patients to enhance safety.
- Do not use weighted (Maloney) bougies with blind insertion, because safer dilators are available. Perform dilatation without fluoroscopy for simple strictures.
- Use fluoroscopic guidance to enhance safety during dilatation of strictures that are long, angulated, or multiple.

Complications

There is a low, but clearly defined, morbidity and mortality attached to this procedure. Thus it should only be undertaken as a planned procedure with suitably experienced staff.

Recovery

- Monitor patients for at least 2 h in the recovery room and provide clear written instructions with advice on fluids, diet, and medications after the procedure
- Do not perform imaging and contrast studies routinely after the procedure, unless patients—during recovery—develop persistent chest pain, fever, breathlessness, or tachycardia
- Ensure that patients are well and tolerating water on leaving the hospital.

Further reading

https://gut.bmj.com/content/gutjnl/67/6/1000.full.pdf (Accessed 29/03/2019).

Oesophageal self-expanding metal stent

Insertion of an oesophageal self-expanding metal stent is a therapeutic endoscopic procedure to maintain the oesophageal patency of strictures caused by intrinsic or extrinsic malignant tumours.

Indications

It is usually undertaken as a palliative procedure, but it is rarely used in patients with benign disease.

Contraindications

As for endoscopic dilatation (→ p. 266) plus the following:
• An oesophageal fistula of any type, unless it is covered by a stent
• Long-term use for a benign stricture
• A stricture that cannot be dilated to pass the endoscope or delivery system
• Stent placement within 2 cm of the cricopharyngeal muscle
• Known oesophago-jejunostomy
• Necrotic bleeding tumour—active
• Polypoid lesions.

Equipment

The equipment used is similar to that for OGD (→ p. 266) ± various sized rigid/balloon dilators:
• Before insertion of the stent, the stricture should be assessed endoscopically and radiologically—if necessary, it should be dilated to 12 mm in diameter
• Prosthesis—knitted titanium wire
• Stent (product may differ according to each hospital protocol)
• Guidewire—0.035 in, with a floppy tip
• Silicone lubricant
• Radio-opaque markers—if placed using X-rays.

Procedure

Two experienced nurses, in addition to the endoscopist, are needed.
• Patient is positioned in the ERCP semi-prone position.
• Dilate the stricture—if required (→ p. 266).
• Lubricate the biopsy channel using silicone.
• Pass the guidewire down the endoscope, through the stricture.
• Pass the delivery system over the wire.
• Measure the length of the stricture, using the scope markings and place radio-opaque marks externally if joint endoscopy/radiology placement.
• Observe the proximal end of the stricture with the endoscope.
• Position the delivery system in the stricture using the side-marking ruler with measurements obtained from the endoscopic examination.
• Non-covered stent 3–4 cm longer than the stricture; covered stent 5–6 cm to bridge the stricture, once deployed.
• Deploy the stent. Monitor the release of the stent, either endoscopically or fluoroscopically, keeping it within the measured margins.

- For fluoroscopic placement, use radio-opaque markers non-endoscopically through wire-guided technique; check the manufacturer's guidance.
- Remove the guidewire and/or endoscope slowly, once the stent is fully deployed.
- Use the balloon dilatation of the stent to aid expansion. The procedure is similar to that for balloon dilatation. Never use a rigid dilator because it could dislodge the stent.

Complications

This is a complex procedure that carries a high complication rate, as per dilatation (🠚 p. 266).

Recovery

Care as for any endoscopic dilatation (🠚 p. 266), with the following additions:

- Post-anterior and lateral chest film.
- Analgesia 24–48 h post-insertion.
- Clear fluids post-insertion; see local policy.
- The patient should be NBM if the stent is placed for a fistula—healing must be confirmed.
- The patient should eat in an upright position and drink plenty of fluids during the meal.
- Food should be chewed well.
- The patient should eat slowly and have a fizzy drink following the meal.
- Certain foods should be avoided—chunky, stringy, or fibrous foods (e.g. bread, meat, and raw vegetables).
- Distal oesophageal stents could require acid-suppression therapy.

Prior to discharge home, the nurse should provide dietary advice and contact details.

Further reading

Parthipun A, Diamantopoulos A, Shaw A, Dourado R, and Sabharwal T (2014). Self-expanding metal stents in palliative malignant oesophageal dysplasia. *Annals of Palliative Medicine* 3(2): 92–103.
https://www.esge.com/assets/downloads/pdfs/guidelines/2012_clinical_guideline_for_biliary_stenting.pdf (Accessed 22/03/2019).

Oesophageal varices: sclerotherapy or banding

Oesophageal varices can be treated with a therapeutic endoscopic procedure such as endoscopic sclerotherapy (injection into varix causing thrombosis) and band ligation. Treatment aims to reduce variceal wall tension by obliteration of the varix.

Indications

People who have experienced bleeding complications.

Preparation

As per OGD (➔ p. 250).

Equipment

As per OGD (➔ p. 250) plus:
- Resuscitation equipment and cardiovascular monitoring
- Oxygen and suction
- Documented blood results—cross-match available
- Two sclerotherapy retractable needles
- Warmed sclerosant, drawn up into 5 ml syringes
- Several syringes of sterile water
- Spare suction liners.

Procedure

- The patient's head should be slightly raised.
- Prime the needle with the sclerosant—check the needle length (~5 mm; single use).
- Lubricate the biopsy channel—to prevent kinking of the needle.
- Forward and retract needle by answering to 'needle out/in', respectively.
- Communicate the injection volume to endoscopist every 0.5 ml.
- Retract the needle if it is not injecting.
- Remove and dispose of the needle as clinical sharp waste.

Banding

Follow the manufacturer's instructions for loading and firing the band. Several different kits are available, but they have similar components and placement techniques.
- Variceal ligation—the occluding of the variceal vessel
- Oesophageal banding kit—pre-packed sterile kit.

Recovery

- Bed rest—the head of the bed should be elevated unless the patient is compromised.
- Observe for perforation, rebleeding, or subcutaneous emphysema (chest, abdominal, or pleuritic pain, tachycardia, and pyrexia).
- Cardiovascular monitoring (pulse and blood pressure) should be performed every 30 min initially and then every hour.
- Administer oxygen therapy, as required.
- Take the patient's temperature every 4 h.
- Rehydrate the patient intravenously—NBM and mouth care.
- The patient can receive a soft diet and fluids after medical review once haemodynamic and cardiovascular stability is obtained.

Further reading

https://www.ncbi.nlm.nih.gov/pmc/articles/PMC3399010/pdf/WJGE-4-312.pdf (Accessed 29/03/2019).

Percutaneous endoscopic gastrostomy

Percutaneous endoscopic gastrostomy (PEG) is a therapeutic endoscopic procedure to enable insertion of an enteral feeding tube.

Indications

There are a number of indications for the insertion of a PEG including:
• Swallowing problems
• Severe burns
• Head injury.

Preparation

NBM for 6 h.

Procedure

Three assistants plus an endoscopist are required for this procedure. Place the patient on their left-hand side initially; they can be placed on their back once a normal gastric outlet is established during OGD (➐ p. 250). Tube placement is a sterile technique.

Equipment

Ensure that a tube of the appropriate size and the following relevant accessory items are on the dressing trolley:
• Dressing pack
• Gastrostomy kit
• Needles—various
• Syringes—5–10 ml
• Local anaesthetic
• Cleansing fluid
• Dressing or appropriate spray.

Method of insertion

• The endoscope is directed at the anterior wall.
• Transillumination of endoscopic light must be observed by both the endoscopist and the first assistant on the screen and on the abdominal wall, with finger indentation indicating no organ obstruction.
• The position should be marked and the area cleaned with antiseptic cleanser.
• Local anaesthetic is infiltrated into the skin, subcutaneously, the fascia, and the gastric mucosa.
• Draw syringe plunger back to check for air—to indicate no air-containing organ, i.e. bowel is overlying the stomach.
• A skin incision is made, using a surgical blade, into the subcutaneous fat.
• Insert a needle trocar into the marked site and push through the anterior wall, while the endoscopist observes the procedure on a screen.
• The endoscopist places a snare wire over the area of insertion internally.
• The assistant inserts a silk-like thread/suture down the catheter, which is grasped by the snare wire in the stomach.
• The endoscope and snare wire are removed, leaving the wire at the mouth and abdominal exit site—a cheese-wire effect.

- A PEG tube is tied to the wire at the mouth and pulled back through the anterior abdominal wall.
- The internal flange should be felt under the fingers on the abdominal wall and exit site.
- The tube is marked with numbers, which should be documented on the endoscopy report, i.e. ~2–5 cm, depending on patient's weight.
- The outer flange must not be over-tightened, as this could cause compression necrosis.
- Apply the appropriate connections.
- Use a sterile dressing or surgical spray dressing according to local policy.
- Document the tube size, exit site (in cm), dressing applied, and aftercare required at the stoma site. An appropriate care protocol should be used.

Push technique

In the event of a failed endoscopic procedure, or known oral pharyngeal or oesophageal obstruction, the feeding tube is passed through the abdominal wall rather than endoscopically. These types of procedures can be placed either radiologically or by direct surgical gastrostomy, as per local guidelines.

Complications

The first 36 h after the procedures are the most important, although it takes at least 10 days for the stoma tract to form. Risks are as follows:
- Septicaemia
- Tissue necrosis—over-tight tube
- Peritonitis
- Tube displacement
- Stoma infection
- Gastrocolic fistula/bowel perforation
- Aspiration pneumonia
- Bleeding
- Refeeding syndrome (⊃ p. 348).

Recovery

As per OGD (⊃ p. 250) plus:
- Oral fluids are given only if appropriate.
- Appropriate pain control—if required.
- Observe for abdominal distension.
- Check the wound—if bleeding is present, dress accordingly and observe the wound for haemostasis.
- Vital signs.
- Discharge home for patients needing PEG feeding requires complex planning.
- Any complications will be investigated and treated.

Further reading

Westaby D, Young A, O'Toole P, Smith G, and Sanders DS (2010). The provision of a percutaneously placed enteral tube feeding service. *Gut* 59(12): 1592–605.

Percutaneous endoscopic gastrostomy-jejunostomy

A percutaneous endoscopic gastrostomy-jejunostomy (PEGJ) is a thera-peutic endoscopic procedure to enable enteral feeding.

Indications

A PEGJ is recommended for patients who need enteral feeding tubes but who have gastro-oesophageal reflux (❥ p. 36) or known motility disorders to ↓ the risk of pulmonary aspiration.

Preparation

As per PEG (❥ p. 27).

Procedure

A normal gastrostomy tube will be placed by either PEG technique (endo-scopically or push technique) (❥ p. 272) with an appropriate extension kit available for the gastrostomy tube. Additional equipment, such as long grasping forceps, is also required.

If the procedure is wire-guided, flush the wire port with saline to ease removal once the tube is placed.

- Flush the gastrostomy tube with water and insert the extension tube.
- The tube should be picked up by the endoscopist using forceps and fed into the jejunum by advancing the endoscope and forceps appropriately.
- The first gastrostomy tube assistant slowly feeds the tube down the gastrostomy port, while keeping eye contact with the procedure on-screen.
- Once the tube is down into the jejunum, the endoscopist draws back the endoscope, while pushing in the forceps to maintain the position of the tube.
- The endoscopist views the tube at the pylorus and assesses the need to withdraw any excess tube from stomach.
- The guidewire is removed from the extension tube and the endoscope is removed.
- Extension tube connectors are then placed, with care taken not to dislodge the internal extension tube. The extension tube must be cut to size; accurate measurement for fitting is essential.
- Accurate documentation of the type of tube inserted must be made in the patient's notes.

Complications

As per PEG (❥ p. 273) insertion.

Recovery

As per PEG (❥ p. 273).

Polypectomy

Polypectomy is a therapeutic endoscopic procedure to remove a colorectal polyp (➲ p. 352) in order to prevent cancer.

Indication

Removal of a polyp.

Preparation

As per colonoscopy (➲ p. 246).

Procedure

As per endoscopy (➲ p. 236). Polyps removal can be hot biopsy or snared.

Polypectomy—hot biopsy

- Sessile polyps can be 'hot biopsied', which involves grasping the polyp with biopsy forceps and pulling it away from the colon wall. An electrical current is applied in addition to a short sharp tug on the forceps, which removes the polyp and ensures haemostasis. Hot biopsy is contraindicated in the right colon (use snare).
- Polypectomy—snared.
- Pedunculated polyps require 'snaring', which involves putting a snare around the base of the polyp stalk. The snare is tightened and an electrical current is applied, which severs the base of the polyp and seals the vessels.

Complications

- Haemorrhage from the polypectomy site
- Perforation of the bowel mucosa at the site can occur days after the procedure, with rates varying.

Recovery

Monitoring the patient's vital signs is of paramount importance, both during and after polypectomy. If haemostasis is not achieved, hypovolaemic shock can result. The patient could require IV fluids to replace any blood loss during the procedure, and this must be explained to the patient before the procedure because afterwards they may be recovering from sedation.

Nursing advice prior to discharge includes if the patient experiences excessive abdominal pain or haemorrhage, they should to return to the Accident and Emergency Department.

Follow-up

Depending on the findings at colonoscopy and the histology of the polyps, the patient might require repeat colonoscopy to ensure that there are no further polyps and to check the previous polypectomy sites. For adenomatous polyps, the patient should enter a regular surveillance programme to ensure that there is no further growth of polyps. Surveillance for >3 adenomas (any size), or 1> 10 mm (5 yearly). Surveillance can vary with local policy.

Further reading

https://gut.bmj.com/content/gutjnl/66/7/1181.full.pdf (Accessed online 09/04/2019).

Variceal balloon tamponade

Variceal balloon tamponade is a therapeutic endoscopic procedure to stop bleeding from an upper GI bleeding varix by exerting pressure on identified bleeding vessels, either in the oesophagus or gastric fundal region, after failed endoscopic therapy or drug intervention. Variceal balloon tamponade is rarely used and should only be inserted by an experienced clinician with the help of an anaesthetist to maintain the airway.

Equipment

Balloon tamponade equipment:
- Sengstaken (or Minnesota) tube—kept cold; aids placement (Fig. 11.2)
- Lubrication
- 30 ml syringe
- Gauze swabs
- Four artery forceps
- Drainage bag
- Adhesive tape/bandage
- Sphygmomanometer.

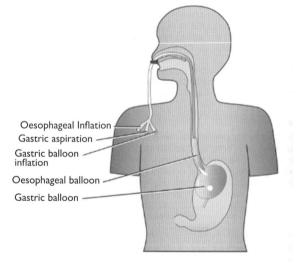

Oesophageal Inflation
Gastric aspiration
Gastric balloon inflation
Oesophageal balloon
Gastric balloon

Fig. 11.2 Oesophageal balloon, with a gastric balloon below. The balloon has three ports: an oesophageal inflation port, a gastric balloon inflation port, and a gastric aspiration port. Sengstaken Blakemore (Minnesota) tube.
Reproduced with kind permission © Burdett Institute 2008.

Procedure

The nurse assistant must ensure the following:
- Check balloons for leaks and deflate completely.
- Label lumens.
- Record the level of gastric balloon inflation using a sphygmomanometer before placement.
- Put the patient in a left lateral position—one nurse must be dedicated to this task.
- Cardiovascular monitoring, suction and oxygen available—there is a high risk of aspiration.
- Lubricate the tube.
- The endoscopist advances the tube through the mouth to 50 cm.
- Secure the tube with the tape or bandage.
- The gastric balloon is inflated. The patient will usually be intubated and paralysed. If not, observe the patient for pain. If the patient is in discomfort, stop, deflate the balloon, and reposition. Slight tension should be applied to maintain the position once the balloon is inflated.
- Measure the balloon pressure, which should correlate with the pre-insertion level.
- Check and record the level of the tube at the patient's incisor.
- Clamp the lumens—using forceps.
- Attach suction to oesophageal aspiration port using low pressure.
- Attach drainage bag to gastric outlet.

Complications

- Aspiration
- Asphyxia—balloon displacement
- Perforation
- Tissue necrosis.

Recovery

- Lay the patient flat, with slight tension on the gastric balloon externally to maintain its position.
- Observe for perforation, rebleeding, or subcutaneous emphysema (chest, abdominal, or pleuritic pain, tachycardia, and pyrexia).
- Cardiovascular monitoring (pulse and blood pressure) should be performed every 30 min initially and then every hour.
- Take the patient's temperature every 4 h.
- Check the balloon pressure every 30 min.
- Deflate the oesophageal balloon for 5 min every hour to prevent tissue necrosis.
- Irrigate the gastric lumen, if required, every 1–2 h with 30 ml of saline.
- Rehydrate the patient intravenously—NBM and mouth care.

Removal

- Disconnect suction.
- Clamp gastric and oesophageal aspirate lumens.
- Deflate the balloons.
- The patient should exhale on withdrawal of the tube.
- The patient should be NBM for 6–8 h.

Nutrition

Nutrition

Nutrition plays a critical role in the physiological and psychological well-being of patients. Healthy food choices are vital in disease prevention, recovery from illness, and in promoting and maintaining health. Nurses are the primary interface between patients and the healthcare system and because nutrition is a part of patient outcomes, nurses play a key part in nutrition education. Since nurses are the main point of contact for patients, they require a thorough knowledge of nutrition to understand how it influences health throughout an individual's lifespan. The gastrointestinal (GI) tract is the organ responsible for ingestion (❯ p. 3), digestion (❯ p. 3), and absorption (❯ p. 3); furthermore, a healthy GI tract is essential in maintaining nutritional health. It is important that the nurse understands the constituents of food and the indications for some of the special diets that may be necessary.

Nutrients

Nutrients are required for growth, maintenance of body tissue, storage of energy for physiological functions, and control of metabolic processes. Nutrients are generally classified into two types:
- Macronutrients—include fats, carbohydrates (starches, sugars, and dietary fibre), and proteins
- Micronutrients, also defined as 'regulatory nutrients'—include water-soluble vitamins, fat-soluble vitamins, macrominerals, and microminerals.

Alcohol is not considered a nutrient. The Department of Health guidelines for the intake of alcohol are that it should not provide >5% of the energy in the diet.

In the United Kingdom, most of the estimated dietary requirements for specific groups of the population are based around advice that was published by the Committee on Medical Aspects of Food and Nutrition Policy (COMA) in 1991 where dietary reference values were set as a series of estimates for energy and nutrition. Since then the Scientific Advisory Committee on Nutrition (SACN) has reviewed the previous recommendations.

Dietary reference values

Dietary reference values (DRVs) describe the requirements for food energy for healthy individuals and were developed for different life stages and sex groups. The DRVs support the maintenance of health in a healthy population and are developed with the principle that the requirements for all nutrients are met. DRVs also serve as the basis for setting reference values in food labelling and in establishing food based dietary guidelines. DRVs include the following categories of estimates derived from the principle that the requirement for a nutrient is normally distributed.
- Estimated average requirements (EARs)—the EAR is an estimate of the 'average' requirement of energy or a nutrient.
- Reference nutrient intakes (RNIs)—the RNI is the amount of a nutrient that is enough to ensure that the needs of nearly all a group (97.5%) are being met.
- Lower reference nutrient intakes (LRNIs)—the LRNI is the amount of a nutrient that is enough for only a small number of people in a group who have low requirements (2.5%), i.e. the majority need more.
- Safe intake is used where there is insufficient evidence to set an EAR, RNI, or LRNI. The safe intake is the amount judged to be enough for almost everyone, but below a level that could have undesirable effects.

Food labelling

The Food Standards Agency is promoting the use of traffic-light labelling to identify for the consumer foods that contain high (red), medium (amber), or low (green) levels of saturated fat, salt, and added sugar.

Further reading

British Nutrition Foundation. https://www.nutrition.org.uk/ (Accessed 24/01/2019).

Committee on Medical Aspects of Food Policy. (1991). Dietary Reference Values for Food Energy and Nutrients for the United Kingdom. London: HMSO.

Scientific Advisory Committee on Nutrition. https://www.gov.uk/government/groups/scientific-advisory-committee-on-nutrition (Accessed 23/01/2019).

Balance of good health

A balanced and healthy diet includes a variety of foods that should provide us with the right amount of energy (calories or kilojoules) to maintain energy balance. Energy balance is where the intake of calories is equal to the calories used by the body. Calories are required for everyday tasks such as walking and for processes such as breathing and blood circulation as well as to aid healing. For this reason, our diets should contain a variety of different foods, to help us get the wide range of nutrients that our bodies need.

Public Health England has formulated documents for healthier eating based around recommendations from the World Health Organization (WHO) and COMA. The documents provide summaries of government dietary advice, nutrient recommendations, and depict a range and amount of foods that are required for a balanced diet. One of the documents uses a pictorial guide dividing foods in to the following groups:

- Bread, other cereals, and potatoes—should make up 37% of daily food intake. Include at least one portion of starchy food at each main meal. This food group provides carbohydrate, calcium, iron, B vitamins, and fibre.
- Fruit and vegetables—eat at least five portions per day (39% of food consumed). This food group provides water-soluble vitamins, carbohydrate, and fibre.
- Milk and dairy products—eat two to three portions per day (8% of food consumed). This food group provides calcium, protein, vitamin B_{12}, and fat-soluble vitamins.
- Meat, fish, and alternatives—eat two to three portions per day (12% of food consumed). This food group provides iron, protein, B vitamins, zinc, and magnesium.
- Foods containing fat and sugar—eat only zero to three portions per day (8% of food consumed). This food group provides fat, carbohydrate, fat-soluble vitamins, and salt.

A balanced diet includes a variety of foods which, if consumed in the above proportions for a period of time, will provide energy and nutrients for the majority of the population to remain healthy.

Guidelines for a healthy diet

- Base each meal on starchy foods.
- Eat plenty of fruit and vegetables.
- Eat more fish.
- Limit the amount of foods containing saturated fat and sugars.
- Eat less salt—no more than 6 g/day.
- Get active and eat the right amount to maintain a healthy weight.
- Drink plenty of water.
- Do not skip breakfast.

Promoting a whole-diet approach to healthy eating is essential because it considers the consequences of the whole diet on health, rather than just individual nutrients or food groups.

Further reading

Public Health England (2014). The eatwell plate: external reference group review. https://www.nhs.uk/live-well/eat-well/5-a-day-portion-sizes/ (Accessed 10/07/2020).

World Health Organization. (2003). Diet, nutrition and the prevention of chronic diseases. http://whqlibdoc.who.int/trs/WHO_TRS_916.pdf (Accessed 22/01/2019).

Nutritional requirements

Establishing nutritional requirements for patients is necessary to enable the appropriate provision of nutritional support.

Energy requirements

Dietary sources of energy (kilocalories) are required to prevent the metabolism of body fat and protein. During periods of inadequate energy intake, catabolism occurs, with the breakdown of body protein. Exogenous sources of fat and carbohydrate are required. Feeding the malnourished patient to meet their predicted energy requirement might cause cardiac, respiratory, renal, metabolic, and neuromuscular complications and initially feeding should be cautious and less than the calculated requirements.

Protein requirements

Protein is the only macronutrient containing nitrogen and therefore protein requirements are often referred to in terms of nitrogen requirements. Protein is not stored within the body: thus, loss of protein has an effect on function. Proteins are continuously synthesized and degraded within a 'pool' that enables the formation of new proteins to meet the changing needs of the body. If the rate of protein synthesis is greater than the rate of protein breakdown, the body is said to be in an 'anabolic' state, with a positive nitrogen balance. If the rate of protein breakdown is greater than the rate of protein synthesis, this is a 'catabolic' state or negative nitrogen balance. To maintain the body in balance in the healthy individual, 0.75 g of protein/kg body weight/day is required. An ↑ protein/nitrogen intake is required in the metabolically stressed patient (e.g. owing to surgery, trauma, or sepsis), although a positive nitrogen balance cannot be achieved in this altered metabolic state. The aim is to limit protein loss. High protein intakes should be carefully monitored and avoided in those with liver and renal impairment.

Fluid and electrolytes

Normal fluid requirements for adults between 18 and 60 years and >60 years are 35 ml/kg body weight/day and 30 ml/kg body weight/day, respectively. Fluid balance can become disturbed during illness. In addition to estimating the fluid requirement on the basis of age and body weight, it is essential to make adjustments according to fluid loss (e.g. diarrhoea, fistula, vomiting, or pyrexia) to prevent dehydration. Overloading of fluids must also be avoided. In addition to impairing cardiac and respiratory function, fluid and electrolyte excess can slow gastric motility. Fluid-balance records, if kept accurately, are a useful tool. A positive fluid-balance chart of ~500 ml/day is desirable because this will account for insensible fluid loss that cannot be measured, such as sweat.

Electrolyte requirements for artificial nutrition support must be calculated on an individual basis. Baseline serum levels should be measured to establish whether requirements are for maintenance or repletion. The National Institute for Health and Clinical Excellence has made recommendations for monitoring electrolytes during artificial feeding.

Investigations

An accurate measurement of the patient's body weight is required because nutritional requirements are related to body composition. There are a number of investigations that can be completed:

- Body mass index (BMI) (➲ p. 306)
- Triceps skin-fold thickness—anthropometric measurements to estimate adiposity
- Mid-arm muscle circumference—muscle mass
- Electrolyte and water composition
- Total body weight.

The goal of nutrition therapy depends on the patient's clinical/metabolic condition. In the management of a stressed patient, the nutritional goal is to minimize depletion. As the patient's condition improves, the goals of nutrition therapy will also change.

Non-essential nutrients

Some nutrients can be made by the body from other nutrients (e.g. vitamin D, some fatty acids, and amino acids) or micro-organisms found in food (e.g. vitamin B_{12}), or the large intestine (e.g. vitamin K). These non-essential nutrients must be included within the diet, especially in the unwell person as their manufacture only occurs in optimal health and normal metabolic processes.

Within digestion (➲ p. 3), the term 'metabolism' is used to describe the mechanisms by which nutrients are processed in the body (i.e. how they are assimilated and incorporated into tissue or detoxified and excreted). Metabolism includes:

- Catabolism—broadly, the breakdown of complex substances.
- Anabolism—the synthesis of complex substances from simple substances.
- Basal metabolic rate (BMR)—the rate at which the body uses energy at rest. This measurement is dependent on age, sex, and body weight.
- Physical activity level—used to estimate an individual's daily activity level as a multiple of BMR, which varies from 1.4 (light energy expenditure in work, with non-active leisure pursuits) to 1.9 (energy-demanding work and leisure-time activity).
- Energy—the kilocalorie (kcal) is the unit of energy used to measure the energy value of food. Guidelines for the intake of energy are based on activity levels of the UK population. Fat, protein, carbohydrate, and alcohol provide energy.

Further reading

British Nutrition Foundation. http://www.nutrition.org.uk (Accessed online 01/02/2019).

Carbohydrates

Carbohydrates are constructed from carbon, oxygen, and hydrogen atoms. Carbohydrates are key components in the diet containing sugars, starches, and fibres found in fruits, grains, vegetables, and milk products. Though often maligned in trendy diets, carbohydrates—one of the basic food groups—are important to a healthy life. Carbohydrates are macronutrients, meaning they are one of the three main ways the body obtains energy or calories. At least half the energy in our diets should come from carbohydrate, mostly as starchy carbohydrates.

The body's tissues require a constant supply of glucose, which is used as a fuel. The main source of glucose is dietary carbohydrate, but it can also be synthesized from protein. If the diet is low in carbohydrate, a greater percentage of dietary protein is used to provide glucose, which means less is available for the growth and repair of body tissues. Thus, carbohydrate in the diet has a protein-sparing effect.

Classification

Carbohydrates can be classified as follows.
- Monosaccharides or simple sugars—cannot be hydrolysed to smaller units
- Disaccharides—two parts of monosaccharides
- Oligosaccharides—short chains of varying monosaccharides joined by covalent bonds
- Polysaccharides—long chains of monosaccharide units (from several to 100 repeating units of glucose or different types of monosaccharide).

Metabolism

Metabolic pathways are regulated according to the need for energy. Pathways of carbohydrate use and storage include the following:
- Glycogenesis—conversion of glucose to glycogen (e.g. in liver and skeletal muscle).
- Glycogenolysis—conversion or breakdown of stored glycogen to glucose.
- Glycolysis—breakdown of glucose (intercellular) to the metabolic intermediate pyruvate. Under anaerobic conditions, pyruvate is used to provide energy by production of lactate; under aerobic conditions, pyruvate enters the Krebs cycle (within mitochondria) and is oxidized to release energy.
- Gluconeogenesis—reversible reaction of glycolysis, resulting in the synthesis of glucose from non-carbohydrate sources (usually occurs in the liver but, during starvation, the kidney contributes to glucose production). Non-carbohydrate sources include lactate, pyruvate, glycerol (from the breakdown of triglycerides), and specific amino acids.

Health implications

- Intrinsic sugars (sugars that are naturally incorporated into the cellular structure of foods) and lactose do not have harmful effects on health; although they can cause ↑ gut transit if consumed in large quantities.
- Non-milk extrinsic sugars contribute to dental caries.
- Consumption of non-milk extrinsic sugars is energy dense (although less so than fats and alcohol) and often associated with excess calorie intake and ∴ is associated with weight gain.
- Intake of sucrose >200 g/day can be associated with ↑ cholesterol and blood glucose.
- Starches should be consumed in preference to other energy-producing foods (fat and alcohol).

Further reading

British Nutrition Foundation. https://www.nutrition.org.uk/ (Accessed 10/07/2020).

Fibre

Dietary fibre is a term that is used for plant-based carbohydrates that if eaten reach the caecum unchanged, unlike other carbohydrates (such as sugars and starch), meaning that they are not digested in the small intestine. Dietary fibre is found in fruit, vegetables, and wholegrain cereal foods.

Functions

Although dietary fibre cannot be broken down by human digestive enzymes, it has important physiological effects and can be broken down by the bacteria in the large bowel. Fibre has the following properties:

- Bulking—delayed gastric emptying, enhanced satiety, reduced intestinal transit time, ↓ intraluminal pressure, and ↑ frequency of defaecation
- Cholesterol ↓
- Delays glucose absorption
- ↑ bile acid excretion
- Fermentation provides energy (in colon).

Classification

There are two main categories of non-starch polysaccharide:

- Soluble—some hemicellulose (found in the cell walls of plants, e.g. bran and whole grains), pectin (found in the cell walls of plants, e.g. apples and citrus fruits), gum (also known as 'hydrocolloid'; found in oatmeal, barley, and legumes)
- Insoluble—some hemicellulose (found in the cell walls of plants, e.g. bran and whole grains), lignin (non-carbohydrate component of root vegetables, wheat, and fruit), and cellulose (found in the cell walls of bran, legumes, peas, apples, and root vegetables).

There is some suggestion that these terms are no longer appropriate. However, what is important to remember is that fibre-rich foods typically contain both types of fibre.

Health implications

- Low-fibre diets are associated with diverticular disease and an ↑ risk of colon cancer.
- Advice to ↑ daily fibre intake should also include advice on an ↑ in daily fluid intake.
- Excessively high intake of fibre can impair the absorption of minerals (cations, e.g. calcium, zinc, and iron). These minerals are released for absorption in the colon if they undergo fermentation.

Further reading

https://www.nutrition.org.uk/healthyliving/basics/fibre.html (Accessed 14/02/2019).

Fats

Fat is obtained from dietary sources in either solid or liquid (oil) form and is also known as 'lipid'. Fat is the most calorific source of dietary energy available and so can influence weight gain. The structure of the building blocks of dietary fat—fatty acids—determines their health effects. Fats provide 1 g of fat per 9 kcal. Some fatty acids are essential components of the diet and are a constituent of cell membranes and steroid hormones as well as a transport for fat soluble vitamins. However, others can be detrimental and as with most nutrients, recommendations exist to help establish dietary balance. Essential fatty acids are precursors to eicosanoids (fatty acids 20 carbon atoms in length), which include the physiologically potent groups of substances called prostaglandins and thromboxane (intracellular messengers regulating blood pressure, diuresis, immune function, and platelet aggregation), in addition to leukotrienes (chemical mediators of hypersensitivity and inflammatory reactions).

Classification

Dietary fats are usually consumed in the form of triglycerides, which are composed of a glycerol molecule attached to three fatty acid molecules. Fatty acids are made up of a hydrocarbon chain, which varies in length. The physical properties of fats are influenced by the combination of fatty acids that comprise the triglyceride. Fatty acids are classified by their chemical make-up. Naturally occurring fatty acids are either 'saturated' or 'unsaturated'

Saturated fatty acids

Characteristically, these fats are solid at room temperature and found primarily in animal products. They get their name because the carbon atoms in the fats are highly saturated with hydrogen. Diets high in these foods are linked to an increased risk of chronic diseases, especially coronary artery disease.

Monounsaturated fats

Fats that only have a single double-bonded carbon atom are known as monounsaturated fats. Liquid at room temperature, monounsaturated fats are found in foods like olive oil, sesame oil, avocados, nuts, peanut butter, and sunflower oil. Fats of this nature can reduce the risk of stroke and heart disease, lower bad cholesterol levels, and provide high levels of vitamin E, an important antioxidant, when eaten in moderation.

Polyunsaturated fats

Fats with at least two double-bonded carbons are known as polyunsaturated fats. Good sources of these fats include safflower oil, corn oil, soybean oil, and fatty fish like trout, salmon, herring, and mackerel. When eaten moderately in place of saturated fats, polyunsaturated fats can be a healthy choice. They can lower the risk of heart disease and also reduce cholesterol levels in the blood. This group of fats includes essential fats that cannot be produced by the body, like omega-3 and omega-6 fatty acids. The only way to get these essential fats is from your diet. Omega-3 and omega-6 are essential for brain function and healthy body development and growth.

Trans fatty acids

Processed foods are often loaded with trans fatty acids, by-products of a chemical process known as hydrogenation. Foods high in these harmful fats include animal products, cooking oils, margarine, shortening, and foods that contain these ingredients. Fats that are altered to a 'trans' configuration, are known to contribute to an increase in low-density lipoprotein cholesterol and an increased risk of coronary heart disease.

Metabolism

Short- and medium-chain fatty acids are directly absorbed. Long-chain fatty acids are packed into chylomicrons which travel through entero-cytes into the lymphatic system, entering the circulation via the thoracic duct. Triglycerides in chylomicrons are broken down into glycerol and fatty acids by lipoprotein lipase, which is found on the surface of cells. This enables the fatty acids and glycerol to enter the cells. Fat metabolism is regulated by catabolic hormones (epinephrine, glucagon, glucocorticoids, and thryroxine) and the anabolic hormone insulin.

Fatty acids and glycerol have the following functions:

- Broken down for energy (oxidation)
- Rebuilt into triglycerides for storage (anabolism) within adipose tissue.

Health implications

A diet high in unsaturated fats has a negative impact on health by increasing serum cholesterol levels leading to a higher risk of coronary heart disease. Monounsaturated and polyunsaturated fats, on the other hand, have a more positive effect on the serum lipid profile, which leads to a decreased low-density lipoprotein (LDL)—oxidation and encouragingly influence the metabolism of diabetics, as well as play a role in heart health. To gain the benefits, it is essential that these fats are mainly supplied by plant oils, such as rape seed or olive oil, and not by foods that are simultaneously rich in saturated fatty acids.

Further reading

www.nutrition.org.uk/nutritionscience/nutrients-food-and-ingredients/fat.html?start=5   (Accessed on 08/02/2019).

Proteins

Proteins are functional components within every cell of the body and are included in a wide range of metabolic interactions, therefore they are essential for growth and repair and the maintenance of good health. Proteins provide the body with approximately 10–15% of its dietary energy and are the second most abundant compound in the body, following water. A large proportion of this will be muscle (43% on average) with significant proportions being present in skin (15%) and blood (16%).

Classification

This is determined by the quality of amino acids contained in the protein source. The body makes some amino acids through a process of transamination, which is possible if the diet contains 'essential' (also known as 'indispensable') amino acids. These amino acids contain an amino group that, if broken down, can be transferred to form other types of amino acid. Some non-essential amino acids become essential under specific physiological conditions and are classed as conditionally essential.

Metabolism

Proteins are large complex molecules made up of many different amino acids. Protein metabolism signifies the various biochemical techniques involved in the synthesis of proteins and amino acids (anabolism) and also the breakdown of proteins (catabolism). Dietary proteins are first broken down to individual amino acids by various enzymes and hydrochloric acid present in the GI tract. To ensure that a balance is achieved, protein metabolism is a continuous process of catabolism and anabolism. A balance is achieved if the amount of protein made is equal to the amount used. A positive nitrogen balance occurs if the protein synthesized exceeds the amount broken down (e.g. in tissue repair and muscle building/growth). During starvation and the associated loss of fat-free mass, the body has a negative nitrogen balance.

Functions

- Growth, development, and repair of body structures and tissues.
- Source of energy (recommended 10–15% food intake): 1 g protein = 4 kcal.
- Dietary protein is used for growth and repair, rather than as a source of energy. However, it will be used as an energy source if none other is available. The functional role of proteins is determined by their structure and organization.

Categories of proteins include the following:
- Enzymes—responsible for catalysing chemical reactions required for normal physiological processes, e.g. digestion, cellular energy production, coagulation, and neuromuscular activity.
- Peptide hormones—responsible for the regulation of body functions by directing the production or activity of enzymes, e.g. insulin, glucagon, thyroid hormones, and many other hormones.
- Transport proteins—these proteins can combine with substances so that the substances can be carried in the bloodstream, e.g. haemoglobin, transferrin, and retinol-binding protein.

- Immunoproteins—produced by white blood cells (B lymphocytes). They bind to antigens, to recognize and inactivate them.
- Structural proteins—including the fibrous proteins (elastin, keratin, and collagen) found in connective tissue, skin, hair, and nails, in addition to the contractile proteins of muscle (actin and myosin).

Implications for health

A higher protein diet can be valuable for health, especially for maintaining muscle mass, losing weight, and lowering the risk of obesity. Although, high protein diets may help weight loss, it may only be a short-term effect, meaning that excess protein is usually stored as fat whilst the surplus of amino acids is excreted. This can lead to weight gain over time, especially if too many calories are consumed while trying to increase your protein intake. There are also safety concerns about very high protein diets that involve cutting out other food groups and caution should therefore be exercised in promoting them. Conversely, a poor intake of protein will contribute to malnutrition. However, excessive amounts of protein in the diet can cause an ↑ loss of calcium, which ↑ the risk of bone disease. Additionally, high intake of protein over a period of time is thought to contribute to impaired renal function in vulnerable individuals, particularly people with diabetes.

Further reading

https://www.nutrition.org.uk/ (Accessed 10/07/2020).

Vitamins

Vitamins are required by the body in small amounts for normal growth and maintenance of health. The body requires differing amounts because each vitamin has a different set of functions. Requirements vary according to age, sex, physiological state, e.g. pregnancy, and state of health. Initially vitamins were given letters (A, B, C etc.) but are now more commonly referred to by their names, e.g. folate, riboflavin.

Classification

Vitamins are classified as micronutrients because they are normally required in small amounts. Vitamins are classified as either water soluble (B_1, B_2, niacin, B_6, folic acid, B_{12}, biotin, and C) or fat soluble (e.g. A, D, E, and K). Most vitamins cannot be synthesized by the body so must be obtained by the diet. An exception is vitamin D which can be synthesized by the action of sunlight on the skin. Small amounts of niacin (a B vitamin) can be made from the amino acid, tryptophan.

Functions

Vitamins contribute to the following fundamental processes:
- Growth
- Metabolism
- Maintenance of health
- Co-factors in enzyme activity
- Antioxidants (prevent damage from free radicals)
- Pro-hormone (only vitamin D).

Metabolism

The two groups of vitamins are processed differently by the body.

Water-soluble vitamins:
- Absorbed into the portal bloodstream
- Carried in the blood by transport proteins
- Cellular uptake facilitated by vitamin-specific enzymes
- Storage in the body tissues is limited—except vitamin B_{12} and biotin
- Toxicity is rare because these vitamins are excreted if the plasma level reaches the renal threshold.

Fat-soluble vitamins
- Transport requires chylomicrons in the lymphatic system and then the general circulation
- Stored in body fat
- If taken in large doses over long periods, toxicity can develop as they are excreted more slowly than water-soluble vitamins.

Implications for health

If insufficient amounts of vitamins are available to the body because of a poor diet medical condition, such as malabsorption disorders deficiency disease can develop. Vitamin deficiency diseases are rare in the UK but still occur in some parts of the world.

Further reading

https://www.nutrition.org.uk/nutritionscience/nutrients-food-and-ingredients/vitamins.html?limit=1&start=12 (Accessed 08/02/2019).

Minerals

Essential minerals and trace elements are inorganic elements with important physiological functions and are acquired as part of the diet. Some minerals are needed in larger amounts, e.g. calcium, phosphorus, magnesium, sodium, potassium, and chloride. Others are required in smaller quantities and are sometimes called trace minerals, e.g. iron, zinc, iodine, fluoride, selenium, and copper. Although only necessary in small amounts, minerals are important in the diet.

Classification

- Minerals—required from the diet in milligram quantities per day, including sodium, potassium, calcium, magnesium, phosphorus, iron, zinc, and chloride.
- Trace elements—required from the diet in micrograms quantities per day, including copper, selenium, iodine, manganese, molybdenum, nickel, silicon, vanadium, arsenic, and boron,

Functions

Each essential mineral and trace element has one or more physiological function. The quantity needed of each element varies; the body has different requirements for each essential element. For optimal function, the concentration of the element falls within a range. Levels outside this range lead to deficiencies or toxicities that impair physiological functioning and might result in death. Minerals have the following functions:

- Structural component of bones, teeth, and other body tissues
- Constituents of body fluids
- Nerve function
- Enzyme function
- Cell membrane stability and transport.

Implications for health

Most people do not show signs of mineral deficiency. However, adolescent girls, women of childbearing age, and some vegans/vegetarians are more susceptible to low iron status as their dietary intake may not match their requirements. Minerals are often absorbed more efficiently by the body if supplied in foods rather than as supplements. Eating a varied diet will help ensure an adequate supply of most minerals for healthy people.

Further reading

www.nutrition.org.uk/nutritionscience/nutrients-food-and-ingredients/minerals-and-trace-elements.html?limit=1&start=1 (accessed 08/02/2019).

Water

Water is the most abundant component of the human body where regular fluid intake is essential for our bodies to function correctly. The amount of fluid required varies between people and according to age, time of year, climatic conditions, diet, and levels of physical activity. Water can be obtained from several sources, such as plain water and other drinks, as well as the food we eat. The water content of an adult remains relatively constant. Men generally have a higher composition of water, which is related to the greater fat-free mass.

Total body water is divided into two main reservoirs:
- Intracellular compartment (water contained within cell membranes—30 litres).
- Extracellular compartment (water found outside cell membranes—15 litres; 3 litres of this is from the intravascular space, the remainder is fluid surrounding the cells or interstitial fluid).

Electrolytes contribute to the osmolality of body fluids and help to maintain body fluids in the appropriate compartment. Monovalent electrolytes—sodium, potassium, and chloride—are found mainly in the extracellular compartment, while potassium, magnesium, and phosphate are found in the intracellular fluid.

Function

The vital functions of water include:
- Regulation of body temperature
- Lubricant
- Solvent and transport medium for nutrients ions and molecules
- Medium for chemical (metabolic) reactions
- Transport medium for the excretion of osmotically active solutes (e.g. urea, sodium (Na^+), chloride (Cl^-), and potassium (K^+).

Requirements

The amount of water and other fluids required each day varies from person to person, depending on age, time of year, climatic conditions, diet, and the amount of physical activity we do. In health, the need for fluid is approximately 30–35 ml/kg. Dietary intake of water includes liquid sources (beverages, fruit juice, squash, carbonated drinks, and milk). About a third of our water intake is from the food we eat (fruit and vegetables have high water content). In health, fluid intake is influenced by factors (social influences/habit, consumption of food) in addition to thirst. Fluid losses include:
- Regulation of body temperature (sweating)
- Respiration (as water vapour)
- The elimination of waste products (the kidneys remove solute from the blood for elimination as urine; water is also lost from the GI tract in faeces).

Regulation

Thirst is experienced as the result of a water deficit and is a mechanism for the regulation of fluid intake. This water deficit (dehydration) will cause an increase in osmolality of all body fluids. Increased osmolality of plasma circulating through the hypothalamus will cause the sensation of thirst (prompting an increase in fluid intake) and the release of the antidiuretic hormone vasopressin. Vasopressin acts on the area for water absorption (renal tubule), increasing the water-absorbing capacity and therefore conserving body water and concentrating the urine.

Health implications

Fluid imbalance is not a problem in healthy individuals with unregulated access to water. Loss of as little as 1% of body water can cause physiological impairment and performance responses. The body has precise systems to maintain our body water. However, consideration should be given to children and older people who may not recognize the sensation of thirst so easily, to ensure they consume enough fluids. A large amount of caffeine in fluids has a diuretic effect. Large amounts of carbonated drinks (especially in the young) should be reduced as they may contain high levels of sugar and are known to affect bone metabolism. It can be dangerous to drink too much water as water intoxication can lead to hyponatraemia.

Further reading

https://www.nutrition.org.uk/nutritionscience/nutrients-food-and-ingredients/liquids.html
(Accessed 08/02/02019).

Influence of diet on health

There are many negative influences of diet on health. There is increasing evidence that the population run the risk of chronic diseases in adult life because of poor dietary choices. Diet-related chronic diseases are attributed to an unbalanced (not always excessive) intake, genetic predisposition, and ↓ levels of physical activity. Diet-related diseases include the following:

- Alcoholism—alcohol provides 7.1 kcal/g in energy. If consumed in moderation, alcohol may have a protective effect against cardiovascular disease. If taken in excess, it can become addictive. Consequences of alcoholism include weight gain and, in extreme cases, malnutrition, which is associated with poor nutritional intake and malabsorption, damage to the liver (❥ p. 302), brain, and heart, also with an ↑ risk of cancer.
- Obesity (❥ p. 306–7)
- Metabolic syndrome is associated with an increased risk of type 2 diabetes mellitus and cardiovascular disease. It is characterized by insulin resistance, dyslipidaemia, abdominal obesity, and hypertension. The disease process involves several metabolic pathways. Nutrition is thought to have a key role in the development of this syndrome because obesity (❥ p. 306–7) is an underlying causative factor.
- Cardiovascular disease is the most common cause of death in the UK. Dietary factors contribute to the risk of atherosclerosis and thrombosis. It is thought that reducing the total amount of fat consumed can be a preventative measure. Changing the ratio of saturated fats to mono and polyunsaturated fats and also increasing soluble fibre can help to regulate cholesterol levels. Essential fatty acids, such as *n*-3 fatty acids, can decrease the level of triglycerides and have anti-thrombotic properties. This enables the synthesis of prostaglandins, therefore regulating body processes, such as cardiovascular function and the immune system, and maintenance of the musculoskeletal system. Additionally, achieving healthy body processes can be helped by decreasing weight, reducing salt intake, increasing physical activity, and cessation of smoking.
- Type 2 diabetes mellitus is typically associated with central abdominal obesity. This can result in a partial or complete lack of insulin production, which directly affects glucose and fat metabolism. Health advice should emphasize weight loss, maintenance of a normal blood sugar level, and ↑ physical activity. Some patients with type 2 diabetes will require insulin therapy if drug and diet therapies are unsuccessful. Uncontrolled diabetes leads to an increased risk of heart disease, renal failure, neuropathy, and blindness.
- Cancer (❥ p. 352)—eating a healthy, balanced diet is important in keeping a healthy weight, because obesity is the second biggest preventable cause of cancer after smoking. Some processed foods, red meats, and salt preserved foods can increase the risk. Whilst foods such as soluble and insoluble fibres can reduce the risk.

Food intolerance/allergy

Food intolerance

Food intolerance is associated with food hypersensitivity or non-allergic food hypersensitivity and refers to difficulty in digesting certain foods. It is important to note that food intolerance is different from food allergy. There is a wide interpretation to what constitutes food hypersensitivity because individuals vary in their tolerance.

Here are the eight most common parts of the diet that cause food intolerances:

- Dairy—lactose is a sugar found in milk and dairy products.
- Gluten—is the general name given to proteins found in wheat, barley, rye, and triticale.
- Caffeine.
- Salicylates—chemicals that have salicylic acid as their base and can be found in fruits, vegetables, and spices.
- Amines—naturally occurring chemicals in certain foods which, like salicylates, are cumulative in the body. Over a period of time, these can build up in your system causing reactions that mimic allergies.
- FODMAPs—fermentable oligosaccharides, disaccharides, monosaccharides, and polyols—complex names for a collection of molecules found in food, that can be poorly absorbed by some people.
- Sulfites—substances that are naturally found in some foods. They are also used as an additive to maintain food colour and shelf-life, and prevent the growth of fungi or bacteria.
- Fructose—a simple ketonic monosaccharide found in many plants, where it is often bonded to glucose to form the disaccharide sucrose. It is one of the three dietary monosaccharides, along with glucose and galactose that are absorbed directly into blood during digestion.

Common symptoms include:

- Diarrhoea
- Bloating
- Rashes
- Headaches
- Nausea
- Fatigue
- Abdominal pain
- Runny nose
- Reflux
- Flushing of the skin.

Elimination diets are usually tried with an aim to remove foods most commonly associated with intolerances for a period of time until symptoms subside. Foods are then reintroduced one at a time while monitoring for symptoms. This type of diet helps people identify which food or foods are causing symptoms.

Food allergy

Food allergy is an allergic reaction to a food that can be described as an inappropriate reaction by the body's immune system to the ingestion of a food. Allergic reactions to foods vary significantly in the severity of the related symptoms and the extent of time for which they persist. An example of this can be seen in a peanut allergy which is more often a lifelong problem and can cause severe, life-threatening, anaphylactic reactions to small amounts of peanut protein. Food allergy is rare, affecting an estimated 1–2% of people in the UK. It is more common in children than adults and is often wrongly used as a general term for intolerances to food.

Further reading

British Nutrition Foundation https://www.nutrition.org.uk/ (Accessed online 24/01/2019).
www.foodcanmakeyouill.co.uk/food-intolerance-handbook.html (Accessed online 03/02/2019).

Undernutrition

Undernutrition refers to insufficient intake of energy and nutrients to meet an individual's needs to maintain good health.

Symptoms

Symptoms of undernutrition can include unintentional weight loss and can result in:

- Muscle weakness—↓ mobility and associated complications, fatigue, ↑ risk of respiratory infection, and impaired cardiac function.
- Impaired immune function—↑ susceptibility to infection.
- Impaired wound healing.
- ↓ tolerance to cytotoxic drugs and chemotherapy.
- Malnutrition is also associated with depression, anxiety, a ↓ ability to concentrate, and an ↑ perception of pain (requiring ↑ analgesia). These factors significantly affect the individual's perception of their quality of life.
- Additionally, ↑ morbidity results in a prolonged hospital stay and an associated economic burden.

Causes

Causes of undernutrition can include:

- Physical problems resulting in a poor nutritional intake—inability of a person to purchase, cook, and/or self-feed. Also, there may be problems with mastication, swallowing, or a ↓ appetite (possibly due to anxiety, depression, or taste changes associated with medication or malignancy). Furthermore, there may be eating disorders such as anorexia nervosa (➋ p. 308) or impaired mental function.
- ↑ metabolism and nutrient requirements—associated with surgery, trauma, sepsis, and pathology, affecting energy expenditure (e.g. malignancy) and reflecting an acute change in the protein–energy status.
- Nutrient losses—poor gut absorption (possibly due to active Crohn's disease, enteropathy, gut atrophy, or ↓ bowel length) and loss of protein from wound exudate, a fistula, or dialysis.

Treatment

Treatment can include a range of possible interventions, from improving the quality of food taken by mouth to artificial nutrition support.

Functional foods

Functional foods and supplements are terms used to describe food and drinks that are augmented with specific nutrients or substances that have the ability to positively impact health over and above their basic nutritional value, e.g. stanol/sterol-enriched; reduced/low fat spreads; dairy products containing probiotic bacteria; folic acid fortified bread or breakfast cereals; omega 3 fatty acids from fish oils added to bread or baked beans. It is important to know that functional foods should never be considered as an alternative to a varied and balanced diet and healthy lifestyle. Legislation exists to protect consumers from any misleading claims and/or information within the European Union with regulation from the European Food Safety Authority (EFSA) ensuring that health claims are subject to scientific assessment.

Examples of functional foods are as follows:

Probiotics

Probiotics are defined as live microorganisms, mostly good bacteria. For many years, probiotics have been developed for promoting health. The action of probiotics is complex. However, for any health benefit to happen it is vital for the bacteria to survive well in the gut. Specific strains, such as *Lactobacillus* and *Bifidobacterium*, have been found to survive throughout the gut and therefore are able to thrive and grow in numbers in the large bowel, and thus influence the components of the gut flora.

Although more research is necessary, studies have shown that probiotics may exert the following on health:

- Reduce infectious diarrhoea
- Prevent antibiotic-associated diarrhoea
- Decrease irritable bowel symptoms.

Prebiotics

Prebiotics are described as non-digestible food ingredients that can promote the growth and/or activity of 'friendly' bacteria by encouraging a healthy environment in the colon and therefore possibly have health benefits. They also inhibit the growth of bacteria that are potentially harmful to intestinal health, e.g. bacteria that produce toxins such as Clostridia and *Escherichia coli*.

Although more research is necessary, studies have shown that prebiotics may exert the following on health:

- Aiding mineral absorption, e.g. calcium
- Improve immune function
- Reduce cholesterol levels
- Relieve irritable bowel syndrome symptoms
- Have a positive effect on intestinal flora in infants.

Plant sterols and stanols

Sterols

Sterols are fundamental elements of cell membranes, with a key role in controlling membrane fluidity and permeability. They are present naturally in small quantities in many fruits, vegetables, nuts, seeds, and legumes.

Stanols

Stanols are chemically like sterols. They occur in similar sources such as nuts, seeds, and legumes but in smaller quantities than sterols.

The structure of plant sterols and stanols are very similar to that of cholesterol and therefore they are thought to reduce the absorption of cholesterol when included in the diet. The EFSA suggests that foods such as yoghurts, milk, cheese, fat spreads, mayonnaise, salad dressing, and other dairy products are the most appropriate for providing the cholesterol-lowering effects.

Further reading

https://www.nutrition.org.uk/nutritionscience/foodfacts/functional-foods.html?start=7 (Accessed 13/02/2019)

Obesity

Consuming high amounts of energy, particularly fat and sugars, and not burning off the energy through exercise and physical activity, causes a surplus of energy, which in turn is stored by the body as fat. Obesity is linked to a number of chronic diseases, including cardiovascular disease, cancer, type 2 diabetes, and osteoarthritis.

Obesity often occurs as a result of energy intake exceeding energy expenditure over a period of years. It is described in adults as a BMI above 30. Data in the UK from the Health Survey for England 2006 showed that 24% of adults (both men and women) were obese and an additional 44% of men and 34% of women were overweight.

Classification

The BMI scale can be used to identify if a person is a correct weight for their height. BMI ranges do not apply to pregnant women.
- Less than 18.5—Underweight
- 18.5 to 25—Desirable or healthy range
- 25 to 30—Overweight
- 30 to 35—Obese (Class I)
- 35 to 40—Obese (Class II)
- Over 40—Morbidly or severely obese (Class III).

Reasons for obesity:
- Lack of regular exercise
- Sedentary occupation
- Irregular eating activity and snacking behaviour
- Availability of high-calorie convenience foods
- ↑ alcohol intake
- Genetics/ethnicity.

Effects on health

Obesity has been found to be associated with mortality and morbidity, with a significant dietary risk factor for a range of chronic diseases:
- Some cancers, including colorectal cancer (➋ p. 352)
- Cardiovascular disease
- Type 2 diabetes
- Gallstones (➋ p. 198–9)
- Osteoarthritis
- High blood pressure—increasing the risk of stroke
- Complications during and after in pregnancy
- Hiatus hernia.

Reducing obesity

When reducing obesity, the aim is to maintain body weight within the healthy BMI range; this can be achieved by:
- Reducing energy intake with a balanced and varied diet
- Seeking advice from a doctor or dietitian
- Changing behaviour
- Avoiding yo-yo dieting
- Pharmacological intervention—if the above fails
- Surgery—when all other treatments have been tried and failed.

Further reading:

https://www.nutrition.org.uk/nutritionscience/obesityandweightmanagement.html (Accessed 14/02/2019).

https://www.nutrition.org.uk/nutritionscience/obesityandweightmanagement/obesity-and-overweight.html?start=2 (Accessed 14/02/2019).

https://www.gov.uk/government/collections/tackling-obesities-future-choices (Accessed 14/02/2019).

https://www.nice.org.uk/guidance/cg189/chapter/1-Recommendations#identification-and-classification-of-overweight-and-obesity (Accessed 14/02/2019).

Eating disorders

Eating disorders are severe illnesses that can affect someone physically, psychologically, and socially. The acknowledged eating disorders are anorexia nervosa (→ p. 308), bulimia nervosa (→ p. 309), and binge eating (→ p. 310). People with eating disorders should be assessed and receive treatment at the earliest opportunity.

Anorexia nervosa

Anorexia nervosa is an eating disorder characterized by:
- Low weight
- Fear of gaining weight
- Strong desire to be thin
- Food restriction/counting calories
- Individuals see themselves as being overweight
- Use of laxatives
- Vomiting
- Amenorrhea
- Social withdrawal
- Dental erosion.

Impact on health
- Infertility
- Decreased oestrogen levels leading to osteoporosis and poor bone health
- Electrolyte imbalance leading to cardiovascular events, seizures
- Gastroparesis
- Endocrine with type 2 diabetes.

Treatment
- Psychoeducation about the disorder
- Psychological support—psychotherapy, cognitive behavioural therapy (CBT)
- Reach healthy weight/weight gain
- Mineral and vitamin supplements—with a balanced diet.

Further reading
https://www.nationaleatingdisorders.org/health-consequences (Accessed 14/02/2019).
https://www.nice.org.uk/guidance/ng69/chapter/Recommendations#identification-and-assessment (Accessed 14/02/2019).
https://www.nutrition.org.uk/nutritionscience/life/teenagers.html?start=7 (Accessed 14/02/2019).

Bulimia nervosa

Bulimia nervosa sufferers are preoccupied with the dread of gaining weight. There is a persistent association of eating large amounts of food, usually followed by self-induced vomiting, taking laxatives or diuretics, and/or purging. People with bulimia often feel a lack of self-control and have an excessive concern with their bodyweight and shape, although this is often within a healthy range.

Bulimia nervosa is characterized by:

- Being secretive about bulimic episodes
- Disappearing soon after eating
- Mood swings and anxiety
- Depression and low self-esteem
- Swelling of the hands and feet
- Amenorrhea or irregularity
- Weight fluctuations
- Poor dental health.

Impact on health

As per anorexia (➔ p. 308).

Treatment

As per anorexia (➔ p. 308).

Further reading

https://www.nationaleatingdisorders.org/health-consequences (Accessed 14/02/2019).
https://www.nice.org.uk/guidance/ng69/chapter/Recommendations#identification-and-assessment (Accessed 14/02/2019).
https://www.nutrition.org.uk/nutritionscience/life/teenagers.html?start=7 (Accessed 14/02/2019).

Binge eating

People who have binge eating may regularly eat very large quantities of food, typically faster than normal or even if they are not hungry, in a short period of time, and experience a loss of control, guilt, and disgust after doing so. The periods of binge eating are not followed by purging to control bodyweight. The binge eating periods are usually planned and take place in secret and can include 'special' binge foods. Binge eating disorder may also be associated with overweight or obesity.

Binge eating can be characterized by:
* Lack of control once one begins to eat
* Depression
* Grief
* Anxiety
* Shame
* Disgust or self-hatred about eating behaviours.

Impact on health

As per anorexia (➜ p. 308).

Treatment

* Guided self-help programmes
* CBT.

Further reading

https://www.nationaleatingdisorders.org/health-consequences (Accessed 14/02/2019).
https://www.nice.org.uk/guidance/ng69/chapter/Recommendations#identification-and-assessment (Accessed 14/02/2019).
https://www.nutrition.org.uk/nutritionscience/life/teenagers.html?start=7 (Accessed 14/02/2019).
https://www.nhs.uk/conditions/binge-eating/ (Accessed 14/02/2019).

Chapter 13

Clinical nutrition

Clinical nutrition

Definition of clinical nutrition

Nutrition support includes a range of interventions, including:

- Improve food intake (oral diet)
- Fortification (energy and nutrient content) and modification (consistency) of the diet
- Sip-feeds can provide a complete oral liquid diet if consumed in sufficient quantity (nutritionally complete preparations) or supplement an inadequate dietary intake
- Artificial nutrition support is the provision of nutrients by artificial means—enteral or parenteral.

Enteral nutrition

Enteral nutrition (EN) ($\bigodot$ p. 316–17) is delivery of feed via the gastrointestinal (GI) tract. It is used to supplement an inadequate dietary intake or provide the patient's total nutritional needs. EN can be used to introduce nutrients to the GI tract while weaning from parenteral nutrition.

Parenteral nutrition

Parenteral nutrition (PN), also known as intravenous nutritional support, is used to provide nutrients and fluid to patients with intestinal failure or if enteral tube access cannot be obtained. Supplemental PN might be used if enteral tube feeding is being introduced but is not meeting the patient's nutritional requirements. EN is generally considered to be more physiological and poses less risk to the patient.

Artificial nutrition support

All patients who are malnourished or are at risk of becoming malnourished should be referred for nutritional support. Following a nutritional assessment, which includes an estimation of the patient's nutritional requirements, the route of nutrition support will be advised. The level of intervention depends on the patient's clinical condition (cause of nutritional depletion and disease process), function of the GI tract and potential accessibility for artificial feeding. Whenever possible, the patient should be involved in decision-making relating to artificial feeding which includes withholding and/or withdrawing nutrition support. Careful delivery and monitoring is essential as normal regulatory mechanisms are bypassed and complications associated with overfeeding, such as hyperglycaemia, hyperlipidaemia, fatty liver, and fluid and electrolyte disturbances, can be fatal.

Withholding and withdrawing nutrition support

The principles surrounding the decision-making process for withholding or withdrawal of nutrition are derived from ethical (autonomy, beneficence, non-maleficence, and justice) and legal principles.

Treatment or care

The provision of fluid and diet by mouth and any assistance that might be needed are considered 'basic care'. Whereas enteral tube feeding and PN are methods of artificial nutrition support and ∴ considered to be medical treatments. The consultant responsible for the patient's care will need to decide if artificial nutrition is appropriate. On initiating artificial nutrition support, treatment goals should be clearly stated. The provision of nutrition support might be intended to do the following:

- Impact on the disease process
- Prolong life by allowing time for recovery
- Improve quality of life
- Provide compassionate care for the relief of symptoms.

Autonomy

In respect of deciding about withdrawal or withholding of nutrition there are a number of autonomous considerations. Competent patients have the right to refuse treatment. Patients can make their wishes known regarding the advanced refusal of life-sustaining treatment; this might be done in anticipation of losing the ability to make treatment choices. Advance decisions, also known as 'advanced directives' or 'living wills', must fulfil specific criteria to be legally valid.

When people are unable to make this decision for whatever reason, for example, lack of capacity, the medical team should consult the family and carers of patients. Doctors are required to make treatment decisions in the 'best interest' of patients who lack the capacity to make their own decisions. This may not be in accordance with the family's wishes, if it is determined that their choice is not in the patient's best interest. Guidelines to assess competence have been produced jointly by the British Medical Association and the Law Society.

Beneficence

Lack of adequate nourishment will cause the physical decline associated with malnutrition. Methods of artificial nutrition support should be considered in those who cannot take enough food by mouth, but also take into account the potential net benefits. The provision of artificial nutrition support might be beneficial in terms of maintaining the body's systems, but, in conditions such as persistent vegetative state, it will not contribute to a recovery. Doctors are not expected to provide treatment if it is deemed to be futile and against their clinical judgement. If the futility of treatment is unknown, the following is expected:

- A second opinion is sought, perhaps from a clinical ethics team.
- A time-limited trial of nutrition should be provided.

Non-maleficence

It is the medical team's responsibility to discuss the risks and burdens (including discomfort) of treatment, in addition to the potential benefits, with the patient and, if relevant, the patient's family. To avoid harm to the patient receiving nutrition support, care should be provided by competent practitioners.

Justice

There is no legal or ethical basis for withholding or withdrawing nutrition support on the grounds of limited resources (equipment or appropriately trained personal). If care cannot be safely provided, the patient's care should be transferred to another hospital/care environment.

Nursing considerations

- Nurses should be aware that the authority to artificially feed, withhold, or withdraw nutrition lies with the consultant.
- Discussions regarding the provision, withdrawal, or withholding of artificial nutrition support should include the patient and their family, in addition to the nursing team.
- The nurse has a significant role in helping the patient to understand the need for the therapy, its potential risks and benefits, and the alternatives (including the consequences of not accepting the treatment) and in functioning as a patient advocate.
- Hospital nutrition support policy and procedure documents should contain guidelines on withholding and withdrawing nutrition support.

Enteral nutrition

EN is the provision of nutrition into the GI tract via tube feeding. EN can be used as the sole route for nutritional therapy or to supplement inadequate oral intake. The benefits of starting EN should outweigh any potential risks and follow the ethical principles of benefit, non-harm, justice, and autonomy (➲ p. 314–15). A risk assessment should be carried out and documented according to local guidelines.

Indications

Patients requiring enteral tube feeding are:
- Unable to take diet safely by mouth, such as unconscious patients, patients at risk of aspiration owing to dysphagia, or patients who have an upper GI pathology
- Unable to take enough diet by mouth to maintain their body weight and nutritional status and ∴ need supplementary enteral tube feeding
- Underweight and/or malnourished and cannot take enough diet by mouth to meet their ↑ nutritional requirements.

Enteral feeding tube access

Enteral feeding tubes can access the GI tract through the mouth (orogastric tube), nose (nasogastric tube, nasojejunal tube, or nasoduodenal tube), or the skin (gastrostomy tube, gastrojejunostomy tube, or jejunostomy tube) (Fig. 13.1). The choice of access depends on the proposed period of feeding, clinical condition of the patient, anatomy of the patient, patient choice, and expertise of the personnel available to insert the tube. Feeding via a tube inserted through the abdominal wall tend to be a longer-term feeding option.

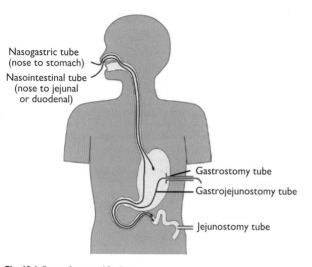

Fig. 13.1 Routes for enteral feeding.
Reproduced with kind permission © Burdett Institute 2008.

Further reading

https:// pathways.nice.org.uk/ pathways/ nutrition- support- in- adults/ parenteral-
nutrition#path=view%3A/ pathways/ nutrition-support-in-adults/ enteral-tube-feeding.
xml&content=view-index (Accessed 12/02/2020).

Short-term enteral feeding

Short-term feeding is usually defined as an anticipated period of feeding for up to 4 weeks.

Indications

There are several possible indications for short-term enteral feeding:

- A short trial (1–2 weeks) of nasogastric (NG) feeding may be used for people who have had a stroke, to maintain nutritional state and hydration, while establishing the possibility of recovery and assess the benefits of feeding, with the option of withdrawing tube feeding.
- NG tube feeding for a patient with oropharyngeal dysphagia following a stroke, while awaiting the recovery of swallow function. The patient might progress to a modified-consistency diet, with supplemental NG feeding, or require alternative long-term enteral access, if there is little or no improvement.
- Malnourished patients in preparation for surgery or in the post-operative period.

Short-term feeding routes

There are several short-term feeding routes:

Orogastric

The feeding tube is placed through the mouth into the stomach by direct vision in the critical care setting. Used when a NG tube placement is contra-indicated, such as basal skull or facial fractures. Tube position should be checked according to the NG tube protocol.

Pharyngostomy and oesophagostomy

A pharyngostomy and oesophagostomy can be placed at the time of laryngectomy but is rarely used. Tube position should be checked according to the NG tube protocol.

Nasogastric

NG tubes are the most common and appropriate route for short-term EN (<4 weeks). Alternatively, a NG tube can be used as a long-term enteral option if alternative methods are unsafe or not possible.

Nasointestinal

Nasointestinal feeding tubes are also referred to as post-pyloric feeding (placed beyond the pylorus of the stomach), such as nasoduodenal (ND) and nasojejunal (NJ) tubes. This option may be selected if there are concerns about gastro-oesophageal reflux causing aspiration into the lungs, delayed gastric emptying, or if intragastric feeding is contraindicated. NJ is required for patients with pancreatitis.

Short-term feeding tubes

Short-term feeding tubes are usually described according to how they are inserted into the GI tract and the distal tip location where the feed is de-livered, for example NG.

Ryles tubes: polyvinylchloride tubes
- Ryles tubes are large-bore tubes, mainly used for gastric decompression, but they can be used for short episodes of orogastric or NG feeding.
- Because of acid hardening, these tubes should be replaced within 10 days.

Fine-bore feeding tubes: polyvinylchloride (6–8FG)
- Fine-bore feeding tubes are usually non-guide-wire assisted.
- Used for short periods of feeding or if the patient is self-intubating on a daily basis.

Long-term enteral feeding

Long-term feeding is the term used for any patient requiring enteral feeding for >6 weeks. By this time, the benefits of continuing to feed are clearly established according to the goals of nutritional therapy. Although the use of gastrostomy tubes is advocated for the majority of patients requiring long-term feeding, this may not always be the case.

Long-term feeding tubes

Long-term feeding tubes are generally made from material that is more pliable (polyurethane and silicone) and therefore more comfortable for the patient. There are a number of fine-bore feeding tubes, made from polyurethane (6–8FG). These tubes are resistant to acid hardening and ∴ can stay in place for >4 weeks, as per the manufacturer's guidelines. Insertion of long-term feeding tubes is usually guidewire assisted. Long-term feeding tubes might have a double lumen for patients at risk of aspiration of gastric contents. This is to enable aspiration of stomach contents (Fig. 13.2) through one port and permit feeding into the duodenum or intestine through a distal port (nasointestinal route). These feeding tubes can be placed at the bedside but may need endoscopic or radiological placement.

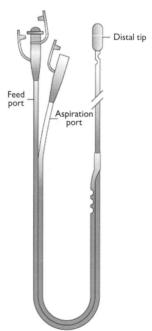

Fig. 13.2 Double-lumen feeding tube.
Reproduced with kind permission © Burdett Institute 2008.

Needle catheter jejunostomy

- A needle catheter jejunostomy is placed at the time of upper GI surgery in patients who are malnourished, where post-pyloric feeding is indicated, and secured with sutures or with a Dacron® cuff.
- Usually <12 FG thus avoid drug administration and take care with flushing as blocked tubes will need to be removed.

Gastrostomy tubes and gastrojejunal tubes

Gastrostomy tubes and gastrojejunal tubes are the most common method for long-term enteral feeding. Tubes have variable durability; some deteriorate more quickly due to interaction with some anti-epilepsy drugs, and micro-organisms such as *Candida*.

Drug administration and enteral nutrition

Patients requiring artificial nutrition support through enteral feeding tubes will often require administration of medication through the feeding tube. The nurse must be aware of the professional and legal issues relating to this aspect of care.

Professional and legal issues

Licensed drugs become 'unlicensed' if not prepared and administered in accordance with the manufacturers' specifications. This has particular relevance to crushing tablets, opening capsules, or delivering the drugs via an enteral tube, although, it is possible to prescribe medication for 'unlicensed' use, stating an alternative to the preparation or administration. In this situation, the nurse who will administer the drug must use his/her professional judgement according to current knowledge and skills in preparation and administration or omission of medication. It is reasonable for the nurse to seek further advice from the pharmacy drug information department regarding the suitability of the drug for enteral-tube administration, preparation, and dosage. The nurse must ensure that protocol is followed if the patient cannot receive their usual medication in situations whereby the feeding tube is blocked, damaged, or unintentionally removed; it is unacceptable to simply omit the drug.

Practice guidelines

The enteral feeding guidelines of the hospital should be followed to include consideration of:
- If safe to do so, drugs should be taken orally.
- Drugs might need to be given during a break in the continuous infusion if the drug is known to interact with the feed and there is a decrease in the efficacy of the drug, e.g. antacids (➋ p. 407), or drug absorption, e.g. carbamazepine, theophylline, or phenytoin.
- Certain drugs might not be absorbed at the site of delivery.
- Enteric-coated tablets, hormones, cytotoxic drugs, and sustained-release capsules should never be crushed.
- Liquid suspensions should be used in preference to crushing tablets or administering syrups.
- A 50 ml catheter-tip syringe should be used.
- Drugs should never be added to the feed solution.
- Measures to ↓ the risk of microbiological contamination should be adhered to.
- Before administration, ensure that the tube is correctly positioned.
- The tube should be flushed with 30 ml of water, to remove residual feed and ↓ the risks of drug–feed interactions, prior to drug administration, 10 ml of water between drugs, and 30 ml to flush the tube after drug administration.

Nasogastric tubes

NG tubes are inserted into the nose and pass down to the stomach for liquid feed +/− medication to be inserted via a non-oral route. There needs to be a clearly documented rationale for the insertion of an NG tube. Referral to the dietetic team should be timely to ensure that the patient has a nutritional assessment, feeding schedule, or prescription.

Cautions and contraindications

NG tube insertion is not always possible or carries ↑ risks associated with insertion or feeding. Careful assessment of the risks and benefits is necessary (Table 13.1).

Table 13.1 Contraindications for NG tube placement or feeding

Condition	Risk
Basal skull fracture	Intracranial placement
Altered mental state	Misplaced tubes
Severe gastro-oesophageal reflux	Aspiration pneumonia
Oesophageal perforation	Misplaced tube
Pathology of the nasopharynx, oropharynx, or oesophagus	Trauma/misplaced tube
Gastroparesis/poor gastric motility (high gastric aspirates)	Regurgitation/aspiration pneumonia
Severe acute pancreatitis	Exacerbation of pancreatitis

Placement of NG tube

The nurse should refer to their hospital policy for guidance on NG tube insertion. Documentation needs to include:
• Type of tube
• Length of tube inserted
• Method used to confirm tube position
• Planned replacement date
• Any difficulties encountered during the insertion.

The NG tube insertion can be undertaken by a competent registered nurse or student nurse under direct supervision of a competent nurse. If bedside placement of the feeding tube is not possible, alternative routes of tube placement, such as orogastric for patients with a history of basal skull fracture or NG placement using fluoroscopic methods should be considered. If the risks are associated with feeding, a plan of care should reflect actions to ↓ these risks.

Using the NG tube

There is a risk that NG tubes can be misplaced on insertion or during use. It is, therefore, necessary to verify where the distal tip is before each use. Regardless of the type of NG tube used, verification of the position should be made according to hospital policy.

NG tubes should be flushed with water before and after use. Flushing should occur before and after feeding or drug administration via the NG tube. It is also important to flush the NG tube before and after each drug if multiple doses are required to be administered via the NG tube.

Care of NG tubes

NG tubes should be secured to prevent pressure necrosis.
- Regular inspection of the nostril should be undertaken.
- Patients should be assisted with oral hygiene.

Care must be taken when assisting a patient to mobilize or reposition to ensure that the NG tube is not dislodged or accidentally removed.

Tube removal

Care should be taken when removing NG tubes. The feeding tube should be flushed and capped prior to removal. If the patient reports pain during tube removal, the procedure should be stopped and investigated for possible knotting of the NG tube. It should be clearly documented that the tube has been removed and noted if the tube is intact.

Gastrostomy tubes

Gastrostomy tubes (Fig. 13.3) are inserted through the abdominal wall into the stomach to enable insertion of liquid feed +/- medication. Gastrostomy tube feeding should be considered if EN is needed for >4 weeks. Occasionally, gastrostomy tubes are placed to facilitate gastric drainage, as a long-term alternative to NG tube placement. The principles of tube and site care are the same.

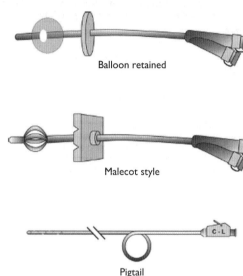

Balloon retained

Malecot style

Pigtail

Fig. 13.3 Gastrostomy tubes.
Reproduced with kind permission © Burdett Institute 2008.

Assessment

A pre-procedure patient assessment should be carried out with the following aims:
• Review of the appropriateness of artificial nutrition
• Assessment of the risks of the procedure.

It is also necessary to inform the patient and relevant carers of the procedure, risks, and aftercare.

Gastrostomy tube placement

Gastrostomy tubes can be placed endoscopically, radiologically, or surgically. Endoscopic and radiological gastrostomy tubes are associated with fewer complications than surgically placed tubes. Gastrostomy tubes are generally placed with concomitant antibiotic prophylaxis.

Percutaneous endoscopic gastrostomy

Percutaneous endoscopic gastrostomy (PEG) tubes are inserted with sedation and local anaesthetic to the abdominal wall There is a disc or flange retained internally (Fig 13.4)—lifespan of months to years.

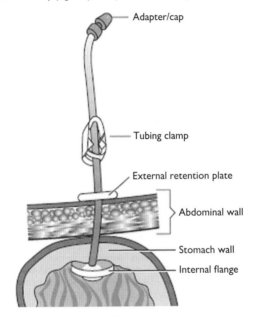

Adapter/cap

Tubing clamp

External retention plate

Abdominal wall

Stomach wall

Internal flange

Fig. 13.4 Cross-section showing a PEG.
Reproduced with kind permission © Burdett Institute 2008.

Surgical gastrostomy

Surgical gastrostomy (SG) tubes require a mini-laparotomy. The tubes are retained using a balloon or Malecot (Fig. 13.5) and there are deep abdominal sutures to secure the stomach to the abdominal wall. The balloon volume needs monitoring weekly.

Radiologically inserted gastrostomy

A radiologically inserted gastrostomy (RIG) requires sedation and local anaesthetic to abdominal wall. The RIG is retained with a Malecot, pigtail, or balloon (Fig. 13.2); for long-term tubes there can be a Dacron cuff, with a lifespan of months to years. The balloon volume needs monitoring weekly. There are deep abdominal sutures (T fasteners) to secure the stomach to the abdominal wall.

Low-profile gastrostomy tube

Low-profile replacement tubes are favoured in young adults and patients with active lifestyles (Fig. 13.5); also referred to as button gastrostomies. A balloon retained device is commonly used but Malecot style catheters are available and have the advantage that they have a longer durability. The balloon volume needs monitoring weekly. The replacement tubes are usually funded through the patient's primary care trust. The replacement procedure is undertaken by appropriately trained members of the nutrition team, the district nursing team or the patient.

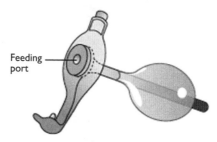

Feeding port

Fig. 13.5 Low-profile balloon gastrostomy.
Reproduced with kind permission © Burdett Institute 2008.

Post-procedure care

Local guidelines must be followed, include monitoring the patient for procedure-related complications, gastrostomy site (stoma) care, and the introduction of the enteral feed preparation.

Using gastrostomy tubes

Enteral feeding tubes should be flushed regularly, even if not in use. As a minimal standard there should be a flush before, between, and after any medicines or feed using a 50 ml syringe. In hospital, sterile water tends to be used for flushing for practical reasons, but at home freshly drawn tap water or cooled boiled water is more practical and not associated with any ↑ infective complications.

Care of gastrostomy

Gastrostomy stomas should be cleaned daily as part of daily hygiene. Initially the site should be cleaned with saline and gauze. Dressings are only indicated if the site is oozing or infected. Once healed the site can be cleaned with soap and water (refer to local policy) to reduce the risk of infection. As a general rule, gastrostomy tubes should be rotated through 360° daily. This is done by pushing the tube ventrally (inwards) 3–5 mm, rotating the tube and then carefully pulling the tube until it is felt against the abdominal wall. Then the external retention plate should be secured. This prevents internal tissue necrosis as well as internal and external over-granulation.

Replacement of gastrostomy tubes

A tract (fistula) develops over time (2–6 weeks), in addition to the adhesion of the anterior abdominal wall to the stomach. This is an important consideration in planning to replace the tube or if the tube falls out prematurely. An established tract enables tubes to be changed safely. PEG tubes should be replaced using the manufacturer's advice. Balloon and Malecot tubes (Fig. 13.1) can be replaced through the tract by competent trained personnel. The balloon volume needs monitoring weekly.

Enteral feeding complications

Complications associated with enteral feeding can be categorized as metabolic, mechanical, infective, or GI (Table 13.2).

Table 13.2 Summary of enteral nutrition complications

Complication	Examples of specific complications
Metabolic	• Hyperglycaemia (➔ p. 332), hypoglycaemia • Over-hydration, under-hydration • Electrolyte imbalance (➔ p. 332) • Drug–nutrient interactions (➔ p. 280) • Refeeding syndrome (➔ p. 348–9)
Mechanical	• Rhinitis, otitis, pharyngitis, oesophagitis (NG) • Mucosal erosion (➔ p. 333) • Tube blockage (➔ p. 333) • Tube displacement (➔ p. 333) • Colon perforation (PEG) • Buried bumper syndrome (PEG, PEG-J, PEJ)*
Infective	• Colonization of stoma site (➔ p. 334) • Aspiration pneumonitis (➔ p. 334)
Gastrointestinal	• Abdominal cramping, distension, nausea, and vomiting • Oesophageal reflux (➔ p. 36–7) • Malabsorption • Diarrhoea (➔ p. 335) • Constipation (➔ p. 335)

* PEG-J percutaneous endoscopic gastro-jejunostomy; PEJ percutaneous endoscopic jejunostomy.

Metabolic complications of enteral nutrition

Hyperglycaemia

Hyperglycaemia is usually related to insulin resistance and might require hyperglycaemic medication or insulin regimens.

Electrolyte imbalance

Electrolyte imbalance can result from over- or under-hydration, refeeding syndrome, medicine administration, or critical illness. Daily biochemical testing is required if electrolyte levels are abnormal or unstable. Intravenous (IV) or enteral correction might be necessary, depending on local.

Drugs–nutrient interaction

Medicines and feed can each affect the absorption of one another, which can, in turn, alter physiological processes and sometimes cause toxicity or deficiency of either therapeutic medicine levels or nutrients. Interactions are usually predictable and the pharmacist can advise on all medicine preparations and administration through feeding tubes.

Refeeding syndrome (➲ p. 348–9) is another complication under this category.

Mechanical complications of enteral nutrition

Mucosal erosion

Contact between a tube and the mucosa of the GI tract can lead to ulceration, pressure necrosis, and infection. Assess the site of the tube daily, for example, the nostrils for NG/NJ tubes and abdomen site for other tubes. If erythema, soreness, induration, or discharge are noted, the nutrition team needs to be contacted to review.

Blockages

Tube blockages are a common occurrence in enterally fed patients. Prevention is the best cure and ∴ flushing the tubes (to ensure no feed or medication is left in the tube) and administering medicines in the correct form are essential. If blockage is apparent, treatment should include checking the tube is not coiled or kinked under the dressing. Treatment should be as per local policy, which is to flush the tube:

- Use a 30 ml syringe and the push–stop technique—smaller syringes might rupture fine-bore feeding tubes.
- Use warm water as the first line of treatment.
- Other unblocking agents include sodium bicarbonate solution or pancreatic enzymes.

Displacement

Ensuring that feeding tubes are securely fixed to the skin will prevent most displacements. Daily checks should be encouraged. The use of nasal loops to prevent accidental NG/NJ tube removal has been successful and is becoming more widely used.

Infective complications of enteral feeding

Patients who are malnourished have an increased vulnerability to infection.

Infected stoma site

Stoma sites can become colonized without being infected. Check the site daily and take action if there are signs of an infection (red, hot, sore, indurated, or exuding pus).

Prevention

To prevent infection, it is important to follow local policy such as changing administration sets daily, and paying attention to hand-washing before accessing the feeding tube will minimize contamination.

Treatment

Treatment should be as per hospital policy but may include:

• Topical cleansing with antiseptics. Alcohol-based cleansers should be used with caution, to ensure they are compatible with the feeding tube.
• Systemic antibiotics must be given in severe cases.
• Topical antibiotics are generally avoided; as they can cause damage to the feeding tube.
• Silver-impregnated charcoal dressings may be useful to ↓ PEG-site colonization and ↓ in the incidence of clinically infected PEG sites.

Aspiration

Aspiration into the lungs can occur in any patient with dysphagia or compromised swallow function, regardless of the route of feeding. Minimizing risk includes:

• Careful assessment of gastric residual volumes in patients with upper GI dysmotility or delayed gastric emptying
• Careful use of prokinetic agents (➜ p. 412)
• Ensuring the patient is sitting up at an angle of at least 30°
• Preventing constipation.

Gastrointestinal disturbances of enteral feeding

Abdominal cramping, abdominal distension, nausea, and vomiting are not uncommon in the early stages of EN. Symptoms may be reduced by ↓ the rate of feed or reviewing medication.

Diarrhoea

In most circumstances, diarrhoea (➋ p. 412) is unlikely to be caused by EN and other causes should be investigated. Unresolved diarrhoea can ↑ nutritional requirements, lead to malabsorption of certain nutrients, or vitamins/minerals and affect fluid balance. In addition to infective agents, diarrhoea can be caused by:

- Medicines, such as antibiotics, which can alter gut flora and may increase gut motility or cause *Clostridium difficile* (C diff).
- Feed, although this is unlikely to be the cause, there may be concerns with osmolarity or malabsorption.

Constipation

Patients receiving EN might develop constipation (➋ p. 204–5), thus bowel activity should be monitored and recorded daily, according to local policy. Constipation can occur as a result of dehydration, a lack of fibre, certain medical conditions, or medicines. Regular assessment of fluid requirements is necessary, especially in hot weather.

Home enteral nutrition

Once the person is medically stable within the hospital environment it is important to continue to provide nutritional support at home or within residential care: this is termed home enteral nutrition (HEN). There are >20,000 adults in the UK who have made the transition from hospital to receiving their tube feed in the community. If appropriate the patient should be supported to be self-caring (42% of patients are independent) with the feeding tube and feeding regime. Alternatively, family, significant others, or healthcare professionals can assist.

Feed, medication, tubes, and feeding pumps are delivered as per local policy, plus ancillaries, such as syringes and giving sets. It is also important to have contact numbers and guidelines to follow if a complication occurs for example.

The majority (43%) of people being sent home with new enteral feed are patients with cancer, the majority being head and neck cancers. Other reasons for home enteral feed include patients with central nervous system problems such as cerebrovascular disorders and neuro-degenerative disorders. Most people with HEN have a gastrostomy tube. There is a patient support group: Patients on Intravenous and Nasogastric Nutrition Therapy (PINNT).

Further reading

https://www.bapen.org.uk/nutrition-support/enteral-nutrition/home-enteral-nutrition (Accessed 12/02/2019).
https://www.nice.org.uk/guidance/cg32 (Accessed 12/02/2019).
https://pinnt.com/Home.aspx (Accessed 12/02/2019).

Parenteral nutrition

PN or intravenous nutrition (IVN) refers to the administration of nutrients into the circulatory system, bypassing the GI tract. In American literature, the term used is 'intravenous hyperalimentation' (IVH) or 'hyperalimentation'. The terms 'parenteral nutrition' is used in preference to the term 'total parenteral nutrition' or 'TPN'. The term TPN is no longer used as the complete range of nutrients cannot always be safely administered in the PN solution; also, nutritional therapy is likely to include some oral or enteral intake. PN is expensive and complex therapy with the risk of potentially life-threatening complications.

Indications

The GI tract is the best route for nourishing the patient and should be used if safe but PN is indicated for a minority of patients who require artificial nutrition support (Table 13.3). The table can be used as a decision-making guide. The two categories of patients who might require PN are:
- Intestinal failure (IF)—if the absorptive function of the intestine is impaired and persisted for >5 days and it is anticipated that there will not be a significant improvement. IF might be acute or chronic.
- Inaccessible GI tract—if the ingestion of nutrients or the safe placement of enteral feeding tubes is impossible and this has persisted or is likely to persist for 5 days or more.

Table 13.3 Examples of indications for PN

Intestinal failure	Example	Considerations
Acute	Prolonged postoperative ileus. Gut rest following upper GI surgery	Careful pre-operative assessment for upper GI surgery, considering possible enteral access during surgery, e.g. NJ or surgical jejunostomy tube placement instead of PN
Chronic	Extreme small bowel resection, radiation enteritis, visceral myopathy, scleroderma, high-output fistula	Try to minimize symptoms and maximise enteral intake, in addition to home PN
Inaccessible gastrointestinal tract	Severe mucositis, severe pancreatitis, oesophageal perforation, oesophageal pouch, oesophageal stricture	Consideration of pathology and clinical conditions that prohibit a normal oral intake and there are risks associated with enteral tube placement and feeding

Further reading

The National Nurses Nutrition Group http://www.nnng.org.uk
https://pathways.nice.org.uk/pathways/nutrition-support-in-adults/parenteral-nutrition#path=view%3A/pathways/nutrition-support-in-adults/parenteral-nutrition.xml&content=view-index (Accessed 15/02/2019).

Parenteral nutrition: central venous catheter access

The decision regarding the route of PN will mainly depend on the risks associated with potential infection and mechanical complications. The patient's clinical condition, current venous access, nutritional requirements, anticipated duration of therapy, patient comfort, and management of the device should also be considered.

Central venous catheters

Central venous catheters (CVCs) are designed to provide access to the thoracic vessels, returning blood to the right-hand side of the heart (Fig. 13.6). The catheter tip should lie at the junction of the superior vena cava and the right atrium of the heart, as the flow and volume of blood are greatest; thus, infused fluids are diluted, enabling large volumes of potentially irritant solutions to be infused.

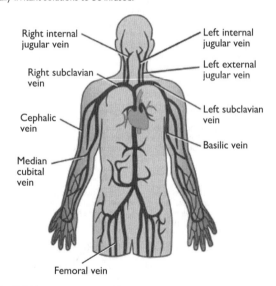

Fig. 13.6 Venous access sites.

Reproduced with kind permission © Burdett Institute 2008.

Catheter material

There are a variety of different types of catheters, which are chosen for their physical characteristics associated with the type of plastic from which they are manufactured. Important considerations should include:

- Strength
- Pliability
- Thromboresistant properties
- Compatibility with the infusion agent
- Visibility on X-ray
- Durability.

Number of lumens

National guidelines advocate the use of single-lumen catheters for the administration of PN. Multi-lumen catheters are acceptable if a port can be dedicated to the use of PN. Advanced planning for patients anticipated to require multiple therapies (chemotherapy or long-term antibiotic therapy) warrants the placement of long-term multi-lumen CVCs.

Tunnelled catheters

Tunnelled catheters can be sutured to secure the catheter for short-term use. Catheters intended for use for more than three weeks are recommended to have a Dacron cuff that is positioned on the catheter within the subcutaneous tunnel. Fibrosis of the cuff anchors the catheter to the subcutaneous tissue within 21 days. This type of catheter has the advantage of ↓ the risk of colonization, avoiding the need of external fixation and ∴ is more comfortable for the patient.

Non-tunnelled catheters

Catheters should preferentially (if not contraindicated) be placed in the subclavian vessel; then consider the jugular vessel and finally femoral sites.

Peripherally inserted central catheters (PICCs)

Access the central venous system through the basilic, median cubital, or cephalic veins. Complications associated with the conventional placement of CVCs are avoided, but they are not indicated for patients requiring long-term PN who will be responsible for catheter care.

Totally implanted devices

Also known as 'implantable ports' (Port-a-Cath®). Rather than having an external component, the catheter has a titanium reservoir (single or double chamber) that is placed surgically in the subcutaneous pocket of the chest wall, abdomen, or forearm (peripheral vein access). Although promoted to ↓ the issue of altered body image, the placement and removal procedures are surgical procedures that carry the risk of greater scarring compared with conventional central catheter placement.

Surgical implant

A transthoracic approach to placement of central catheters (superior vena cava or right atrium) might be considered if the central vessels cannot be safely accessed. This requires referral to a vascular surgeon.

Parenteral nutrition: peripheral vein catheter access

Peripheral access is indicated in patients who are anticipated to need PN for <14 days. PN administration through the peripheral veins is limited by high infusion rates and the need for high levels of electrolytes and hypertonic solutions.

Standard peripheral cannula

Peripheral cannulae (18 Fr) are commonly placed in the peripheral veins of the hand. They require vigilance and regular replacement (24–48 h) to prevent thombophlebitis. This site should usually be avoided for the administration of PN, as vessels are too small.

Midline catheters

Fine (18–23 Fr) polyurethane–hydromer-coated radio-opaque catheters 15–20 cm long. They are described as midline or medium-vein catheters because they are intended to be placed in the medium veins of the antecubital fossa. These catheters are promoted for peripheral use because they are less thrombogenic and tend to have a lifespan of 5–28 days. They should be removed promptly at the first signs of phlebitis.

Further reading

Hamilton H (ed.) (2000). *Total Parenteral Nutrition: A Practical Guide for Nurses*. Churchill Livingstone, Edinburgh.

Parenteral nutrition: catheter insertion

Catheters are commonly placed percutaneously but can be placed as a surgical procedure (described as a 'cut-down procedure'). For non-tunnelled catheters, accessing the subclavian vein is the first choice for placement, followed by the jugular vessel, and then the femoral vessel. Techniques for cannulating the vessel include insertion of a catheter through the needle, over the needle, through a cannula, and over a guidewire. The technique used will be dictated by the make of catheter and operator preference. Catheters are often placed under ultrasound guidance or fluoroscopy (to ensure successful placement and ↓ potential life-threatening complications) in vascular suites of the radiology department. Patients having long-term catheters inserted should be consulted about the preferred exit site. Observe the following for placement of CVC:

- Maximal sterile precautions—sterile gown, gloves, and large drapes must be used.
- Skin preparation—chlorhexidine gluconate (2–5%) in 70% isopropyl alcohol.
- Patients are usually sedated and ∴ require oxygen therapy.
- The patient will be placed in the Trendelenburg position (to ↓ the risk of air embolism) unless contraindicated.

Complications

Fewer complications will occur if the operator is experienced, but complications related to central catheter insertion include:

- Malpositioned catheters (↑ the risk of thrombosis and arrhythmias)
- Haemorrhage
- Pneumothorax
- Air embolism
- Nerve damage
- Infection.

Parenteral nutrition: catheter care

In the immediate post-insertion period, it is important to monitor the patient as per local policy. This will include appropriate dressings to the insertion site. It is important to observe for signs and symptoms of procedure-related complications as listed in Table 13.4. (◑ p. 342).

Table 13.4 Central catheter complications

Later complications	Comments
Catheter-related infection (exit-site, tunnel, bloodstream infection)	Following protocols will ↓ the risk of infection. Careful monitoring of the patient's condition will detect potential problems, making early interventions more likely to succeed. Exit-site infection can be successfully treated using antibiotic therapy and frequent dressing changes. Infection of the subcutaneous tunnel warrants catheter removal. Salvaging catheters should only be attempted for long-term central catheters following consultation with the microbiologist, according to evidence-based protocols
Central vein thrombosis	Caused by catheter-tip position (proximal location in the superior vena cava) and the composition of the infusion. Symptoms include neck and face swelling (more noticeable in the morning following infusion) which should prompt upper limb venography. Treat using infusion of thrombolytic therapy
Catheter occlusion	Causes include luminal deposits of fibrin, lipid amorphous debris, or kinking. Catheter-care protocols should limit blood sampling, routine withdrawal of blood, and meticulous flushing technique. Ethanol (70%) solution lock can be used to treat lipid occlusions and fibrinolytics can be used to treat blood-related occlusions (identified by recent history of flashback or withdrawal occlusion)
Catheter damage	A damaged catheter puts the patient at risk of air embolism, in addition to infection. Damage might be caused by flushing using excessive pressure, incompatible connections, friction between the clavicle and first rib (subclavian catheters), or wear and tear of long-term catheters. Accidental fracture is rare. Patients should be trained to use atraumatic clamps for immediate first-aid management. Long-term catheters can be repaired

Flushing

Catheters should be flushed with 0.9% sodium chloride solution using a push–pause technique and positive-pressure clamping.

Accessing the catheter

Appropriate cleaning solutions should be used for hub decontamination. Furthermore, catheters should not be used routinely for blood sampling.

Parenteral nutrition: formulation

PN solutions are highly complex chemical mixtures that might contain >50 different ingredients. Strict compounding procedures must be followed to ensure that the ingredients are compatible and remain stable in the infusion bag. PN provides energy (in the form of glucose or combined with lipid), nitrogen (as amino acids), water, electrolytes, and micronutrients.

Many hospitals rely on commercially produced solutions and emulsions (containing lipid) that have a long shelf life. Standard or 'off-the-shelf bags' are used for convenience and can be suitable for patients who do not have unusual electrolyte or fluid requirements.

Additions should never be made outside the aseptic unit. This is to avoid compatibility problems and introducing infection.

Parenteral nutrition—infusion

A volumetric pump with alarms for ↑ pressure and air must be used. Accumulation of air in the giving set can be ↓ by allowing the feed to reach room temperature before administration (it must never be artificially warmed).

Change the giving set every 24 h. Continuous infusion over a 24 h period is required on commencement of PN therapy. Infusions should not hang for >24 h (the time starts on removal of the bag from the refrigerator).

Cyclical infusions

Cyclical infusion is advocated to ↓ the risk of abnormal liver function and fatty liver. It will also improve the patient's ability to mobilize and participate in usual activities.

The infusion is delivered over a period of 10–20 h. This type of infusion is used if:

- The patient's condition allows.
- The patient has an appropriate intravascular device.
- The patient can tolerate the ↑ hourly fluid and nutrient delivery.

There are a number of potential complications:

The most common problems associated with PN are fluid and electrolyte abnormalities, with high faecal losses possibly associated with an underlying GI condition. Retention of fluid might be associated with renal, cardiac, or hepatic failure, alternatively an over-prescription of fluid and salt. Fluid retention will further impair gastric and intestinal motility and delay the progression to oral/enteral intake. The risk of refeeding syndrome should be considered before commencing and during PN. Hyperglycaemia, resulting from insulin resistance, is common in the stressed patient. If the patient is hyperglycaemic and not receiving excess macronutrients, they will need an IV insulin infusion. Additionally, care is needed to ensure vulnerable patients do not suffer hypoglycaemia when cyclical infusions are discontinued. Patients who are malnourished at the start of therapy or take little by mouth in the long term are potentially at risk of micronutrient deficiencies.

Effects of PN on other systems

Abnormalities associated with the hepatobiliary system will also be affected by malnutrition, underlying disease (e.g. inflammatory bowel disease, sepsis, or malignancy), drug therapy, and a limited oral intake (predisposing to biliary sludge). The infusion of excess lipid or glucose will cause hepatic steatosis—in this situation there should be a temporary omission of lipid from the infusion, cyclical feeding, and a review of the feed prescription. Investigations and biochemistry (ultrasound and biopsy) are rarely indicated. Metabolic bone disease is more of a consideration for patients receiving long-term PN, especially if they have a history of malnutrition or corticosteroid therapy. Intestinal permeability (with associated bacterial translocation) and intestinal atrophy are concerns for patients who do not take an oral diet.

Home parenteral nutrition

Home parenteral nutrition (HPN) is undoubtedly a life-saving therapy for patients with IF or patients for whom attempts to establish enteral feeding access have failed. Although continuing PN therapy in the community is expensive, HPN is a considerably cheaper alternative to a prolonged hospital stay, but it is a complex therapy, with several potentially life-threatening complications. Additionally, patients with IF are likely to have a chronic intestinal condition. HPN was first described in 1970. The number of patients on HPN in 2012 was over 1000, and the number of patients on HPN dramatically increased subsequently. Although most new patients are aged between 41 and 60, a proportion of patients receiving HPN are aged between 70 and 90.

Patients might need HPN for different periods of time:
- Short term—weeks for patients requiring palliative care for example.
- Medium term—months to years for patients with resolving IF or awaiting reconstructive surgery.
- Long term—decades for patients with type III chronic IF.

Discharge planning

The majority of patients can be taught how to safely care for their CVC and IV infusion. The time needed to learn the aseptic techniques is ~4–6 weeks. All patients on HPN will need 24 h telephone access to their clinical team, monitoring in a nutrition clinic, information about the national patient support group (PINNT), and an awareness of the availability of social and psychological support.

Further reading

https://www.bapen.org.uk/nutrition-support/parenteral-nutrition/home-parenteral-nutrition (Accessed 16/02/2019).
https://pinnt.com/Home.aspx (Accessed 17/02/2019).

Refeeding syndrome

Refeeding syndrome is a combination of potentially life-threatening complications associated with too rapid reintroduction of feeding in patients who are malnourished, after a period of starvation, or have had a poor dietary intake. The syndrome is characterized by life-threatening micronutrient deficiencies, fluid and electrolyte imbalance, and organ and metabolic dysfunctions. Thus, extreme care should be taken in initiating nutrition support. This might cause cardiac, respiratory, neurological, neuromuscular, renal, haematological, hepatic, and metabolic problems.

Causes

The reason that refeeding syndrome may occur is during starvation, insulin production is ↓ because the intake of carbohydrate is ↓. Catabolism of protein and fat stores provides energy, with the loss of intracellular electrolytes. On feeding, carbohydrate becomes the main energy source, resulting in ↑ secretion of insulin. This, in turn, causes a metabolic shift, with the cellular uptake of electrolytes (phosphate, potassium, and magnesium) causing a rapid ↓ in serum electrolyte levels. There is ↑ demand for electrolytes and micronutrients.

Patients are at risk of refeeding syndrome if they have two or more of the following:

- Body mass index (BMI) <18.5 kg/m²
- Unintentional weight loss of >10% of body weight in the previous three to six months
- Little or no intake for more than five days
- History of alcohol abuse, chemotherapy, antacids, or diuretics.

People are at a higher risk of refeeding syndrome with the following:
- BMI <16 kg/m²
- Unintentional weight loss of >15% of body weight in the previous three to six months
- Little or no intake for >10 days
- Low serum potassium, phosphate, or magnesium before feeding.

Treatment

It is recommended that:

- All patients must be screened on admission, to identify their nutritional risk and referred to the nutrition and dietetic services.
- Seriously ill patients and those who have eaten little for >5 days, should have their artificial nutrition support started at no greater than 50% of their estimated need and ↑ gradually.
- All patients at risk should have baseline biochemical monitoring, with frequent monitoring while the feed is introduced.
- Patients at high risk of refeeding syndrome and those at risk of Wernike–Korsakoff syndrome should receive a high dose of thiamine and vitamin B complex supplementation before and during the first 10 days of feeding.

- People at high risk should have feed introduced at a rate of 5–10kcal/kg body weight/day, ↑ slowly over a period of seven days.
- Pre-feeding serum electrolyte levels are usually within the normal range; correction of low levels can only be successfully achieved once feeding has commenced.
- Daily requirements for potassium, phosphate, and magnesium are ↑.

Off-the-shelf PN formulations must not be used without appropriate additions.

Wernike–Korsakoff syndrome

Wernike–Korsakoff syndrome is a life-threatening complication associated with feeding patients who are malnourished or have had a poor dietary intake. Neurological symptoms of this syndrome include apathy, depression, ataxia, eye movement disorders, and short-term memory impairment. Alcoholics and those with chronic vomiting disorders are at risk. This is caused by an acute thiamine deficiency secondary to an ↑ demand for thiamine as the body reverts to carbohydrate metabolism.

Thus, extreme care should be taken in initiating nutrition support. Micronutrient deficiencies as well as fluid and electrolyte shifts can occur if too much feed is given, feed is given too quickly or the feed is unbalanced. This might cause cardiac, respiratory, neurological, neuromuscular, renal, haematological, hepatic, and metabolic problems.

Distal limb feeding (fistuloclysis)

The term distal limb feeding, also known as fistuloclysis, is an uncommon method of infusing nutrients into a 'defunctioned' bowel. The bowel might be 'defunctioned' because of a fistula or a loop stoma for example. It is important to have a clear goal to determine the purpose of the distal limb feeding. Distal limb feeding may be used to increase absorption and to help prevent atrophy of the distal portion of bowel. The distal limb feeding may be supplementary nutrition support or the sole method of gaining nutrition. In some cases, it is possible to stop PN if distal limb feeding is successful and there is adequate bowel length and bowel function.

Feed is provided by insertion of a feeding tube into the distal segment of the fistulated bowel. The feeding tube will be inserted through the stoma or fistula appliance. Care must be taken to secure the tube so that it cannot migrate into or out of the bowel.

The 'feed' can be enteral formula or the output from the gut (stoma or fistula) and is termed chyme. Furthermore, the feed can be a bolus or continuous. Continuous is more commonly used to reduce the need for PN. Bolus infusions are less likely to have this benefit. Chyme might contain particles and thus might need to be sieved to remove any particles that might block the feeding tube; but it has the benefit of containing some of digestive enzymes.

To be considered for distal limb feeding there is generally considered that 100 cm of healthy small bowel is necessary.

Side effects of distal limb feeding include:
- Diarrhoea
- Nausea and vomiting
- Abdominal pain.

Chapter 14

Colorectal cancer

Colorectal cancer

Most colorectal cancers (>90%) arise from adenomatous polyps (adenomas) that become adenocarcinomas. Adenomas are common and seen in many of the UK population. The process of an adenoma changing to a carcinoma is seen in Fig. 14.1. This process is in general slow, taking up to 10 years for a cancer to develop.

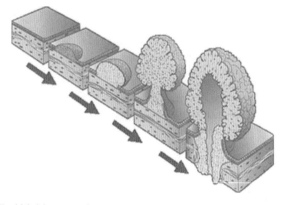

Fig. 14.1 Adenoma–carcinoma sequence.
Reproduced with kind permission © Burdett Institute 2008.

Most colorectal cancers are sporadic rather than hereditary. Sporadic cancers occur as a result of a genetic mutation which can occur by chance but is increased by exposure to risk factors, such as smoking. Hereditary means that there is a genetic mutation passed from parent to child in the DNA (deoxyribonucleic acid), accounting for about 5% of all colorectal cancers. Hereditary colorectal cancers include familial adenomatous polyposis (FAP) (➲ p. 92–3).

Colorectal cancer—staging

Colorectal cancer, also termed bowel cancer, can be seen as the uncontrolled growth of cells within the colon and/or rectum that have the ability to spread to other parts of the body. There are a number of ways to stage colorectal cancer: using the TNM staging system, stages 1–4, or the Dukes staging system.

TNM staging system:

T denotes the tumour.

N denotes spread to nearby lymph nodes.

M denotes metastasis.

The TNM staging system is graded as follows:

Tumour:

- T1—the tumour is within the inner layer of the bowel
- T2—the tumour has spread from the inner layer to the muscle layer of the bowel wall
- T3—the tumour has spread into the muscle layer of the bowel wall
- T4—the tumour has spread through the outer layer of the bowel wall.

Nodes:

- N0—no tumour has spread into the lymph nodes
- N1—there is cancer spread into 1–3 lymph nodes
- N2—there is can cancer spread into 4 or more nearby lymph nodes.

Metastases:

- M0—no cancer spread to other organs
- M1—cancer has spread to other parts of the body.

Whereas using number staging:

Stage 1—the cancer is within the bowel or rectal lining but not past the muscle wall (T1N0M0 or T2N0M0)

Stage 2—the cancer has spread beyond the bowel muscle +/− into nearby local surfaces (T3N0M0 or T4N0M0)

Stage 3—the cancer has spread to nearby lymph nodes (any TN1M0 or any TN2M0)

Stage 4—the cancer has spread to a distant organ, commonly the liver (anyTanyNM1); also termed advanced cancer.

In Dukes staging system:

Dukes A—cancer is in the inner lining of the bowel +/− a little spread into the muscle layer.

Dukes B—cancer has spread through the muscle layer of the bowel

Dukes C—cancer has spread to at least one nearby lymph node

Dukes D—cancer has metastases to other parts of the body such as the liver.

Grading

Grade I—well differentiated—similar to normal cells and less likely to spread

Grade II—moderately differentiated—appears more abnormal

Grade III—poorly differentiated—appears very abnormal and more likely to spread.

Colorectal cancer—symptoms

Many people have no signs of colorectal cancer but symptoms include:
- Rectal bleeding
- Change in bowel habit
- Abdominal discomfort
- Abdominal bloating
- Abdominal pain
- Unplanned weight loss.

There are many other reasons that these symptoms can occur, such as bleeding haemorrhoids.

More advanced cancer can present with bowel obstruction, with symptoms of:
- Absence of bowel action, occasionally severe, worse after eating
- Abdominal pain
- Unintentional weight loss
- Abdominal swelling
- Vomiting.

Abdominal obstruction requires urgent medical attention.

Colorectal cancer—causes

The exact cause of colorectal cancer is not fully understood but there are some risk factors making it more likely to develop:

• Polyps in the bowel lining can become cancerous, but this process, if it does occur, often takes several years.
• Other risk factors include:
  • Age over 60
  • Family history—a first-degree relative (mother, father or sibling) diagnosed with colorectal cancer under 50 years of age
  • Diet—high in red and processed meat
  • Smoking
  • Excessive consumption of alcohol
  • Obesity, particularly in men
  • Lack of physical exercise
  • Long-term, extensive inflammatory bowel disease (➋ p. 368–9)
  • Genetic conditions, such as FAP (➋ p. 92–3), carry an almost certain cancer risk by age 50.

Protective factors include a diet high in fibre.

Most colorectal cancers (more than 90%) develop from adenomatous polyps (adenomas).

Colorectal cancer—incidence

About 1 in 20 people develop colorectal cancer, making it the 4th most common cancer diagnosed in the UK. In 2015, there were about 42,000 new cases of colorectal cancer diagnosed in the UK, which accounts for about 12% of all cancers diagnosed that year. Incidence is largely unchanged since the early 1990s but is anticipated to reduce as a result of bowel screening (➲ p. 365).

There is a higher number of men (55%) diagnosed than women (45%) in the UK.

Most people in the UK are diagnosed as stage II, III, or IV.

Almost 90% of cases are diagnosed in people aged 60 or more.

The most common area for a colorectal cancer to develop is the rectum: a third in men and a quarter in women. This increases to two-thirds of men and half of women when the sigmoid colon and rectum are considered together.

There are higher incidences of colorectal cancer in developed countries than areas such as Asia and many parts of Africa.

Further reading

https://www.cancerresearchuk.org/health-professional/cancer-statistics/statistics-by-cancer-type/bowel-cancer/incidence (Accessed 10/04/2019).

Colorectal cancer—investigations

There are a number of investigations that might be carried out by the GP for someone with a suspected colorectal cancer, including:
- Digital rectal examination (DRE)
- Blood tests—for iron deficiency anaemia.

Additional tests in hospital to diagnose a colorectal cancer may include:
- Endoscopy—flexible sigmoidoscopy (● p. 249), colonoscopy (● p. 246–7), +/− biopsy
- Computed tomography (CT) colonography (● p. 220); also termed virtual colonoscopy (VC)
- CT scan (● p. 220) for bowel obstruction.

If a colorectal cancer is diagnosed, there are some further tests that might be carried out:
- CT scan of the chest and abdomen (● p. 220)—to check for spread to the liver or lungs
- Magnetic resonance imaging (MRI) (● p. 222)—for rectal cancer to provide imaging for the surrounding organs.

Colorectal cancer—treatment

Coordination of cancer treatment is undertaken in the UK by the multidisciplinary team. This team will include, at a minimum, a surgeon, oncologist, radiologist, and specialist nurse. There are three main treatment options for colorectal cancer: surgery, chemotherapy, and/or radiotherapy, with surgery being most common. Treatment will depend upon which part of the bowel is affected and the staging of the cancer. Ideally treatment aims to cure the cancer but treatment can be palliative to control symptoms or slow the spread of the cancer. If all of the cancer is removed during surgery, this is termed an R0, as there is no residual tumour left. If all visible cancer is removed but microscopic cancer cells are left this is called an R1 resection. Whereas if there is visible tumour left in situ at the end of the operation, this is an R2 resection margin. The more advanced the cancer, the less chance of a cure; this is also the case if there are any macroscopic or microscopic cancer cells remaining.

Colorectal cancer—surgery

For early cancers that have not spread, it is possible to have a local excision of the cancer: simply taking a small area of the bowel lining. In some centres this can be undertaken endoscopically or transanally (via the anus).

If the cancer is within the bowel walls, such as the muscle layer (⊃ p. 358–60), then a section of the colon and/or rectum may need to be removed. This can include colonic operations, such as a left hemicolectomy (⊃ p. 488–9) or a right hemicolectomy (⊃ p. 488–9). Rectal surgery can include an anterior resection (⊃ p. 482), TME (total mesorectal excision) (⊃ p. 482), or an abdominoperineal resection of the rectum (⊃ p. 478–9).

Chemotherapy

Chemotherapy is the use of systematic medication to shrink or kill the cancer cells. Chemotherapy is systemic and will affect healthy as well as cancerous cells but it can also treat local and metastatic disease. Medication can be in the form of tablets (oral chemotherapy) and/or intravenous chemotherapy. Chemotherapy given before surgery is termed neoadjuvant, whereas chemotherapy given after surgery is termed adjuvant, and finally there is palliative chemotherapy to slow the spread of the cancer or it may be used for symptom control. The length of time needed for chemotherapy depends upon a variety of issues such as response and can last for up to six months.

Side effects

The side effects of chemotherapy include:
- Fatigue
- Nausea
- Vomiting
- Diarrhoea
- Mucositis (⊃ p. 48)
- Altered sensations such as numbness, tingling and burning in feet, hands, and neck (palmar/plantar syndrome)
- Pancytopenia (deficiency in red blood cells, white blood cells, and platelets).

These side effects usually resolve when the chemotherapy ends. It should be noted that hair loss is uncommon when associated with chemotherapy for colorectal cancer. Chemotherapy also weakens the immune system, increasing the risk of infections. Furthermore, chemotherapy can affect fertility, temporarily damaging sperm and eggs. Sometimes changes in treatment dose are required if side effects are intolerable.

Nursing advice

The nurse should advise the need for rest interspersed with activity. Antiemetics can be advised to treat/prevent nausea and vomiting and to try small frequent meals. Diarrhoea can be reduced with medication such as Loperamide and regular sipping of drinks throughout the day. To help mucositis, keep lips well moisturized and encourage teeth cleaning after each meal with a soft toothbrush. Importantly, the nurse should advise the patient to seek medical assistance if they notice signs of an infection, such as pyrexia or feeling generally unwell. Also advise the use of a reliable contraceptive during and for a time after chemotherapy.

Radiotherapy

Radiotherapy is the use of radio waves to treat cancer, potentially reducing the tumour size or eradicating all tumour cells. There are two types of radiotherapy: external radiotherapy and brachytherapy (internal radiotherapy). External radiotherapy beams radio waves at the rectum; it is often given daily for five days each week. Treatment is often given for between 1 and 5 weeks for up to 15 minutes a session. Alternatively, brachytherapy is the insertion of a small amount of radiation into the rectum, through the anus. Brachytherapy may be undertaken after radiotherapy and prior to surgery and may involve several sessions. Palliative radiotherapy often is given for up to 10 days.

Radiotherapy can be used before surgery to shrink a rectal cancer, increasing the chance of a complete removal of the cancer. Radiotherapy might shrink the cancer so well that there is nothing visible at the end of the treatment. In this case, it is uncertain whether to resect that area; some centres choose a 'watch and wait' option for certain people. Alternatively for people who cannot have surgery, radiotherapy might be useful for an early rectal cancer. For people with advanced cancer, it might be useful to have palliative radiotherapy to control symptoms or slow the spread of the cancer.

Side effects

There are a number of side effects of radiotherapy that include:
- Nausea
- Fatigue
- Diarrhoea
- Localized skin irritation, that feels like sunburn
- Frequent urination
- Burning sensation on urination.

In general side effects resolve after radiotherapy ceases. There are potential long-term side effects of radiotherapy that include:
- More frequent passage of urine and faeces
- Passing blood per rectum or urethra
- Infertility (consider egg or sperm storage)
- Erectile dysfunction.

Biological treatments

Biological treatments have been more recently used to treat, but not cure, advanced colorectal cancer rather than chemotherapy or radiotherapy. Biological treatments are also termed monoclonal antibodies. Monoclonal antibodies are antibodies from laboratory-manufactured clones that are derived from a single cell and bind to a specific protein in the body, such as on a cancer cell. This can help to treat cancer in a number of ways: stimulating the body's own immune system or carrying substances directly to the cancer cells, such as drugs, toxins, or radioactive substances. Sometimes this type of treatment is called targeted therapy. Biological treatments can be used alone or in combination with other treatments for cancer.

Side effects

There are a number of side effects that are associated with biological treatments, such as:
- Fatigue
- Nausea
- Anorexia
- Sore mouth
- Anaemia.

Colorectal cancer—prevention

It is not possible to prevent a colorectal cancer from occurring but it is possible to have a healthy life-style that will reduce the risks of developing cancer. Risk factors that can be modified include:

- Smoking
- High alcohol consumption
- Being overweight/obese (→ p. 306–7)
- High consumption of red meats
- High consumption of processed meats
- Physical inactivity.

Other risk factors include:

- Increasing age, over 50 years
- Personal history
- Family history of colorectal cancer
- Inflammatory bowel disease (→ p. 368–9)
- Type II diabetes.

Another way to prevent colorectal cancer is to undertake bowel cancer screening (→ p. 365).

Colorectal cancer—prognosis

Colorectal cancer survival is currently increasing, but the UK remains be-hind many other similar countries. Survival has more than doubled from 22% to 57% in 40 years. The survival rate at 1 year from diagnosis is 76%, dropping to 59% at 5 years and remaining fairly static at 10 years. Rates are fairly similar for both men and women.

10-year survival for colorectal cancer ranks as 10th highest in England and Wales.

Further reading

https://www.cancerresearchuk.org/health-professional/cancer-statistics/statistics-by-cancer-type/bowel-cancer/survival [Accessed 16 April 2019]

Colorectal cancer—survivorship

Treatment for cancer can unfortunately result in temporary or permanent changes. Thus it is important for the nurse to be aware of these potential issues. Depending upon how much colon or rectum is resected, there can be frequency or urgency of the bowels. Frequency means that several trips to open the bowels are needed in a short time period, often in the morning. Urgency means that the trip to the toilet cannot be delayed for long and if it is not possible to access the toilet quickly then faecal incontinence can occur. Alternatively there can be changes in bowel function that can lead to concerns that the cancer has recurred. Frequent bowel actions can result in perianal soreness (➲ p. 454). The nurse can advise that many of these symptoms resolve within about 12 weeks of surgery as the remaining bowel adapts. However persistent symptoms may require further investigation.

There can be pelvic pain, particularly with men.

Rectal cancer treatment might result in nerve damage that can temporarily or permanently affect urination or sexual function. As treatments improve these risks decrease, but they are not completely eradicated, although it should be noted that most people are able to have sexual relations after colorectal cancer treatment.

It is worth the nurse reminding the patients that prescription costs are free for all medications for 5 years after a cancer diagnosis, for eligible people.

Bowel screening

To prevent development of colorectal cancer, there are a number of government initiatives within the UK. These are bowel scope and bowel screening, designed to detect cancer at an early stage and thus improve survival rates, as it is known that cancer takes often takes time to develop from an adenoma. Bowel screening began in 2006 and is now a national programme. The aim of bowel screening is to detect colorectal cancer before symptoms occur and thus enable treatment, if necessary, to be established sooner than waiting for symptoms. The test is posted to people every two years and requires faeces to be smeared onto a test, which is then posted back to the laboratory for testing. Since introduction the age of people sent the test has reduced to 60 years old. The return rate of the screening kit is poor, particularly in some ethnic groups and people with learning disabilities.

Faecal occult blood test

The screening test was initially the faecal occult blood test (FOBt); which is cheap and non-invasive. People with a positive test for guaiac (haemoccult) will be sent for further investigation: a colonoscopy (➔ p. 246–7). FOBt is used to detect blood in the faeces and can give a false positive in people who consume high levels of red meat for example. Alternatively, some cancers do not bleed and this can result in a false negative.

Faecal immunochemical test

FIT (faecal immunochemical test) is a more expensive and sophisticated faecal test for blood. Due to some of the drawbacks of the FOBt, the FIT was phased in to replace it in the UK from 2017. This test is easier to complete than the FOBt and thus it is expected to have a better uptake. Furthermore, it is more specific than the FOBt and thus less likely to give false positives as it is able to detect human blood rather than blood from other sources.

Bowel scope screening

Bowel scope screening is an examination using an endoscope (➔ p. 365) to visualize the lining of the rectum and sigmoid. Preparation is an enema, self-administrated by the patient at home prior to the procedure. During the procedure any polyps can be removed, preventing them to potentially develop into cancers. This examination is being rolled out across England and currently offered to men and women as a one-off test when they are 55. The majority (95%) will have a normal result, with less than 1% having a cancer found and less than 5% having further investigations such as a colonoscopy because polyps were found and removed. The nurse needs to advise patients that a small amount blood passed per rectum after the procedure is normal but this should not last more than a day and there should not be pain; if either is noted the person should contact their GP or the centre where the bowel scope screening was undertaken.

Inflammatory bowel disease

Inflammatory bowel disease

Inflammatory bowel disease (IBD) is an umbrella term for inflammatory diseases of the bowel that include ulcerative colitis (➲ p. 370) and crohn's disease (➲ p. 377). IBD is incurable but treatable. IBD is not to be confused with irritable bowel syndrome (➲ p. 96–8).

Symptoms

- Symptoms of IBD are unpredictable; symptoms may relapse and remit. There are common symptoms to both diseases that include diarrhoea, abdominal pain, anaemia, and fatigue.
- Additionally, patients may have an extra-intestinal manifestation (➲ p. 392–3) of their IBD. Extra-intestinal manifestations can affect joints, skin, eyes, and the liver.
- People with IBD have an increased risk of developing colorectal cancer (➲ p. 352). The cancer risk increases with the extent and duration of IBD and a family history of colorectal cancer.

Causes

- The exact cause of IBD is unknown, but it is related to a defective immune system, genetics, and environmental issues.

Incidence

- The global of incidence of IBD is increasing. In the UK the prevalence is estimated to be up to 1% of the population: thus, there are about 620,000 people in the UK with a diagnosis of IBD. Most commonly IBD occurs in adolescence or young adulthood.

Treatment

The principle aim of treating IBD is to induce and maintain clinical remission. Treatment will be determined by the symptoms and issues such as:
- Disease severity
- Disease site
- Lifestyle
- Previously effective and ineffective medication
- Side effects of medications
- Patient choice and compliance.

Living with inflammatory bowel disease

Although most patients will be completely well between relapses, active IBD can cause many problems and be very disruptive, with symptoms potentially restricting activities. Additionally, planning activities can be difficult as disease flares can occur at any time. Further concerns include:
- Body image (➲ p. 526–7).
- Relationships—when unwell, there might be an inability to participate in usual activities. Low self-esteem and embarrassment could make it difficult to form new relationships.

- Sexuality and fertility—illness and poor body image can cause a loss of libido. Women wanting to become pregnant or who are pregnant might have concerns about the possible adverse effects of their medication. Fertility ↓ in ♂ taking sulfasalazine (➲ p. 421). Pregnancy must be avoided by people on methotrexate (➲ p. 421) because of its teratogenicity (possible damage to developing foetus) and other medications. In general, many medications should be continued, but advice should be sought from an IBD specialist. Contraceptive advice is crucial and possibly a discussion about sperm/egg banking and possible later in vitro fertilization (IVF) in patients with incomplete families.
- Education/career—IBD can occur when the individual is often trying to finish education or start a career. There might be problems with repeated absences, especially if diagnosis has not been disclosed.
- Financial issues—some patients are unable to work periodically or permanently. Those with severe disease may be eligible for monetary support from the government.
- Holidays—care must be exercised to guard against gastrointestinal infections, which could trigger an IBD relapse. It is vital that travel insurance covers IBD.

Although most patients have the support of family and friends, the fact remains that IBD affect body parts and causes symptoms that can be embarrassing. Membership of a support organization, such as the National Association for Colitis and Crohn's Disease (NACC) might be useful.

Further reading
Kemp K, Dibley L, Chauhan U, et al. (2018) Second N-ECCO Consensus statements on the European nursing roles in caring for patients with Crohn's disease or ulcerative colitis. *Journal of Crohn's and Colitis* 12(7): 760–76.

Ulcerative colitis—definition

Ulcerative colitis (UC) is seen as inflammation of the mucosa and sub-mucosa of bowel. UC affects the colon and rectum, starting in the rectum and extending proximally, sometimes including the whole colon with the area of inflammation being continuous. UC can be described as:

• Pancolitis/extensive colitis—affects the whole of the colon and rectum (19% of patients)
• Left-sided colitis—affects the descending colon and rectum (33% of patients)
• Distal colitis—affects the rectum and sigmoid colon
• Proctitis—affects the rectum only (48% of patients).

One of the longest used tools within UC is the assessment tool that defines severity by Truelove and Witts (Table 15.1). This tool includes observations, blood results, and bowel function.

Table 15.1 Assessing UC severity

Feature	Mild	Moderate	Severe
Motions/day	<4	4–6	>6
Rectal bleeding	Small	Moderate	Large amounts
Temperature	Apyrexial	Intermediate	37.8°C on >2 out of 4 days
Pulse rate	Normal	Intermediate	>90bpm
Haemoglobin	>11 g/dl	Intermediate	<10.5 g/dl
ESR	<20 mm/h	Intermediate	>30 mm/h

There is also endoscopic grading (Table 15.2). Endoscopic surveillance (➲ p. 377) for colorectal cancer is recommended for people with pancolitis after about 8 years since diagnosis and about 15 years for left-sided ulcerative colitis.

Table 15.2 Endoscopic appearance of UC

Mild	Moderate	Severe
Diffuse erythema	Granular mucosa	Intense inflammation
Loss of vascular pattern	Petechial haemorrhage	Purulent exudate
Contact bleeding	Spontaneous bleeding	Discrete ulcers

Ulcerative colitis—symptoms

Symptoms include:
- Rectal bleeding
- Passage of mucus
- Abdominal pain
- Diarrhoea
- Faecal urgency
- Possibly faecal incontinence
- ↑ bowel frequency
- Occasionally constipation
- Loss of appetite
- Lethargy.

UC is associated with extra-intestinal manifestations including:
- Primary sclerosing cholangitis
- Arthralgia
- Colorectal cancer
- Uveitis/iritis
- Erythema nodosum
- Pyoderma gangrenosum.

Ulcerative colitis—cause

The cause of UC is unknown, but a number of genetic, physiological, immunological, and environmental issues are considered to be risk factors.
- 15% of patients diagnosed with UC have a family member with IBD—UC occurs at a younger age in familial cases (28 years compared with 35 years for familial and non-familial traits, respectively).
- More common in Jewish than non-Jewish communities.
- The colonic mucosal barrier is impaired, leading to ↑ intestinal permeability and an ↑ inflammatory response because the gut mucosa allows antigens into the submucosa (Fig. 15.1).
- When the disease is active, the lamina propria of the mucosa becomes heavily infiltrated with a mixture of acute and chronic inflammatory cells. There is a predominant ↑ in IgG within the mucosa, resulting in the release of numerous cytokines and amplification of the inflammatory process.
- Ex-smokers are three times more likely to have UC than smokers. This is attributed to the effect of nicotine in suppressing the inflammatory response.
- The removal of the appendix at an early age has been associated with a preventative effect on the development of UC.
- Anti-inflammatory drugs (⊃ p. 406) can trigger exacerbations of UC.

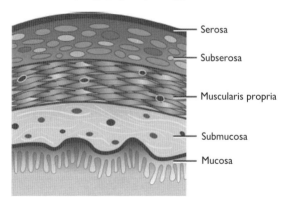

— Serosa

— Subserosa

— Muscularis propria

— Submucosa

— Mucosa

Fig. 15.1 Diagram of bowel wall.

Ulcerative colitis—incidence

The prevalence of UC is ~100–200 cases/100,000 population.

It is estimated that 50% of patients with UC will relapse in any given year and it is likely that a significant number of patients will have frequently relapsing or continuous disease. It is estimated that 20–30% of patients will need a colectomy at some point, although this is delayed by the advent of improved medical therapy. Many patients remain fully capable of work.

Ulcerative colitis—investigations

Investigating UC enables confirmation of diagnosis, assessment of disease severity, extent of the UC, and detection of any complications.

A full assessment (➲ p. 202) should be undertaken when first presenting, including:
- Recent travel
- Medication
- Smoking
- Family history of IBD
- Observations—pulse, blood pressure, temperature, and weight.

Additional assessment should include a bowel history:
- Stool frequency
- Stool consistency
- Urgency
- Rectal bleeding +/− mucus.

Further assessment includes:
- Abdominal pain
- Pyrexia
- Weight loss
- Malaise
- Any extra-intestinal manifestations (➲ p. 392–3).

There should also be a physical examination of the abdomen and anorectum to include:
- Abdominal masses or tenderness on palpation
- Oral ulceration
- Anal skin tags
- Anal fistulae
- Postprandial pain (pain after eating) might indicate obstruction
- Anaemia.

Other investigations include:
- Blood tests—full blood count, urea and electrolytes, liver function tests, C-reactive protein (CRP), and erythrocyte sedimentation rate (ESR) (levels of ESR and CRP may be normal in distal UC)
- Stool sample—to exclude infective sources—culture and sensitivity, ova, and parasites
- Colonoscopy (➲ p. 246–7) and biopsy—may need to be deferred if clinically unwell due to the risk of perforation (biopsy typically reveals acute inflammatory reaction with neutrophil infiltration, crypt abscesses, and goblet cells depleted of mucus—these are highly suggestive of UC but not unique to the disease).

For an acute presentation, it might be advisable to order:
- An abdominal X-ray—to assess for toxic dilation, perforation, or obstruction.

Ulcerative colitis—medical treatment

Treatment for UC is guided by the extent of disease.

Proctitis

The use of prednisolone (➲ p. 428) or mesalazine suppositories (➲ p. 375) is usually effective. Severe proctitis that has not responded to suppositories will usually require treatment with a reducing dose of oral prednisolone (➲ p. 428).

Left-sided disease

Foam or retention enemas used nightly +/– suppositories, can induce remission. Water-based retention enemas, containing steroids (➲ p. 428) or mesalazine (➲ p. 375) can be messy and difficult for patients to retain in their rectum.

Oral 5-ASA (5-aminosalicylic acid) preparation, such as mesalazine (➲ p. 375), the dose can be ↑ in conjunction with topical treatment for mild to moderate disease flare up.

Severe left-sided disease or a disease flare up that has not responded to the above medications will usually require treatment with a reducing dose of oral prednisolone (➲ p. 428).

Pancolitis

A mild disease flare up might respond to an ↑ in oral 5-ASA +/– topical treatment, but typically will require treatment with a reducing dose of oral steroids.

Severe or fulminant disease, defined by a high bowel frequency in association with fever, tachycardia, ↑ inflammatory markers (e.g. ESR), anaemia, low serum albumin level, or systemic symptoms such as malaise, will require hospital admission and treatment with intravenous (IV) steroid therapy (➲ p. 428). Additionally, IV fluids may be necessary for dehydration and treatment for anaemia may be necessary. If symptoms do not settle, treatment with IV ciclosporin (➲ p. 408) or biologics (➲ p. 421) should be considered. When IV steroids are failing, it is advisable to discuss surgery.

The majority of disease flares will respond to therapy within two weeks. Then treatment can be tapered, and maintenance regimens commenced or recommenced.

Immunosuppressant therapy

Patients who present with severe or fulminating disease, or who have steroid-refractory or steroid-dependent disease, despite maintenance therapy with oral 5-ASA (➲ p. 375), should be counselled and started on immunosuppressant therapy to achieve improved remission. Standard immunosuppressant therapies include azathioprine (➲ p. 421) and mercaptopurine (➲ p. 421) and these should be first-line choices.

Any patient commencing immunosuppressant therapy must be counselled regarding the side effects of this group of drugs, including the risk of neutropenia (about 1 in 300 risk). Measurement of thiopurine methyl transferase (TPMT) prior to commencing therapy can identify patients at higher risk of this effect. An agreement to undertake regular monitoring of blood counts must be undertaken by the patient and healthcare provider, with implementation of robust systems for checking the results.

Ulcerative colitis—surgical treatment

Surgery is needed for UC if medical treatment fails. If patients have severe or fulminant colitis, surgery is indicated if there are signs of toxic megacolon (➲ p. 105) developing despite intensive treatment with IV steroids (➲ p. 408) and ciclosporin (➲ p. 408). Rarely, surgery is needed as emergency management for perforation of the colon or severe haemorrhage. Surgery is also recommended for chronic symptoms with steroid dependence and/or lack of efficacy or intolerance of immunomodulatory drugs. Chronic UC can lead to poor overall health and a much-reduced quality of life. About 25–30% of patients with extensive colitis will require surgery. Occasionally, surgery is performed for severe dysplasia or high-risk presence of colorectal cancer (➲ p. 352).

Even if UC is not present throughout the colon, it is advisable to remove it all, in an operation termed a total colectomy. Initially, most patients will have a total colectomy and temporary ileostomy, leaving a rectal stump in situ. After a period of recovery, there are three options:

- An ileo-pouch anal anastomosis (➲ p. 488–9)
- Proctectomy (➲ p. 508) with a permanent ileostomy (➲ p. 508)
- Leave the rectal stump *in situ* and keep under surveillance for cancer, with an ileostomy (➲ p. 508).

Colorectal cancer surveillance

People with UC are at higher risk of developing colorectal cancer (➔ p. 352) than the general population: 2% at 10 years, 8% at 20 years, and 18% at 30 years since onset of UC. People at a higher risk include people with:

- Extensive disease
- Family history colorectal cancer
- Primary sclerosing cholangitis.

To prevent development of colorectal cancer, colonoscopic surveillance is recommended.

Crohn's disease

Crohn's disease is an inflammatory bowel disease, seen as inflammation of the bowel lining in any area of the gastrointestinal tract from the mouth to the anus. This inflammation can be transmural (affecting all layers). Inflammation is intermittent and the areas of healthy mucosa between areas of disease are called skip lesions. There can be areas where the bowel lumen is narrowed due to scarring (fibrosis) and are termed strictures or where the bowel lumen is almost no longer patent which is termed stenosed. The bowel can also develop a hole within it, which is termed a fistula—that is, the Crohn's disease penetrates the bowel mucosa and is connected with other structures. This can include the bladder, vagina, small bowel, or skin, such as the perianal area.

Crohn's disease—symptoms

Symptoms vary depending on the area and severity of the disease, but usually all sites of Crohn's disease include symptoms of:
- Abdominal pain
- Diarrhoea
- Weight loss
- Anorexia
- Pyrexia
- Lethargy.

Rectal bleeding is not always present.
   Small bowel Crohn's disease may present with:
- Nausea and vomiting
- Bloating and abdominal distention
- Aphthous ulcers
- Duodenal ulcers
- Abdominal pain
- Abdominal mass, potentially palpated in the right iliac fossa.

Colonic Crohn's disease may present with:
- Severe diarrhoea
- Rectal bleeding
- Mucus per rectum
- Toxic megacolon.

Perianal Crohn's disease may present with:
- Recurrent perianal fistulae, abscesses, and anal skin tags
- Severe rectal pain
- Alternating bowel habit.

Symptoms for people with a stricture/stenosis will have obstructive type symptoms including:
- Nausea
- Vomiting.

Crohn's disease—causes

The cause of Crohn's disease is unknown, but risk factors include:
- A family member with a UC or Crohn's disease diagnosis (15% of people with Crohn's disease)
- Genetics.

A number of genetics have been identified such as *NOD2* (*CARD15*), thought to be associated with small bowel disease and stenosing disease. With a greater knowledge of genetics comes the potential for screening, prevention, and early intervention.

Modifiable environmental factors include:
- Smoking cigarettes—there is also a likely worse disease course if continued.

Crohn's disease—incidence

The prevalence of Crohn's disease in the UK is up to 1 in 1000 people, with 4 to 11 new cases being identified in every 100,000 people each year. The most common age of presentation is between 20 and 60 years, with more women affected than men.

Crohn's disease—investigations

A full assessment (❍ p. 202) should be undertaken when first presenting, including:
- Recent travel
- Medication
- Smoking
- Family history of IBD (❍ p. 202)
- Observations—pulse, blood pressure, temperature, and weight.

Additional assessment should include a bowel history:
- Stool frequency
- Stool consistency
- Urgency
- Rectal bleeding ± mucus.

Further assessment includes:
- Abdominal pain
- Pyrexia
- Weight loss
- Malaise
- Any extra-intestinal manifestations (❍ p. 392–3).

There should also be a physical examination of the abdomen and anorectum, including:
- Abdominal masses or tenderness on palpation
- Oral ulceration
- Anal skin tags
- Anal fistulae
- Postprandial pain (pain after eating) might indicate obstruction
- Anaemia.

Other investigations include:
- Blood tests—full blood count, urea and electrolytes, liver function tests, serum B12, iron, folate, CRP, and ESR
- Stool sample—to exclude infective sources—culture and sensitivity, ova, and parasites
- Ultrasound scan (❍ p. 227)—looking for thickened bowel loops, inflammatory masses, and collections/abscesses
- Computed tomography (CT) scan (❍ p. 220)—looking for complications of Crohn's disease, such as thickened bowel loops, strictures, and fistulae
- Magnetic resonance imaging (MRI) (❍ p. 222)—looking for fistulae tracts, such as in perianal disease.

To assess the colon and rectum:
- Colonoscopy (❍ p. 246–7) ideally—looking for patchy inflammation within the colon, inflammation at the terminal ileum, or rectal sparing (disease-free rectum)
- Biopsy from the endoscopic procedure—looking for transmural infiltration (inflammation penetrating the bowel mucosa), lymphocytic infiltration (evidence of inflammatory response), and granulomas.

To assess the small bowel and upper parts of the gastrointestinal tract:
- Gastroscopy (➲ p. 250) assessment of the oesophagus and stomach
- Barium meal (➲ p. 217)
- Barium follow-through (➲ p. 216)
- Capsule endoscopy (➲ p. 245).

For an acute presentation:
- An abdominal X-ray—to assess for toxic dilation, perforation, or obstruction might be advisable.

Scoring systems for Crohn's disease

A commonly used scale is the Crohn's disease activity index (CDAI) that provides a method of assessment.

Crohn's disease—dietary treatment

Dietary therapy can be a primary treatment or a supportive treatment.

Supportive dietary treatment during a disease flare-up can often assist with:
• Poor appetite
• Nausea
• Food intolerances
• Partial or complete bowel obstruction.

This might be the addition of vitamin and mineral supplements, high-calorie drinks, or supplemental feeding with liquid diets. Very occasionally, parenteral nutrition (PN) is used if oral diet is not possible or there is very extensive small bowel disease or resection. If there is subacute obstruction, a low-residue or liquid diet is needed until the obstruction is resolved through medical/surgical management. Patients may need to be referred to a specialist dietitian.

Primary dietary treatment

A liquid diet can be a primary treatment for Crohn's disease that can induce remission without side effects. This is of particular benefit for the undernourished and children. A liquid diet can be elemental, semi-elemental, or polymeric, and needs to be taken for several weeks. After this time, food can be gradually reintroduced. The benefits of a liquid diet include possible disease remission without steroids (❸ p. 428). However, patients need to be well motivated to not eat with all the social and psychological issues associated with not eating. Some patients find the liquid diet to be unpalatable; this is potentially resolved by nasogastric tube feeding. In rare cases, such as oesophageal Crohn's disease, percutaneous endoscopic gastrostomy (PEG) tube (❸ p. 272–3) feeding can be utilized for longer-term feeding. Furthermore, some people report that the liquid diet causes osmotic diarrhoea, resolved by taking the liquid diet more slowly or more diluted. Patients report that the most common symptom-provoking foods include dairy products, wheat, and caffeine.

Crohn's disease—medical treatment

In established Crohn's disease, the site of disease can help with treatment choice.

Ileocaecal Crohn's disease

Mild-to-moderate disease exacerbation—oral budesonide (❍ p. 428) is recommended over prednisolone (❍ p. 428). If remission is not achieved, treatment with a standard tapering dose of prednisolone is recommended.

Moderate localized disease—antibiotics such as ciprofloxacin (❍ p. 408) and metronidazole (❍ p. 408) may be required if there is a suspicion of septic complications. However, side effects and limited tolerability by patients restrict antibiotic use.

Severe disease—oral prednisolone (❍ p. 428) is advocated with early introduction of immunosuppressant therapy (❍ p. 421) for patients who relapse on dose ↓ or withdrawal. Biologics (❍ p. 360) are indicated for those patients who prove immunosuppressant intolerant or unresponsive, although surgery should also be discussed at this time.

Colonic Crohn's disease

Colonic Crohn's disease can be managed in a similar fashion to UC (❍ p. 370), with the use of steroids (❍ p. 428) and 5-ASA therapy (❍ p. 421), depending on distribution of disease, including rectal treatments. Immunosuppressant therapy (❍ p. 421) should be considered early in patients with relapsing disease, although the slow action of this group of drugs does not promote their use as first-line therapy in active disease. Biologics (❍ p. 360) can be used, as appropriate, in patients who prove refractory to other treatments or situations in which surgery is contraindicated.

Small bowel Crohn's disease

Active disease can require a tapering dose of oral steroid therapy (❍ p. 428) and early consideration of the introduction of immunomodulatory therapy (❍ p. 421). The use of a liquid diet (❍ p. 382), such as polymeric or elemental diets, can provide an alternative for patients who want to avoid steroids. Liquid diet is effective in children and adults with mild disease. Biologics should be considered in refractory patients who do not respond to first-line therapy.

Fistulating/perianal disease

The use of antibiotics such as ciprofloxacin (❍ p. 408) and metronidazole (❍ p. 408) can be beneficial in the presence of sepsis or abscesses, often for an extended period of time. Many patients relapse when the drugs are withdrawn and there are side effects associated with long-term use, particularly paraesthesia (tingling and sensory loss) with metronidazole. Immunosuppressants, such as azathioprine (❍ p. 421) and mercaptopurine (❍ p. 421), can be effective in perianal disease, although the response can be very slow. Biologics (❍ p. 360) may be effective, but sepsis needs to be excluded prior to commencing treatment. Topical therapy may be effective.

Other medication considerations

- If oral corticosteroids are used, it is considered good practice to prescribe concomitant calcium (➲ p. 295) as a bone protector.
- If required, oral steroid courses should be kept as short as possible, with alternatives used wherever feasible. Give the patient a steroid card.
- If the patient has small bowel disease or an ileostomy, avoid enteric-coated medication as it may be poorly absorbed.
- Extreme caution in relation to pregnancy (both genders).

Crohn's disease—surgical treatment

Surgery may be necessary for people with Crohn's disease who do not improve with medical treatment or to address sepsis or other complications. About 80% of patients will need surgery at some point, although with the newer medications such as biologics (❷ p. 360), surgery is often delayed. Half of people undergoing surgery will require more surgery, with recurrence of inflammation at the surgery site and/or elsewhere. Thus, resections should be conservative as extensive resections can result in intestinal failure (❷ p. 70–3). Surgery is therefore not a cure for Crohn's disease, as it is for UC (❷ p. 376).

Indications for surgery

- Emergency—bowel perforation or severe haemorrhage
- Acute—small bowel inflammatory obstruction or inflammation that is unresponsive to medical management
- Chronic—small bowel obstruction due to fibrostenotic stricture
- Repair of fistula or abscess (perianal or internal)
- Severe dysplasia or malignancy (rare).

The surgical procedures include:
- Ileocolic resection—for terminal ileal/colonic inflammation
- Ileal resection
- Colonic resection
- Ileorectal anastomosis
- Pan proctocolectomy with ileostomy
- Laying open of perianal fistula
- Insertion of seton suture—to keep a fistula open and prevent abscess formation
- Drainage of perianal or abdominal abscess
- Dilation of stricture
- Strictureplasty—for ileal strictures (Fig. 15.2).

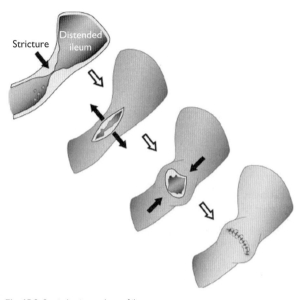

Fig. 15.2 Surgical stricturoplasty of ileum.
Reproduced with kind permission © Burdett Institute 2008.

Indeterminate colitis

Indeterminate colitis (also termed IBD unclassified) is an inflammatory bowel disease, but diagnosis is not possible due to a lack of histopathological distinction between UC (→ p. 374) and Crohn's disease (→ p. 380–1). It is uncertain if indeterminate colitis is a separate disease, but about half of people do progress to a diagnosis of UC or Crohn's disease.

Incidence

About 10% of people with IBD (→ p. 388) are diagnosed as indeterminate colitis.

Investigations

Investigations include:
• Colonoscopy
• Biopsy.

Treatment

Treatment for people with indeterminate colitis is in general the same as for UC.

The main concern of indeterminate colitis is when medical management fails, and surgery is necessary. It appears that this group of patients who require surgery do worse than people with UC but better than people with Crohn's disease.

Microscopic colitis

Collagenous colitis and lymphocytic colitis are forms of microscopic colitis. In microscopic colitis, the endoscopic appearance is normal, but biopsies show changes. There is an increase in lymphocytes when there is inflammation. In collagenous colitis, a thicker collagen layer develops within the colonic lining, and there may be an increase in lymphocytes. With lymphocytic colitis, there is an increased number of lymphocytes within the bowel lining. Microscopic colitis may be misdiagnosed as irritable bowel syndrome (→ p. 96–8).

Symptoms

The main symptom of microscopic colitis is chronic watery diarrhoea that may occur suddenly, but blood is rarely seen. Diarrhoea may also be explosive and severe, resulting in dehydration. Furthermore, it can occur over night disrupting sleep. Other symptoms can include:
- Abdominal pain—cramping or dull
- Weight loss
- Fatigue
- Faecal incontinence
- Joint and muscle pain
- Bloating
- Flatus.

Causes

The cause of microscopic colitis is unknown, but there are people with microscopic colitis who have a greater number of other autoimmune diseases compared to the rest of the population. These autoimmune diseases include coeliac disease, rheumatoid arthritis, thyroid disorders, and type I diabetes. There are also several drugs associated with microscopic colitis that include:
- Non-steroidal anti-inflammatory drugs (NSAIDs) (→ p. 406)
- Some proton pump inhibitors (PPIs)
- Aspirin
- Ranitidine
- Statins.

Not all studies confirm all the above potential causes. Finally smoking seems to be linked with an increased risk of microscopic colitis.

Incidence

The incidence of lymphocytic colitis is slightly higher than that of collagenous colitis, but both are relatively rare with just a few people in every 100,000 people being diagnosed with microscopic colitis. However, due to an increased awareness of the disease, the incidence is increasing. Microscopic colitis is most commonly diagnosed in people in their 60s, but about quarter will be diagnosed in people under 45 years of age, and rarely it is seen in children.

More women are diagnosed than men with microscopic colitis. There is some evidence that there is a hereditary component to microscopic colitis.

Investigations

Diagnosis is made by:
- Colonoscopy to enable biopsies to be taken
- Blood tests to eliminate coeliac disease.

Treatment

Many people do not require treatment and symptoms will often resolve independently. If the cause is drug-related, stopping the medication may help to resolve symptoms. When medication is required, it is related to symptoms. Mild symptoms may require anti-diarrhoeal medication (➔ p. 411) to reduce symptoms of diarrhoea. Worse symptoms may require a steroid, although many people will have a flare-up of symptoms once the drug is discontinued. If this is ineffective, drugs that can assist in the control of IBD (➔ p. 375) can be used, with advice from the IBD team.

There is no real evidence that a change in diet will be beneficial, although logically reducing caffeine may help.

Prognosis

About three-quarters of people will be able to achieve long-term remission of their microscopic colitis. There does not seem to be a risk of progression of microscopic colitis developing into IBD (➔ p. 368–9) or colorectal cancer (➔ p. 352).

Extra-intestinal manifestations

There are a number of extra-intestinal manifestations; these are symptoms of IBD that are not within the gastrointestinal tract. Some of these extra-intestinal manifestations are related to active disease and others are not (see Table 15.3). Up to 25% of patients with IBD suffer from extra-intestinal manifestations. It is not fully known why these extra-intestinal symptoms occur. It is a possibility that the inflammation in the colon is only another manifestation of what is a systemic disease.

Table 15.3 Extra-intestinal manifestations

Disease activity	Common (5–20%)	Uncommon (<5%)
Related to disease activity	Aphthous ulcers	Pyoderma gangrenosum
	Erythema nodosum	
	Finger clubbing	
	Ocular	
	Conjunctivitis	
	Episcleritis	
	Iritis	
	Arthritis	
	Osteoporosis	
Unrelated to active disease	Gallstones	Liver disease
		Fatty liver
	Sacroilitis	Primary sclerosing cholangitis
		Ankylosing spondylitis
	Arthralgia	Renal stones
		Osteomalacia
	Nutritional deficiency	Sweet's syndrome
		Systemic amylodosis

Musculoskeletal manifestations

- Arthritis occurs in up to 20% of patients—the main types seen in UC are peripheral arthritis, ankylosing spondylitis, and sacroiliitis.
- Peripheral arthropathies—a range of joints could be involved, from large joints, such as knees, to smaller joints, such as fingers. A relapse in bowel symptoms is associated with symptoms of arthritis in 29% of patients. The majority of these symptoms of arthritis are seronegative arthropathies, such as ankylosing spondylitis and reactive arthritis.
- The incidence of finger clubbing is ↑ in Crohn's disease.
- ↓ bone mass density, resulting in osteoporosis or osteopenia, has been reported in 3–77% of patients with IBD; it may be steroid-related.

Skin

- Oral lesions occur in Crohn's disease.
- Erythema nodosum can be seen in UC or Crohn's disease, but occurs most often in Crohn's disease. The presentation of erythema nodosum is raised inflamed bumps or nodules, most commonly on the legs; these are red and very painful to touch. Its appearance generally parallels IBD disease activity and usually responds well to steroid therapy.
- Pyoderma gangrenosum occurs in 5% of patients with UC and 2% of patients with Crohn's disease. It can manifest itself in wound sites post-operatively and looks like large areas of irregular-edged, ulceration, with a dusky purple outline. These ulcers can be very large, painful, and distressing for the patient.

Ocular manifestations

- Episcleritis occurs in 3–4% of IBD patients and causes local, tender inflammation. It can be treated with topical steroids.
- Uveitis is a more serious condition. It can mirror the activity of the colonic inflammation and presents with pain, blurred vision, and photophobia. There is a risk of scarring and possible blindness if it is not treated promptly, so patients complaining of these symptoms need a quick and early diagnosis.

Primary sclerosing cholangitis

- Primary sclerosing cholangitis (PSC) (⊕ p. 200) is linked to UC.
- PSC occurs in 3–10% of patients with UC. It is more common in ♂, and 95% of patients will have extensive disease, leading to an ↑ risk of colorectal carcinoma and the need for regular screening colonoscopy

Renal stones

There is an ↑ incidence of renal stones in Crohn's disease, particularly in patients with ileal disease after surgical resections.

Rarer extra-intestinal manifestations

- Amyloidosis—occurs in <1% of patients; can be fatal
- Pancreatitis—often related to medication such as azathioprine (⊕ p. 182)
- Bronchopulmonary inflammation
- Pleuropericarditis.

Paediatric gastrointestinal care

Duplication cysts

Intestinal duplication cysts are rare birth defects (congenital defects) in which an abnormal part of the intestine is connected to the wall of the stomach or intestines. Duplication cysts are most commonly seen in the small bowel although they can occur anywhere in the gastrointestinal tract.

Cause

It is unclear what the cause may be.

Symptoms

Symptoms depend on location of duplication cyst:
- Vomiting, sometimes with blood
- Abdominal pain
- Gastrointestinal obstruction
- Blood in the stool.

Investigations

Diagnostic procedures may include various imaging studies:
- Abdominal x-ray (➜ p. 230)
- Computed tomography (CT) scan (➜ p. 220)
- Abdominal ultrasound (➜ p. 227)
- Magnetic resonance imaging (MRI) (➜ p. 222).

Treatment

Treatment will usually involve surgery to remove the abnormal part of the bowel.

Hirschsprung's disease

Hirschsprung's disease is a birth defect in which a failure of development of the neural ganglia in the myenteric and submucosal plexus of the colon +/− rectum (nerves are missing from parts of the colon/rectum). This results in a lack of peristalsis and a loss of involuntary relaxation of the internal sphincter. Hirschsprung's disease is typically diagnosed shortly after birth, although symptoms may develop into adulthood.

Causes

It is not completely clear what causes Hirschsprung's; however, it is thought that the following contribute to the problem:
- Short segment—nerve cells are missing or do not form completely in the rectum and sigmoid colon.
- Long segment—nerve cells are missing or do not form completely throughout the colon and sometimes the last part of the small bowel.
- Rarely nerve cells are missing throughout the entire colon and small bowel.
- Disorder may be associated with Down Syndrome.

Symptoms

- Failure to pass meconium within 48 hours following birth
- Constipation (➋ p. 458–9)
- Bowel obstruction
- Distended abdomen, with pain
- Diarrhoea (➋ p. 204)
- Vomiting
- Explosive stool following rectal examination
- Faecal retention.

Investigations

- Rectal examination
- Abdominal X-ray
- Rectoanal inhibitory test on anorectal manometry—measures the relaxation reflex of the internal anal sphincter after rectal distention (not generally available for neonates)
- Rectal suction biopsy—removal of tissue by suction from the rectal mucosa and submucosa
- Full thickness biopsy—removal of a thicker piece of tissue under anaesthetic.

Treatment

Treatment predominantly involves surgery:

- The Swenson procedure was the original surgical procedure where removal of the entire aganglionic segment was resected with an anastomosis.
- Surgery was a laparotomy with deep pelvic dissection and the anastomosis performed from a perineal approach.
- The most commonly used technique is a laparoscopic-assisted transanal pull-through. This can be performed in one or two stages. In a two-stage procedure, a temporary diverting colostomy will be used.

Faecal soiling may occur after a pull-through procedure. This is often as a result of abnormal sphincter function, abnormal sensation, and/or overflow incontinence associated with constipation. Treatments will vary according to symptoms.

Further reading

https://www.sages.org/wiki/hirschsprung-disease-2/ (Accessed 20/05/2019)
https://emedicine.medscape.com/article/178493-treatment (Accessed 20/05/2019)
https://journals.lww.com/jaapa/Fulltext/2016/04000/Surgical_management_for_Hirschsprung_disease__A.4.aspx (Accessed 20/05/2019)
https://www.niddk.nih.gov/health-information/digestive-diseases/hirschsprung-disease (Accessed 20/05/2019)

Imperforate anus

Imperforate anus is a defect that is present from birth (congenital). It is characterized by the absence of the normal opening of the anus. Elimination of faeces may not be possible until surgery is performed.

Causes

Imperforate anus may occur in several forms:
- The rectum may end in a pouch that does not connect with the colon.
- The rectum may have openings to other structures. These may include the urethra, bladder, base of the penis, or scrotum in boys, or vagina in girls.
- There may be narrowing (stenosis) of the anus.
- There may be no anus.

Symptoms

- Failure to pass meconium in the first 24 hours, which should lead to examination of the rectum
- Passing faeces through another opening, e.g. urethra for males and vagina for females
- Distended abdomen.

Investigations

A doctor can usually diagnose an imperforate anus with a rectal examination. However, other investigations may be necessary to reveal the extent of the abnormalities.
- X-ray
- Abdominal ultrasound.

Treatment

Imperforate anus almost always requires surgery. The type of surgery can depend on the precise defect, which includes how far the rectum descends, how it affects the pelvic muscles, and whether there are any fistulas.
- A perineal anoplasty may be performed to close any fistulas and create an anus with normal positioning.
- A pull-through—where the rectum is pulled down and connected to the new anus.

Multiple procedures may be necessary to correct the problem with the formation of a temporary stoma. Anal dilatation of the new anus may periodically be required to prevent any narrowing.

Most children will do well following surgery. However, toilet training can take a little longer and laxatives may be required later in life to relieve constipation. Follow-up care throughout childhood is likely to be beneficial.

Further reading

https://medlineplus.gov/ency/presentations/100030_3.htm (Accessed 20/05/2019

Malrotation

Intestinal malrotation is a birth defect involving a malformation of the intestinal tract that occurs whilst the foetus is forming. Intestinal malrotation is most often recognized in infancy and in the first week following birth. It is rarely seen in older children, and when it does occur, symptoms may be absent or intermittent.

Cause

- Malrotation occurs when the intestine does not make the turns as it should.

Symptoms

The majority of children with malrotation develop symptoms within the first year.

- Acute bowel obstruction
- Vomiting bile
- Abdominal pain
- Distended abdomen
- Diarrhoea (⊃ p. 204)
- Constipation (⊃ p. 458–9)
- Rectal bleeding
- Bloody stools.

Investigations

In addition to a physical examination, diagnostic procedures may include various imaging studies:

- Abdominal X-ray (⊃ p. 230)
- CT scan (⊃ p. 220)
- Barium enema (⊃ p. 214–15).

Treatment

- Intravenous fluids
- Antibiotics
- Nasogastric tube.

Malrotation of the intestines is not always evident until it presents as a volvulus.

Oesophageal atresia

Oesophageal atresia is a rare birth defect that affects the oesophagus. The upper part of the oesophagus does not connect with the lower oesophagus and stomach. It usually ends in a pouch, which means food cannot reach the stomach.

Cause

Although the cause is uncertain it is thought to be a problem with the development of the oesophagus while in the womb.

Symptoms

- May be seen prior to birth
- Difficulty in swallowing
- Difficulty in breathing.

Investigations

- The diagnosis may be suggested prenatally by a small or absent stomach bubble on antenatal ultrasound scan at around 18 weeks gestation.
- All infants with oesophageal atresia should have an echocardiogram prior to surgery. The echocardiogram will define any structural anomaly of the heart or great blood vessels.

Treatment

Treatment consists of surgical procedures to correct the oesophageal atresia.

Toilet training

Toilet training is the procedure of teaching children bladder and bowel control.

Most children usually begin to gain bowel and bladder control between the age of 18 and 24 months. Although, children develop at their own pace and therefore timing can vary from one child to another. This also applies to the length of time it may take to toilet train with most taking between 3 and 6 months for daytime continence, which is often extended from months to years for overnight. There are suggestions that toilet training centres on physical, developmental, and behavioural markers rather than age. As a result, it is not always straightforward to know when the time is right. The consensus is that a child needs to be able to sit themselves on a potty and get up independently as well as be mature enough to communicate and follow instructions. If a child is beginning to show signs of being aware when needing to pass urine and evacuate their bowels they are starting to recognize the signals and therefore are likely to be ready.

There is a great deal of information on how to progress with hints and tips on effective toilet training. Education and resources for improving childhood continence (ERIC) have a website and leaflets containing detailed information to work through the process.

Further reading

https://www.eric.org.uk/Handlers/Download.ashx?IDMF=cad20060-c174-4566-afcd-25f0087614a4 (Accessed 13/08/2019)

Volvulus

A volvulus is when a loop of intestine twists around itself and the mesentery that supports it, resulting in a bowel obstruction.

Cause
• Malrotation.

Symptoms
• As per malrotation (◓ p. 401).

Investigations
• As per malrotation (◓ p. 401).

Treatment

Surgery is required where the bowel will be untwisted. If the bowel is damaged this will be removed and an anastomosis formed, which may involve a temporary stoma, depending on the length of damage to the bowel.

Further reading

https://www.bmj.com/content/347/bmj.f6949 (Accessed 20/05/2019)

Chapter 17

Drugs in gastrointestinal care

Analgesia

Analgesia is medication used to relieve pain.

Drug	Indication	Side effects
Aspirin	Analgesia Prevention of cerebrovascular accident	Dyspepsia (⊃ p. 22–3)
Codeine phosphate	Abdominal pain Diarrhoea	Constipation (⊃ p. 458–9)
NSAIDs (non-steroidal anti-inflammatory drug), such as ibuprofen	Pain Inflammation	Dyspepsia (⊃ p. 22–3) Gastric ulcer (⊃ p. 30–1) Gastritis (⊃ p. 32–3) Haematemesis (⊃ p. 436–7), Duodenal ulcers (⊃ p. 66)
Opioid—morphine	Severe abdominal pain Post-operative abdominal pain	Gastroparesis (⊃ p. 38–9 C2) Nausea and vomiting (⊃ p. 49)
Paracetamol	Pharyngitis Gallstones Fever	Rare

This list is not exhaustive and further enquiry should be made with an up to date British National Formulary (BNF).

Antacids

Antacids help to neutralize acid in the stomach. Antacids can help to relieve symptoms but will not cure them.

Drug	Indication	Side effects
Gaviscon®	Barrett's oesophagus GORD (⊃ p. 36–7 C2) Dyspepsia (⊃ p. 22–3 C2)	Diarrhoea Constipation Aluminium toxicity
Magnesium hydroxide	Barrett's oesophagus GORD (⊃ p. 36–7 C2) Dyspepsia (⊃ p. 22–3 C2)	Diarrhoea Nausea Vomiting
Calcium carbonate	Barrett's oesophagus GORD (⊃ p. 36–7 C2) Dyspepsia (⊃ p. 22–3 C2)	Nausea Vomiting Renal stones Alkalosis

This list is not exhaustive and further enquiry should be made with an up to date BNF.

Antibiotics

Antibiotics are specific for the type of bacteria being treated. Thus antibiotics are ineffective unless a bacterial infection is present, thus they are often ineffective in pharyngitis, for example.

Drug	Indication	Side effects
Ciprofloxacin	Travellers' diarrhoea Anorectal abscess Perianal abscess	Pyelonephritis Arthralgia Myalgia
Metronidazole	Stomach/intestinal ulcers caused by *H. pylori* (➲ p. 42) Small bowel bacterial overgrowth Ischaemic colitis *C.difficile* (➲ p. 34) Perianal abscess Radiation enteropathy	Vomiting Nausea Headache Dizziness
Erythromycin	Gastroparesis (➲ p. 38)	Diarrhoea Dizziness Skin rash/hives/welts Sore throat Vomiting
Amoxicillin	GI infections	Bloating Diarrhoea Dizziness Headache Skin hives/welts Nausea Vomiting
Cefuroxime	Appendicitis	Diarrhoea Nausea Vomiting Abdominal pain
Vancomycin	*C.difficile* Stomach/colon infections	Hypotension Itching Dizziness Indigestion Hives Wheezing

This list is not exhaustive and further enquiry should be made with an up to date BNF.

Anticholinergics/antispasmodics

Anticholinergics prevent contractions, cramps and spasms, such as in IBS (➔ p. 96–8).

Drug	Indication	Side effects
Atropine	To decrease digestion Diarrhoea Mucus secretion	Dry mouth Not to be used by people with constipation
Hyoscine butylbromide	Stomach cramps/bloating (➔ p. 96–8 IBS)	Constipation Dry mouth Nausea
Mebeverine	Stomach cramps/bloating (➔ p. 96–8 IBS)	Indigestion Diarrhoea Constipation Dizziness
Colpermin® (peppermint oil)	IBS	Anorectal discomfort Vomiting GORD Dyspepsia Contains peanut oil as excipient thus allergy risk

This list is not exhaustive and further enquiry should be made with an up to date BNF.

Antidepressants

Antidepressants can help with symptoms of IBS (◑ p. 96–8).

Drug	Indication	Side effects
Amitriptyline	Oesophageal spasm IBS (◑ p. 96–8) pain Abdominal IBS contractions Bloating in IBS Distension in IBS Use in low doses	Dry mouth Constipation Nausea Weight gain Rash and hives
Fluoxetine	Pain in IBS Diarrhoea in IBS Constipation in IBS Bloating in IBS Nausea in IBS Faecal urgency in IBS	Drowsiness Nausea Dry mouth Insomnia Dizziness
Citalopram	Pain in IBS Diarrhoea in IBS Constipation in IBS Bloating in IBS Nausea in IBS Faecal urgency in IBS	Drowsiness Nausea Dry mouth Insomnia Dizziness

This list is not exhaustive and further enquiry should be made with an up to date BNF.

Anti-diarrhoeal

Anti-diarrhoeal medication provides symptomatic relief for diarrhoea. It is important to determine the cause of symptoms; ensuring that other conditions are not masked by use of anti-diarrhoeal medication.

Drug	Indication	Side effects
Loperamide Available as capsules or liquid suspension	Diarrhoea Faecal urgency in IBS (⊃ p. 96–8 IBS) High output stoma Intestinal failure	Constipation Nausea Flatulence Use with caution in gastroenteritis as it may mask other conditions
Bismuth subsalicylate	Diarrhoea Upset stomach	Nausea Vomiting Darkening or blackening of faeces and tongue
Atropine	Diarrhoea	Nausea Vomiting Dizziness Confusion Depression
Codeine phosphate	(⊃ p. 406 to analgesics)	(⊃ p. 406 to analgesics)

This list is not exhaustive and further enquiry should be made with an up to date BNF.

Antiemetic

Antiemetics are used in preventing nausea and vomiting. It is important to understand the cause of the nausea/vomiting and ensure that use of an antiemetic does not mask any other condition.

Drug	Indication	Side effects
Metoclopramide	Nausea Vomiting	Diarrhoea All other medications should be reviewed prior to taking, as may interact with other medicines
Prochlorperazine	Nausea Vomiting	Dry mouth Dizziness Drowsiness Weight gain All other medications should be reviewed prior to taking, as may interact with other medicines
Ondansetron	Nausea Vomiting	Diarrhoea Dizziness Drowsiness Headache Fever
Domperidone	Gastroparesis (➲ p. 38–9 C2) (caution may mask other symptoms)	Diarrhoea Dizziness Drowsiness Headache Rash Itching Hives Leg cramps Insomnia

This list is not exhaustive and further enquiry should be made with an up to date BNF.

Antifungal

Antifungal medications are used to treat fungal infections such as candidiasis (thrush).

Drug	Indication	Side effects
Fluconazole	Oral candidiasis	Diarrhoea
		Heartburn
		Abdominal pain
		Dizziness
		Headache
		Drowsiness

This list is not exhaustive and further enquiry should be made with an up to date BNF.

Antisecretory

Antisecretory medication may be useful to treat symptoms of bowel obstruction. Also upper GI problems.

Drug	Indication	Side effects
Ranitidine	Duodenal ulcer Benign gastric ulcer Ulcers associated with *H. pylori* GORD	Urticaria Diarrhoea Constipation Nausea Abdominal pain
Cimetidine	Inhibits gastric secretion Duodenal ulcer GORD Meal related upper abdominal pain Reduce malabsorption and fluid loss in short bowel syndrome	Diarrhoea Pancreatitis (rare) Skin rash

This list is not exhaustive and further enquiry should be made with an up to date BNF.

Antivirals

Antivirals are drugs used to treat specific viral infections.

Drug	Indication	Side effects
Sofosbuvir	Hepatitis C	May interact with other medications, headache, fatigue, nausea
Ribavirin		
Paritaprevir		
Simeprivir		
Ledipasvir		
Ombitasvir		
Daclatasvir		
Peginterferon alfa	Hepatitis B	May interact with other medications,
Interferon	Hepatitis D	

This list is not exhaustive and further enquiry should be made with an up to date BNF.

Calcium channel blockers

Calcium channel blockers are a group of medications used to reduce the blood pressure. This is achieved by slowing the movement of calcium into the heart cells which reduces the workload of the heart.

Drug	Indication	Side effects
Diltiazem	Anal fissures, although unlicensed	Nausea Vomiting Dizziness Headache
Nifedipine	Achalasia (⮩ p. 18 C2) Improve swallowing Possibly useful in oesophageal spasm (⮩ p. 54)	Headache Nausea Dizziness Heartburn Constipation Cough

This list is not exhaustive and further enquiry should be made with an up to date BNF.

Chelates

Chelates can be used to treat the side effects of radiotherapy, such as enteropathy.

Drug	Indication	Side effects
Sucralfate enemas	Radiation enteropathy	Pain
Sucralfate	Bile reflux post-gastrectomy	Nausea, vomiting, diarrhoea, constipation, itching, headache

This list is not exhaustive and further enquiry should be made with an up to date BNF.

Cytotoxic agents

Cytotoxic drugs affect the growth and action of some cells, they can also be termed anticancer or chemotherapy.

Drug	Indication	Side effect
Podophyllin	Anal warts Note: avoid in pregnancy	Burning Itching Pain Ulceration
Trichloroacetic acid	Genital warts Anal warts Note: avoid in pregnancy	Burning Itching Pain Ulceration

This list is not exhaustive and further enquiry should be made with an up to date BNF.

Diuretics

Diuretics increase the passage of urine.

Drug	Indication	Side effects
Furosemide	Heart failure Liver disease Kidney disease High blood pressure	Nausea Vomiting Diarrhoea Constipation Dizziness Headache Blurred vision Stomach cramps
Spironolactone	Heart failure High blood pressure Hypokalaemia Ascites	Nausea Vomiting Diarrhoea Dizziness Irregular periods Erectile dysfunction Stomach cramps

H₂ receptor antagonists

H_2 receptor antagonist is an antihistamine medication. H_2 receptor antagonist block the action of histamine within the parietal cells of the stomach.

Drug	Indication	Side effects
Ranitidine	Duodenal ulcer Benign gastric ulcer Ulcers associated with *H. pylori* GORD	Urticaria Diarrhoea Constipation Nausea Abdominal pain
Nizatidine	Duodenal ulcer Benign gastric ulcer GORD	Sweating Urticaria
Cimetidine	Inhibits gastric secretion Duodenal ulcer GORD Meal related upper abdominal pain Reduce malabsorption and fluid loss in short bowel syndrome	Diarrhoea Pancreatitis (rare) Skin rash

This list is not exhaustive and further enquiry should be made with an up to date BNF.

Immunosuppressants

Immunosuppressant medication reduces the effects of the immune system.

Drug	Indication	Side effects
Tacrolimus	Liver transplant	Gastrointestinal perforation Bone marrow depression, leucopenia Thrombocytopenia Note: can interact with other medications
Azathioprine	Liver transplant Ulcerative colitis Crohn's disease	Can interact with other medications, bone marrow depression, leucopenia, thrombocytopenia
Infliximab	Ulcerative colitis Crohn's disease	Congestive heart failure Intestinal/perianal abscess Bacterial infections Note: Patients to be monitored for infections before and after treatment

This list is not exhaustive and further enquiry should be made with an up to date BNF.

Laxatives

A laxative is medication that aids defaecation.

Drug	Indication	Side effects
Ispaghula husk (bulk forming)	Low intake dietary fibre	Excess wind Bloating Can cause obstruction with not enough fluids
Sterculia (bulk forming)	Low intake dietary fibre	Bloating Wind Stomach pain
Senna (stimulant)	Acute constipation	Abdominal pain Cramps Diarrhoea Electrolyte abnormalities Melanosis coli Nausea
Bisacodyl (stimulant)	Acute constipation	Abdominal cramping Electrolyte imbalance Excessive diarrhoea Nausea Rectal burning Vomiting
Lactulose (osmotic)	Chronic constipation	Diarrhoea Nausea Vomiting Bloating Wind Belching Stomach pain
Macrogols (osmotic)	Chronic constipation	Nausea Vomiting Bloating Wind Anal discomfort Diarrhoea Electrolyte imbalance
Docusate sodium (softener)	Chronic constipation	Bitter taste Bloating Cramping Diarrhoea Wind Rectal irritation Throat irritation

Drug	Indication	Side effects
Prucalopride	Impaired motility of constipation	Headache Nausea (short lived)
Linaclotide	IBS constipation	Diarrhoea Dizziness Hypotension
Lubiprostone	IBS constipation	Nausea Abdominal pain Flatus Diarrhoea Bloating Vomiting Dry mouth

This list is not exhaustive and further enquiry should be made with an up to date BNF.

Neurotoxins

Neurotoxins are toxins that are destructive to nerves; this can be temporary.

Drug	Indication	Side effects
Botulinum toxin	Relieve symptoms of achalasia Improve swallowing (➲ p. 24 C2) Gastroparesis (➲ p. 38–9 C2) note: these uses are classed as being used off licence Anal fissures	If used in anal fissure can cause faecal incontinence

This list is not exhaustive and further enquiry should be made with an up to date BNF.

Nitrates

Nitrates relax the blood vessels.

Drug	Indication	Side effects
Isosorbide mononitrate (ISMO)	Relieve symptoms of achalasia (⊃ p. 18 C2); Note neurotoxins should always be tried initially	Nausea Vomiting Dizziness Headache
Nitroglycerin	Relieve symptoms of achalasia (⊃ p. 18 C2), Note neurotoxins should always be tried initially Anal fissures (ointment)	Nausea Vomiting Dizziness Headache
Diltiazem (cream)	Anal fissures, although unlicensed	Nausea Vomiting Dizziness Headache

This list is not exhaustive and further enquiry should be made with an up to date BNF.

Oral rehydration solution

For people who are at risk of dehydration it is important to rehydrate them.

Drug	Indication	Side effects
Oral rehydration solution e.g. World Health Organization Dioralyte	Giardiasis (➲ p. 67) Diarrhoea (➲ p. 204)	High blood sodium High blood potassium

The recipe for the World Health Organization can be found at: https://www.who.int/maternal_child_adolescent/documents/fch_cah_06_1/en/ (accessed 16/07/20).

Proton pump inhibitors

Proton pump inhibitors (PPIs) work by blocking and reducing the production of stomach acid.

Drug	Indication	Side effects
Omeprazole	Duodenal ulcers Gastric ulcers Used with antibiotics for H. pylori (❸ p. 42 C2) GORD Oesophagitis Dysphagia (❸ p. 24 C2)	Headache Abdominal pain Constipation Diarrhoea Flatulence Nausea Vomiting Note: can interact with other medications
Lansoprazole	Duodenal ulcers Gastric ulcers Used with antibiotics for H. pylori (❸ p. 42 C2) GORD Oesophagitis Dysphagia (❸ p. 24 C2)	Headache Abdominal pain Constipation Diarrhoea Flatulence Nausea Vomiting Note: can interact with other medications
Pantoprazole	Duodenal ulcers Gastric ulcers Used with antibiotics for H. pylori (❸ p. 42 C2) GORD Oesophagitis Dysphagia (❸ p. 24 C2)	Headache Abdominal pain Constipation Diarrhoea Flatulence Nausea Vomiting Note: can interact with other medications
Rabeprazole	Duodenal ulcers Gastric ulcers Used with antibiotics for H. pylori (❸ p. 42 C2) GORD	Headache Abdominal pain Constipation Diarrhoea Flatulence Nausea Vomiting Note: can interact with other medications

This list is not exhaustive and further enquiry should be made with an up to date BNF.

Steroids

Steroids are anti-inflammatory drugs.

Drug	Indication	Side effects
Oral steroids	Reduce inflammatory conditions including IBD (🔿 p. 368)	Gastric ulcers (🔿 p. 30–1 C2)
Hydrocortisone (IV)	Toxic megacolon (🔿 p. 105) Ulcerative colitis (🔿 p. 370) Crohn's disease (🔿 p. 377)	Gastric ulcers (🔿 p. 30–1 C2) Hypertension Note: elderly people require close supervision
Hydrocortisone cream	Anal fissure (low dose)	Hypersensitivity
Ursodeoxycholic acid	Gallstones Primary biliary cholangitis	Pasty stools Diarrhoea Note: May interact with other medications

This list is not exhaustive and further enquiry should be made with an up to date BNF.

Chapter 18

Gastrointestinal emergencies

Appendicitis

Appendicitis is an acute inflammation of the appendix.

Symptoms
- Nausea
- Vomiting
- Abdominal pain, starting centrally and moving to the right iliac fossa—mild to moderate
- Fever
- Diarrhoea—occasionally
- Generalized peritonitis (➔ p. 442).

Causes
Often the cause of appendicitis is an infection.

Incidence
Appendicitis is common in children and young adults but less common in people over 40 years of age.

Investigations
Investigations should include:
- Observations
- Urinalysis
- Consider pregnancy
- Blood tests—full blood count (FBC)—white cell count is often but not always raised); urea and electrolytes (U&Es).

Treatment
Treatment includes:
- Insertion of intravenous (IV) access
- Analgesia
- IV fluids if dehydrated or awaiting surgery
- IV antibiotics.

Accurate nursing assessment should enable differentiation between patients with localized pain in the right iliac fossa and those with more serious pathology, for example, generalized peritonitis and shock. Assessment should also include investigations that may point to another cause.

Acute abdominal pain

Presentation with acute abdominal pain represents the commonest surgical presentation to the Accident and Emergency department.

Causes

The cause (see Table 18.1) will depend upon factors such as patient history, site of pain, if the pain radiates, and if there are any aggravating factors.

There are other potential non-gastrointestinal causes of an acute abdomen, such as a ruptured ectopic pregnancy.

Table 18.1 Patterns of the common causes of acute abdominal pain

	Site	Radiation	Aggravating factors	Natural history
Appendicitis	Central, right iliac fossa	Nil	Movement	Pain shifts from the centre to the right
Diverticulitis	Left iliac fossa	Nil	Movement	Older patient, recurrent pain
Gut obstruction	Symmetric	Nil	Meals	Severe pain, might start as subacute
Gut perforation	Upper	Nil	Movement	Acute history
Cholecystitis	Right upper quadrant	Left shoulder tip, back	Inspiration	Recurrent bouts of colic
Pancreatitis	Central, upper	Nil	Movement	Severe pain, might be acute or chronic
Renal colic	Flank	Groin	Nil	Acute severe pain

Investigations

Investigations include:
- Routine bloods (including amylase)
- Urine microscopy
- A pregnancy test (if appropriate to exclude ectopic pregnancy).

Imaging might include:
- Erect chest X-ray—if a bowel perforation is suspected—revealing air under the diaphragm
- A supine abdominal X-ray—can exclude renal stones and bowel obstruction
- Ultrasound—to detect free fluid
- Consider computed tomography (CT) scan

Physical examination might reveal features of:
- Peritoneal irritation
- An abdominal mass
- An obstruction, such as secondary to a hernia.

Inflammatory bowel disease

Ulcerative colitis (➲ p. 370) is not commonly associated with severe pain; except in major disease flares.

The presence of acute pain in a patient with Crohn's disease requires blood tests to measure C-reactive protein (CRP) and erythrocyte sedimentation rate (ESR). If these inflammatory markers are elevated, the causes might include an acute inflammatory flare, development of an intra-abdominal abscess, or drug-induced pancreatitis. If these markers are not elevated consider intestinal stricture, adhesion obstruction, peptic ulcer, or renal/biliary colic.

Treatment

Management of acute pain depends on the cause. In general, analgesia should be offered—opiates are often needed for severe pain. If the diagnosis is uncertain, an overnight admission may be needed. Other possible treatment options include:

- Anti-spasmodic (➲ p. 409)—for colicky pain
- Anti-emetics (➲ p. 412)
- Antacid (➲ p. 407)—for epigastric pain
- Antibiotics (➲ p. 408)—if perforation or infection
- IV fluids—if dehydrated, nil by mouth, vomiting, or shocked
- O_2—if shocked
- Consider insertion of a urinary catheter—if shocked to monitor urine output
- Consider nasogastric tube insertion (➲ p. 324–5) if bowel obstruction or perforation is reported.

The nurse also needs to provide support and explanation.

Bleeding of the gastrointestinal tract

Lower gastrointestinal (GI) bleeds are most commonly small and due to bleeding haemorrhoids. An acute lower GI bleed is rare, but can be seen in the elderly due to diverticular disease (→ p. 90–1), inflammatory bowel disease (→ p. 368–9), colorectal cancer (→ p. 352), or ischaemic colitis (→ p. 100). Upper GI bleeds can be seen as haematemesis (→ p. 436–7).

Symptoms

GI tract bleeds (duodenal or above) can present as melaena—seen as black, tarry/sticky stool as a result of the altered blood. Other symptoms can include anaemia or iron deficiency anaemia.

Causes

Most iron deficiency anaemia in men and post-menopausal women is of GI origin.

Investigations

Investigation should include the upper and lower GI tract.

Treatment

Patients may require resuscitation if shocked.

Haematemesis

An acute upper GI bleed, can be seen as haematemesis—vomiting blood. Haematemesis can be an emergency, depending on the volume and type of bleeding.

Symptoms

The appearance of the haematemesis can vary:
- Fresh blood—bright red bleed
- Altered blood—'coffee ground' in appearance has been in the stomach for a few hours
- Altered blood with small flecks of fresh blood—might indicate prolonged vomiting
- Major bleed.

Causes

There are a number of causes for haematemesis:
- Peptic ulcer (➋ p. 30)—50%
- Oesophageal varices (➋ p. 55)—10–20%, although the mortality rate is >50% if secondary to liver cirrhosis
- Gastric erosions—15–20%
- Others—Mallory–Weiss tear; 5–10% (➋ p. 45), gastric erosion, oesophageal erosion or reflux, gastric cancer, pancreatitis, gallstone perforation of duodenum, swallowing blood (e.g. nosebleeds), ingested foreign body (➋ p. 264–5) or poisons, and other rare disorders
- Children—foreign bodies and the possibility of Munchausen's syndrome by proxy.

These causes may be associated with a history of:
- Alcohol abuse
- Liver disease (➋ p. 145–79)
- Medications— non-steroidal anti-inflammatory drugs (NSAIDs) (➋ p. 406), anticoagulants, or steroids (➋ p. 406).

Investigations

A full assessment is required including for signs of shock:
- Hypotension
- Postural hypotension
- Tachycardia
- Collapse.

When the source of the bleeding is uncertain then perform:
- Upper GI endoscopy
- Liver function tests.

Treatments

It might be necessary for emergency fluid resuscitation for a large bleed such as peptic ulcer or oesophageal varices (➋ p. 55). Initiation of a major bleed policy (as per Trust policy) might be appropriate, with advice from a haematologist.
- Consider airway protection—if reduced consciousness, possibly intubation
- O_2—possibly by nasal prongs if vomiting

- IV access with large-bore cannula into large veins—for IV fluids and possibly a transfusion is required
- Consider central access for major bleeds
- Consider urinary catheter insertion to monitor hourly urine output
- Consider nasogastric tube insertion
- Warm the patient
- Consider cardiovascular support—inotropes and vasopressors
- Monitor observations—pulse, respiration rate, oxygen saturation, blood pressure, conscious levels, ECG (electrocardiogram)
- Carefully record fluid balance.

It is ideal to keep the patient nil by mouth until the endoscopy is undertaken. Reassurance is needed from the nurse as this can be alarming for the patient.

Prognosis

The mortality rate is 10% of admissions overall. The elderly and people with comorbidities are at greater risk of dying. The Rockall score, including factors such as age and comorbidities, is used to determine mortality risk.

In 30% of patients, no cause of the bleeding is found.

Treatment

Treatment depends on cause of bleeding and can include:
- Injection sclerotherapy for varices
- Endoscopic band ligation (◆ p. 270–1) for varices
- Injection with dilute adrenaline, thrombin, or fibrin glue—ulcers
- Electrocoagulation—ulcers.

Treatment is also required if there is an underlying problem, such as liver disease.

Prevention of rebleed can include:
- IV omeprazole for ulcers.

Close monitoring of vital signs. Explanation and appropriate reassurance as patient and family likely to be very anxious. Note repeated treatment is required if bleeding recurs.

Obstruction

Intestinal obstruction can be a complete or partial blockage of the bowel. This might mean that the intestinal contents do not move along the GI tract.

Symptoms

There are a number of symptoms of intestinal obstruction:
- Abdominal distension
- Absent bowel sounds or 'tinkling' sounds
- Abdominal pain—when severe may indicate strangulation
- Abdominal cramp
- Vomiting
- Constipation or diarrhoea
- Halitosis
- Signs of shock
- Peritonitis (➋ p. 442)
- Fever.

It should be noted that above the obstruction the bowel can become inflamed, strangulated, ischaemic, and necrotic.

Causes

Small bowel obstruction may be caused by:
- Adhesions
- Crohn's disease (➋ p. 377)—small bowel obstruction can be due to active inflammation (➋ p. 377), fibrosis (➋ p. 377), or strictures (➋ p. 377).

Less commonly:
- A strangulated hernia
- Intussusception (➋ p. 138–9)—telescoping of the bowel within itself.

Colonic obstruction may be caused by:
- Bowel (colonic) cancer (➋ p. 352)
- Sigmoid volvulus (➋ p. 116)
- Diverticular disease (➋ p. 90–1).

In the post-operative period, there might be an ileus/paralytic ileus—when peristalsis (➋ p. 8) ceases.
   An ileus can be caused by:
- Medication—narcotics
- Injury to the blood supply
- Complications of intra-abdominal surgery
- Intraperitoneal infection.

A paralytic ileus in a newborn might be due to necrotizing enterocolitis (➋ p. 76) and is life-threatening.
   Mechanical obstruction may be caused by:
- Hernia
- Surgical adhesions
- Impacted faeces
- Colorectal cancer (➋ p. 352)
- Intussusception (➋ p. 138–9)
- Volvulus—twisted bowel (➋ p. 116)
- Foreign bodies (➋ p. 440–1).

Bowel cancer

About 15% of patients with a colorectal cancer present with acute obstruction of the colon by the malignancy. There is an added risk that the cancer might perforate, leading to peritonitis (◑ p. 442) and a potentially life-threatening situation.

Investigations

Investigations include:
- Observations
- Blood tests for inflammatory markers etc
- Abdominal X-ray—may show distended bowel loops above the obstruction
- Colonoscopy.

Treatment

Treatment depends on the diagnosis. Treatment might include:
- IV access
- O_2
- Analgesia
- Antiemetics
- IV fluids
- IV antibiotics
- Nasogastric tube insertion
- Urinary catheter insertion and monitoring of urine.

Care must be taken to ensure that the obstruction does not occlude the blood supply and cause tissue death, infection, and gangrene.

Surgery might be required if symptoms do not resolve.

Perforation

Bowel perforation (sometimes termed a ruptured bowel) can occur for a number of reasons.

Symptoms

The signs of perforation are commonly pain and peritonitis. Peritonitis is often characterized by the following:
• Fever
• Guarding
• Rebound tenderness
• Rigidity
• Absent bowel sounds.

In inflammatory bowel disease (IBD), these symptoms might be masked by steroids.

Signs to observe for ingested foreign objects in children, people with mental health issues, or elderly are as follows:
• Excessive salivation
• Regurgitation
• Choking
• Distress.

Pain or fever suggests a perforation. Generally, once through the pylorus, the foreign object might pass spontaneously. However, ileocaecal perforation can occur.

Chest pain might indicate a perforation, either after endoscopic removal of the foreign object or following ingestion. A small haematemesis might be due to perforation of a major blood vessel. For either symptom, assessment from a thoracic surgeon should be urgently sought.

Causes

There are a number of potential causes of a perforated bowel including:
• Inflammatory bowel disease
• Diverticular disease
• Ingested matter, such as bones or pins.

Ulcerative colitis

In ulcerative colitis (➜ p. 370), perforation can occur as a complication of toxic dilation, delayed surgery, or colonoscopy during a severe attack.

Crohn's disease

In Crohn's disease (➜ p. 377), the patient with a perforation rarely presents acutely. This is because an abscess cavity often forms and steroids frequently suppress clinical features.

Diverticular disease

In a perforated bowel associated with diverticular disease, there might be signs of peritonitis or a pelvic, paracolic, or subphrenic abscess. However, in the elderly or debilitated, there might be chronic pyrexia, ill health, and weight loss. Perforation of the diverticulum has a high mortality rate because the signs of peritonitis can be minimal. The risk of perforation, and subsequent mortality, is particularly high in the immunocompromised.

Investigations

Useful investigations for determining a bowel perforation are:
- A plain abdominal X-ray—showing free gas
- An erect chest X-ray.

For ingested objects, the following investigations are suggested:
- Looking in the mouth
- X-ray.

Treatment

Treatment can include addressing any symptoms including:
- Analgesia
- Anti-emetic
- IV access
- O_2 therapy
- Blood—U&Es, FBC, liver function tests (LFTs), and also group and save (in case transfusion is needed)
- IV antibiotics
- IV fluids if dehydrated
- Nasogastric tube insertion
- Urinary catheter insertion.

Treatment for a perforated bowel in ulcerative colitis (UC) is with fluid, blood, and electrolyte replacement. When the patient is stable, surgery is indicated—colectomy and temporary ileostomy (p. 504–5).

Treatment for a perforated diverticulum might include surgery, such as a Hartmann's procedure and temporary end colostomy (p. 504–5).

Treatment for ingested foreign objects depends on symptoms and assessment. If the object is impacted in the throat, it can be removed by an ENT (ear, nose, and throat) surgeon. Endoscopy (p. 236) might be able to retrieve objects that have not yet passed into the duodenum.

Peritonitis

Peritonitis is an inflammation of the lining of the abdomen, the peritoneum (➲ p. 5) this can be caused by a bacterial infection secondary to a rupture of an abdominal organ, such as the bowel. Peritonitis can result in death if left untreated.

Symptoms

There are a number of symptoms associated with peritonitis, including:

- Acute, severe abdominal pain, worse on movement or palpation
- Fever
- Tachycardia
- Tachypnoea
- Reduced urine output
- Distention
- Rigid abdomen
- Rebound tenderness
- Absent bowel sounds
- Nausea and/or vomiting
- Anorexia
- Hypovolaemic shock.

Patient may be critically ill with septic shock, although in the elderly or with people with IBD sometimes symptoms are more insidious.

Causes

There are a number of potential causes of peritonitis, including:

- Perforated gastric/duodenal ulcer
- Perforated appendix
- Crohn's disease
- Diverticulitis
- Pancreatitis
- Surgery
- Cirrhosis.

Investigations

There are a number of investigations that are required, including:

- Observations
- Blood tests including FBC, U&Es, amylase/lipase
- Arterial blood gases
- Evaluate for signs of shock—hypovolaemic or septic
- Assess, treat, and monitor pain
- Erect chest X-ray—to show free gas under the diaphragm from an acute perforation
- Abdominal X-ray.

Treatment

Treatment depends upon the severity of the symptoms and infection. Treatment may include IV antibiotics (➲ p. 408). Alternatively, surgery may be necessary: this might be to drain an abscess under local anaesthetic with a needle, or removal of a ruptured appendix or a section of bowel for perforated diverticulum.

Varices

Oesophageal varices are enlarged veins within the oesophagus. The veins often enlarge as a result of the blood flow through the portal vein being obstructed as a result of liver damage. The most common site is the gastro-oesophageal junction.

Symptoms

There are usually no obvious symptoms until bleeding occurs, with bright red blood.

Causes

There is usually a history of alcohol abuse and cirrhosis (♦ p. 152–4) in people with oesophageal varices. In 90% of people, there are oesophageal varices after 10 years with alcoholic cirrhosis.

Incidence

Acute bleeding from oesophageal varices accounts for about 10–20% of acute upper GI bleeds. About 50% of patients with portal hypertension will bleed from their varices.

Investigations

Depending upon the extent of the bleed, urgent endoscopy is needed to inspect and treat the varices.

Treatment

On presentation to the accident and emergency department with a major upper GI bleed, initial treatment is airway maintenance and fluid resuscitation. The major bleed policy, as per Trust protocol, should be followed.

Treatment via endoscopy if possible, to enable ligation (♦ p. 270) or sclerotherapy (♦ p. 270). The latter involves injection into the veins to enable clotting/narrowing of the blood vessel.

If endoscopy is unavailable consider:
• Vasopressin +/− glycerine trinitrate infusion
• Somatostatin, octreotide.

Consider additionally prophylactic antibiotics to reduce mortality and morbidity.

In the majority of people with alcoholic cirrhosis who stop alcohol intake, there is a reduction in the size of the varices, which may totally resolve.

To prevent bleeds, prophylaxis can be propranolol or surgery.

Prognosis

Mortality is high; about 50% of patients die following the first episode of bleeding.

Bowel care

Defaecation

Defaecation is the final act of digestion by which faeces are eliminated from the digestive tract via the anus. The first step occurs when contraction of the circular muscle in the colon triggers a defaecation reflex, which in turn propels the faeces towards the rectum. If a sufficient volume accumulates in the rectum, this will stimulate a reflexive contraction in the rectum where the internal sphincter will relax, and the external sphincter will contract. Defaecation does not occur at this point—it is the urge to defaecate that occurs. Depending on the circumstances, defaecation will either occur or there may be a delay.

Defaecation depends on several factors for the bowel to function and work properly including the following:

• The nerves of the rectum and anus need to be able to send the correct messages to the brain, so that stool (faeces) and flatus can be felt when arriving in the rectum, which in turn can send messages to the external sphincter to hold on.
• The internal and external anal sphincters need to be working correctly.
• Stool should be soft to formed, so that sphincters can cope with holding on.

There is a spectrum of what can be considered normal frequency of defae-cation and is generally anywhere between one to three times a day to three times a week. However, this can vary considerably from one individual to another. There are times when the defaecation reflex does not function appropriately and therefore altered defaecation processes lead to altered bowel function and disorders that are commonly encountered in clinical practice.

Faecal incontinence

Faecal incontinence is defined as involuntary leakage of liquid or solid stool at a socially inappropriate time. The term anal incontinence is generally used as a definition if wanting to include flatus incontinence. Faecal incontinence is a sign or a symptom, not a diagnosis. Therefore, it is important to diagnose the cause or causes for each individual. There is no consensus on methods of classifying the symptoms and causes of faecal incontinence. It is most commonly classified according to symptom, character of the leakage, patient group, or presumed primary underlying cause.

Causes

- Anal sphincter disruption/weakness:
  - Obstetric injury
  - Surgery
  - Idiopathic sphincter degeneration
  - Penetration.
- Anal fissure (➲ p. 120–1)
- Haemorrhoids (➲ p. 126–8)
- Gut motility
- Stool consistency
- Congenital anomalies (➲ p. 395–404)
- Irritable bowel syndrome (IBS) (➲ p. 96–8).

Assessment

Nursing assessment takes time and needs privacy for the patient to be able to relax and provide a full picture of their problem and how this impacts on psychological well-being. Assessment can be used to plan individualized care with a guide to a methodical approach. A general assessment (➲ p. 202 to assessment chapter) should be followed by the following more specific assessment. Investigation of any red flags (such as rectal bleeding) should be undertaken.

- History of the bowel problem and previous bowel habit
- Usual bowel pattern/stool consistency
- Faecal incontinence, how much, how often?
- Urgency/urge incontinence
- Soiling
- Flatus control
- Difficulty evacuating
- Dietary and fluid details
- Prolapse
- Bleeding
- Obstetric history
- Skin problems
- Bladder symptoms
- Effects on lifestyle/relationships/emotions/psychological impact
- Coping strategies.

Patient history/assessment can be supported by patient-reported outcome measures (PROMs) to quantify symptoms and transform individual experiences into objective data. In so doing, this grades the severity of faecal incontinence allowing for monitoring of treatment. An example of a PROM for faecal incontinence is the International Consultation on Incontinence Questionnaire Anal Incontinence Symptoms and Quality of Life Module (ICIQ-B). The ICIQ-B provides a robust measure organized into three domains: bowel pattern, bowel control, and impact on quality of life associated with anal incontinence symptoms.

Physical examination

Physical examination is used when disease is suspected or already identified. It may also be utilized as a screening examination when there is no suspicion/expectation of disease and used as part of the history-taking.

The reasons pertaining to the procedure should be explained to the patient. The procedure itself should be explained and a chaperone should be offered (➲ p. 208–9).

Further reading

NICE (2007). Management of faecal incontinence in adult: CG 49. https://www.nice.org.uk/guidance/cg49 (Accessed 20/7/2020).

Royal College of Surgeons (2017). Faecal Incontinence Commissioning Guidance. https://www.rcseng.ac.uk/library-and-publications/rcs-publications/docs/faecal-incontinence-guide

Faecal incontinence—conservative management

Conservative bowel management is generally regarded as first-line treatment for faecal incontinence, once all necessary investigations have been performed to rule out any organic pathology. Faecal incontinence occurring exclusively secondary to diarrhoea, such as IBD (➜ p. 368–9), colorectal cancer (➜ p. 352), and diverticular disease (➜ p. 90–1), needs to be managed by treating the underlying cause of the diarrhoea first.

People who report or are reported to have faecal incontinence should be offered care, managed by healthcare professionals who have the relevant skills, training, and experience, and who work within an integrated continence service.

Management of faecal incontinence will depend on the patient's symptoms, but can include lifestyle modifications and other approaches.

Patient education

Developing an understanding of the digestive tract and the pelvic floor can improve the individual's compliance with treatment when strategies are clarified. The education about what a normal bowel movement is can be the first part of the process in comprehending and addressing any concerns. It is at this point that results of any investigations can be given and discussed, thereby, improving the patient's understanding of how their bowel functions.

Other conservative bowel management techniques include:
- Diet and fluid management (➜ p. 445–72)
- Medication management (➜ p. 445–72)
- Bowel and muscle retraining (➜ p. 445–72)
- Plugs/inserts (➜ p. 445–72)
- Transanal irrigation (➜ p. 445–72).

Faecal incontinence—diet and fluid management

Diet and fluid modification

The patient may report triggers that worsen their symptoms. Management should be based on the presenting factors of the individual, such as foods and drinks that may exacerbate faecal incontinence:

Fibre

- Wholegrain cereals/bread (reduce quantities)
- Porridge/oats may cause fewer problems than whole-wheat based cereals.

Fruit and vegetables

- Rhubarb, figs, prunes, and plums—consider avoiding these as they contain natural laxative compounds
- Beans, pulses, cabbage, and sprouts
- Spices
- Chilli.

Artificial sweeteners

- May be found in special diabetic products such as chocolate, biscuits, conserves, and in some sugar-free items including many nicotine replacement gums.

Alcohol

- Especially stout, beers, and ales.

Lactose

- Some patients experience a lactase deficiency. While small amounts of milk, for example in tea, or yoghurt are often tolerated, an increase of milk in the diet may cause diarrhoea for some.

Caffeine

- Excessive intake of caffeine may loosen stool and thus increase faecal incontinence in some patients.

Care should be undertaken to not exclude essential foods from the diet, and assistance from a dietitian may be necessary.

Faecal incontinence—medication management

Consistency of stool can greatly impact on faecal incontinence and severity of symptoms. Some medications can worsen symptoms and require review. When reviewing medication, healthcare professionals may consider alternatives to drugs that could create a looser stool and therefore contribute to faecal incontinence, for example, metformin. Additionally, any over-the-counter medicines may be a factor and may require further review. Should altering/reducing medications that have a diarrhoeal effect not help symptoms, and if all other investigations are negative, then the following can be considered as means to improving stool consistency, thus preventing loose/soft stool, which as a result may improve the faecal incontinence.

Medication to help thicken faeces includes:
- Loperamide (➲ p. 411)
- Bulking agents (➲ p. 422–3)
- Amitriptyline (➲ p. 410).

Loperamide (➲ p. 422–3 to pharmacological chapter)

Patients can be advised to start with a lower dose of 0.5 mg when using liquid form and titrate accordingly to each individual, up to 16 mg when using tablet form. It is preferable for it to be taken 30 min before eating, which will help to reduce the gastrocolic response, allow water from the stool to be reabsorbed and provide a more manageable stool.

Bulking agents (➲ p. 422–3 to pharmacological chapter)

Bulking agents work by increasing the bulk of the stool and therefore provides a firmer stool that is more manageable in faecal incontinence, for example Fybogel. Can take 2–3 days to work and will need titration according to the individual's symptoms.

Amitriptyline (➲ p. 410 to pharmacological chapter)

Other medications, such as amitriptyline, may help to improve stool consistency by decreasing rectal contractions and therefore reducing rectal sensation and urgency.

Faecal incontinence—bowel and muscle retraining

Biofeedback

Biofeedback is a re-education tool using instruments, such as a computer or video with sensors, which provides information on the function of the pelvic floor that is displayed visually +/− sound. Consequently, the individual can train their pelvic floor muscles as a result of the feedback gained.

Pelvic floor exercises

The principal goal of pelvic floor exercises is to improve the pelvic floor and anal sphincter muscle strength, tone, endurance, and coordination to create a positive effect in function with a decrease in bowel symptoms. Patients are generally taught through rectal or vaginal examination and are taught to contract, which may involve endurance contractions and fast-twitch contractions. A programme of pelvic floor exercises is set to individual attainment and advised to practice each day to strengthen the pelvic floor. Alternatively exercises can be advised by likening the pelvic floor to a lift, which is able to stop at different floors as it ascends and descends. The length of time for positive results varies from person to person and is usually discussed with the therapist from assessment. It should be noted that if patients have difficulty in performing a muscle contraction, neuromuscular stimulation with electrodes can be used with a vaginal or rectal probe to enhance awareness of the pelvic floor and aid learning about how to contract these muscles.

Urge resistance

Patients with faecal incontinence often experience urgency in spite of an adequate pelvic floor contraction, although this is seldom maintained. Resisting the urge through the use of varying instruments, for example, an air inflated balloon can be used in a clinic setting. The balloon is inserted rectally and inflated with air until the urge to defaecate is felt. The patient is then taught to contract the pelvic floor in the correct manner and therefore maintain a longer contraction, which in turn will diminish the symptoms of urgency.

Further reading

DeBevoise TM, Dobinsky AF, McCurdy-Robinson CB, et al. (2015). Pelvic floor physical therapy: More than Kegels. *Women's Healthcare* May 2015: 34–9. http://npwomenshealthcare.com/wp-content/uploads/2015/05/Pelvic_M15.pdf (Accessed 25/06/2019).

Johannessen H, Wibe A, Stordahl A, et al. (2017). Do pelvic floor muscles exercises reduce postpartum anal incontinence? A randomised controlled trial. *British Journal of Obstetrics and Gynaecology* 124 (4): 686–94. https://obgyn.onlinelibrary.wiley.com/doi/10.1111/1471-0528.14145 (Accessed 16/07/2020).

Scott KM (2014). Pelvic floor rehabilitation in the treatment of fecal incontinence. *Clinics in Colon and Rectal Surgery* 27(3): 99–105. https://www.ncbi.nlm.nih.gov/pmc/articles/PMC4174224/ (Accessed 16/07/2020).

Faecal incontinence—plugs and inserts

Occasionally having a physical barrier can help to reassure the patient. The concept behind plugs and inserts are to act as a barrier in preventing leakage. They are easily inserted into the rectum, can be removed and disposed of allowing for replacement with a fresh product. There are two products currently on the market that are recognised for such use.

Coloplast anal plug

This device is a porous absorbent material that lets air in and blocks the leak offering the patient freedom from faecal incontinence/leakage and therefore improving quality of life.

Renew insert

This device is made from supple silicone that adapts to the body for a soft and comfortable fit. They are safe to wear day and night and inserted with a fingertip applicator.

Further reading

https://www.continenceproductadvisor.org/products/faecaldevices/analplugs
https://renew-medical.uk/products/renew-insert/

Faecal incontinence—transanal irrigation

Transanal irrigation (TAI) is the instillation of water to produce a bowel action to provide better control over bowel function. When conservative management such as diet, medication, and exercises have failed to adequately improve symptoms the next step in treatment is generally considered to be TAI.

TAI is performed by instilling warm water into the bowel, via the anus, producing expulsion of water and faeces. Irrigation products can use either low volumes of instilled water, e.g. approximately 70 ml of water to clear the rectum. Alternatively high volume products can instil up to 800 mls of water clearing the rectum and proximal colon.

Regular use of TAI can aid emptying of the bowel and thereby re-establish a more predictable evacuation and control of bowel function by choosing a suitable time for the individual to defecate. Effectively emptying the rectum +/− colon is likely to reduce symptoms of faecal incontinence and therefore enable active management.

Follow-up for the first month after training on irrigation is crucial to support the patient and address any problems that may occur. This empowers the patient to become independent.

Companies who supply TAI systems are:
- Aquaflush
- BBraun
- Coloplast
- Qufora
- Wellspect.

Most companies have support that can complement the healthcare professional in their support and follow-up. Ensuring that the patient has contact details and information for ordering products can strengthen a smooth transition to independence.

Further reading

Emmanuel AV, Krogh K, Bazzocchi G, et al. (2013). Consensus review of best practice of transanal irrigation in adults. *Spinal Cord* 51(10): 732–8.

Faecal incontinence—stimulation options

Percutaneous tibial nerve stimulation

Percutaneous tibial nerve stimulation (PTNS) is the use of external neuromodulation to stimulate the nerves related to continence. The aim of PTNS is to achieve a neuromodulatory effect through a minimally invasive route, but its exact mechanism of action is unclear.

A fine gauge needle is inserted just above and medial to the ankle next to the posterior tibial nerve and a surface electrode is placed near to the arch of the foot. The needle and electrode are connected to an external stimulator. Stimulation of the posterior tibial nerve produces a motor (flexion and fanning of the toes) and sensory (tingling in the ankle, toes, or foot) response. Treatment consists of 12 outpatient's visits lasting about 30 min each time, typically a week apart.

Sacral nerve stimulation

Sacral nerve stimulation (SNS) is the use of an internal neuromodulator to stimulate the nerves related to continence. Altering sphincter functioning is possible using the surrounding nerves and muscles by applying stimulation to one of the sacral nerves via an electrode place in the sacral foramen.

Initially the electrode is placed as a temporary measure during a test period. If the temporary SNS improves symptoms then an implantable, permanent device is inserted, with a battery pack placed in the buttock.

Further reading

NICE (2011). Percutaneous tibial nerve stimulation for faecal incontinence (IPG 395). https://www.nice.org.uk/guidance/ipg395/chapter/2-The-procedure (Accessed 27/06/2019).

NICE (2004). Sacral nerve stimulation for faecal incontinence. https://www.nice.org.uk/guidance/ipg99/chapter/2-The-procedure (Accessed 27/06/2019).

Faecal incontinence—stoma formation

A stoma (➲ p. 507–24) is a surgical procedure to bring out part of the bowel to the surface of the abdominal wall to pass faeces into a stoma appliance. A colostomy is the term used when the colon is used to form the stoma. A stoma is usually formed when conservative treatment modalities have failed to improve the patient's bowel dysfunction.

Stoma formation is a good treatment option for some people but not as first-line treatment.

Constipation

Definition of constipation is often seen as infrequent bowel movements, excessive straining, incomplete evacuation, failed or lengthy attempts to defaecate, digital removal of stool, abdominal bloating, and hard stools. Constipation can be classified into two groups: primary and secondary. Primary constipation is sometimes known as functional or chronic constipation. Secondary constipation is caused by another reason such as a side effect of medication.

Causes of primary constipation

Categorized into three main subtypes:
- Slow transit—prolonged transit time throughout the colon
- Evacuation disorder—incoordination of the pelvic floor muscles with a normal transit time or slow transit time
- Idiopathic constipation—constipation with a normal transit throughout the colon.

Causes of secondary constipation

Medications
- Antidepressants (⊃ p. 410)
- Opioids (⊃ p. 406)
- Iron preparations (⊃ p. 295)
- Anticholinergics (⊃ p. 409)
- Diuretics (⊃ p. 419)
- Antispasmodics(⊃ p. 409)
- Antihypertensives (⊃ p. 416)
- Antipsychotics (⊃ p. 410).

Medical conditions
- Endocrine—hypothyroidism, diabetes
- Neurological—Parkinson's, stroke
- Psychiatric—depression, anxiety, dementia
- Pregnancy.

Incidence

Constipation is one of the most common gastrointestinal complaints in the UK.

Assessment

Nursing assessment takes time and needs privacy for the patient to be able to relax and provide a full picture of their problem and how this impacts on their psychological well-being. Assessment can be used to plan individualized care with a guide to a methodical approach. Following a generic assessment (⊃ p. 202) should be the following:
- History of the bowel problem and previous bowel habit
- Usual bowel pattern/stool consistency
- Sensation of incomplete evacuation
- Bloating
- Straining/difficulty evacuating
- Digital evacuation
- Prolapse

- Bleeding
- Dietary and fluid details
- Details of previous and current laxatives
- Effects on lifestyle/relationships/emotions/psychological impact
- Coping strategies.

Investigation of any red flags should be addressed.

Patient history/assessment can be supported by PROMs to quantify symptoms and transform individual experiences into objective data. A PROM that is frequently used for constipation is the patient assessment of constipation symptoms (PAC-SYM).

Physical examination

Physical examination is used when disease is suspected or already identified. It may also be utilized as a screening examination when there is no suspicion/expectation of disease and used as part of the history-taking.

The reasons pertaining to the procedure should be explained to the patient. The procedure itself should be explained and a chaperone should be offered (➲ p. 201–10 to assessment chapter).

Further reading

Collins B and Bradshaw E (2016). *Bowel Dysfunction: A Comprehensive Guide for Healthcare Professionals*. Springer Nature, Switzerland.

Nazarko L (2017). Constipation: A guide top assessment and treatment. *Independent Nurse*. http://www.independentnurse.co.uk/clinical-article/constipation-a-guide-to-assessment-and-treatment/155936/ (Accessed 27/06/2019).

Yiannakou Y, Tack J, Piessevaux H, et al. (2017). The PAC-SYM questionnaire for chronic constipation: defining the minimal important difference. *Alimentary Pharmacology & Therapeutics* 46(11–12): 1103–11. https://www.ncbi.nlm.nih.gov/pmc/articles/PMC5698746/ (Accessed 27/06/2019).

Constipation—conservative management

In patients with no known secondary causes of constipation, conservative non-pharmacologic treatment measures generally are recommended as first-line therapy. These strategies typically include dietary modification, increased fluid intake, and bowel habit training.

Patient education

Developing an understanding of the digestive tract and the pelvic floor can improve the individual's compliance with treatment when strategies are clarified. The education of what is a normal bowel movement can be the first part of the process in comprehending and addressing any concerns. It is at this point that results of any investigations can be given and discussed, enhancing the understanding of bowel function.

Constipation—diet and fluid management

One of the first steps in addressing constipation is to look at diet. For an acute phase, adding in more fibre to the diet may relieve symptoms. However, for chronic constipation, diet may require modification, especially as increasing insoluble fibres in the diet may have an impact, which can increase bloating or flatulence, and produce harder stools. Decreasing insoluble fibres in this group of patients may help to relieve symptoms of bloating and flatulence, although it may not improve transit time.

Insoluble fibres can be found in:
- Wheat bran
- Some vegetables (stalks, skins, and seeds)
- Whole grains.

Referral to a dietitian may be necessary.

Constipation—medication management

There are a number of medications that can be useful for treating constipation. The most common are laxatives.

Laxatives

Laxatives may be required for people who do not respond to other conservative measures such as diet. The type of laxative will depend on individual symptoms.

Type of laxative	Indication
Bulk forming (➲ p. 422–3)	Low intake dietary fibre
Stimulant (➲ p. 422–3)	Short term relief, acute
Osmotic (➲ p. 422–3)	Chronic constipation
Stool softeners (➲ p. 422–3)	Chronic constipation

Other medications that can be useful include:
- Prucalopride (➲ p. 422–3)
- Lubiprostone (➲ p. 422–3)
- Linaclotide (➲ p. 422–3).

Constipation—bowel and muscle retraining

Behavioural treatment enables patients to learn the physiological mechanisms of defaecation. This includes learning how to use their diaphragms, as well as abdominal and pelvic floor muscles, to evacuate the bowel.

Evacuation techniques

The patient should be advised to adopt a squatting type position where feet are placed on a stool to ensure knees are raised higher than the hips. This helps to relax the pelvic floor. A combination of this and bulging out the abdomen creates intra-abdominal pressure and therefore prevents straining.

Constipation—transanal irrigation

Transanal irrigation (TAI) is the instillation of water to produce a bowel action to provide a controlled bowel evacuation. When conservative management, such as diet, medication, and exercises, has failed to adequately improve symptoms, the next step in treatment is generally considered to be TAI.

TAI is where warm water is instilled into the bowel, via the anus, producing expulsion of water and faeces. Irrigation fluid can be up to 800 mls of water to clear the rectum and proximal colon.

Regular use of TAI can aid emptying of the bowel and thereby re-establish evacuation at a suitable time for the individual.

Follow-up for the first month after training on irrigation is crucial to support the patient and address any problems that may occur. This empowers the patient to become independent.

Companies who supply TAI systems are:
• Aquaflush
• BBraun
• Coloplast
• Qufora
• Wellspect.

Most companies have support that can complement the healthcare professional in their support and follow-up. Ensuring that the patient has contact details and information for ordering products can strengthen a smooth transition to independence.

Further reading

Emmanuel AV, Krogh K, Bazzocchi G, et al. (2013) Consensus review of best practice of transanal irrigation in adults. *Spinal Cord* 51(10): 732–8.

Constipation—stoma formation

Formation of a stoma (➔ p. 504–5) can enable passage of faeces from the bowel. This might be a colostomy (➔ p. 504–5) for people with evacuation difficulties or an ileostomy (➔ p. 504–5) for people with transit problems.

Further reading

Collins B and Bradshaw E (2016). *Bowel Dysfunction: A Comprehensive Guide for Healthcare Professionals*. Springer Nature, Switzerland.

Neurogenic bowel dysfunction

Neurogenic bowel dysfunction (NBD) is the inability to control defaecation/evacuation due to a nervous system problem.

Causes

- Spinal cord injury
- Spina bifida
- Cauda equina
- Multiple sclerosis.

Assessment

Assessment is per faecal incontinence assessment (➔ p. 448–9) and constipation assessment (➔ p. 458–9). Additionally the following:

- Hand function
- Balance
- Accessing the toilet independently
- Is a carer required?
- Availability of adapted toilet facilities
- Risk to skin integrity
- General health (i.e. postural hypotension)
- Home circumstances
- Cognitive ability.

Physical assessment

Physical assessment is as per faecal incontinence (➔ p. 449) and constipation (➔ p. 459).

Neurogenic bowel dysfunction—spinal cord injury

Bowel dysfunction caused by spinal cord injury is due to loss of normal sensory or motor control or both, as a result of central neurological disease or damage. This can be classified into two types:

• Upper motor neuron (reflexic) lesion—most commonly occurs with spinal cord injuries at and above T12. The nerve connections between the spinal cord and colon remain intact, thus preserving reflex co-ordination and stool propulsion. This presentation is influenced where the external anal sphincter is unable to relax with an inability to defecate. This results in retention of stool and is typically associated with constipation and faecal retention.

• Lower motor neuron (areflexic) (flaccid) lesion—most commonly occurs with spinal cord injuries at and below L1. For that reason, people with a lower motor neuron lesion lack peristalsis and have slow stool propulsion with a risk of faecal incontinence due to the atonic external sphincter and a lack of control over the levator ani muscle that creates opening of the rectum.

Bowel treatment—spinal cord injury

Treatment programmes can vary from patient to patient and can depend on the level of the spinal cord injury. Additionally, initial bowel management in the acute phase may differ when compared to the long-term bowel management strategy. Therefore, bowel management is multifaceted using a combination of strategies to have a successful outcome.

Reflexic bowel	Areflexic (flaccid) bowel
Aim for Bristol Scale 4 stool	
Daily or alternate days	Once or more daily
Stimulate laxative (➲ p. 422–3) 8–12 hours before planned care if needed	Stimulate laxative (➲ p. 422–3) 8–12 hours before planned care if needed
Rectal stimulant suppository/ microenema	
Abdominal massage	Abdominal massage
Digital rectal stimulation (see Further reading RCN (2015))	Digital removal of faeces (see Further reading RCN (2015))
	Single digital check to ensure rectum is empty 5–10 min after last bowel action

Diet and fluids

Long-term dietary advice is generally around increasing consumption of fruit and vegetables to five each day. Although this will require individual evaluation of consistency of stool and adjusted accordingly.

Suggested fluid intake is 1.5–2.5 litres each day. This is also evaluated according to bladder output and adjusted accordingly.

Further reading

www.spinal.co.uk/wp-content/uploads/2015/08/Bowel-management-Guidelines_Sept_2012.pdf (Accessed 29/07/02019).

www.mascip.co.uk/wp-content/uploads/2015/02/CV653N-Neurogenic-Guidelines-Sept-2012.pdf (Accessed 29/07/2019).

Royal College of Nursing (RCN) (2015). Bowel care, including digital rectal examination and manual removal of stool. Guidance for nurses. RCN, London.

Autonomic dysreflexia

Autonomic dysreflexia is a syndrome in which there is a sudden onset of excessively high blood pressure. It is more common in people with spinal cord injuries of T6 or above.

Cause

Episodes of autonomic dysreflexia can be triggered by many potential causes. Essentially, any painful, irritating, or even strong stimulus below the level of the injury can cause an episode of autonomic dysreflexia. Bladder irritation and faecal impaction/constipation are the most common.

Bladder

- Distended bladder
- A kink in the catheter
- An over-full leg bag
- Blockage or obstruction that prevents urine flowing from the bladder
- Urinary tract infection or bladder spasms
- Bladder stones.

Bowel

- Distended bowel which can be due to a full rectum, constipation, or impaction
- Haemorrhoids
- Anal fissures
- Stretching of rectum or anus, or skin breakdown in the area.

There are potentially many other causes for autonomic dysreflexia.

Symptoms

- A pounding headache
- A flushed face and/or red blotches on the skin above the level of spinal injury
- Sweating above the level of spinal injury
- Nasal stuffiness
- Nausea
- Bradycardia
- Goose bumps below the level of spinal injury
- Cold, clammy skin below the level of spinal injury.

Treatment during an autonomic dysreflexia event:

- Sit up and drop feet
- Loosen any clothing and check nothing is putting pressure on the skin
- Perform a quick assessment to identify the cause so that the stimulus may be removed.

Additional actions for bladder, if a urinary catheter is in situ, are to check the following:

- Is drainage bag full?
- Is there a kink in the tubing?
- Is the drainage bag at a higher level than the bladder?
- Is the catheter blocked/plugged?

After correcting the obvious problem and if the catheter is not draining in 2–3 min, catheter must be changed immediately. If there is no urinary catheter in situ, perform a catheterization to empty the bladder.

Note: A bladder washout should not be attempted, as this may increase blood pressure.

Additional actions for bowel:

- Insert a gloved finger lubricated with an anaesthetic lubricant such as 2% lignocaine gel, into the rectum.
- If the rectum is full, insert some lubricant and wait for a minimum of 3 min. This is to reduce the sensation in the rectum which is important as performing digital stimulation and manual evacuation may worsen the autonomic dysreflexia.
- Gently perform manual evacuation.

Note: If manual evacuation/stimulation was being performed when the autonomic dysreflexia event occurred, stop the procedure and resume after the symptoms subside

Actions for other causes can be found on the spinal injuries' association website (www.spinal.co.uk).

Further reading

All information is taken from the following: https://www.spinal.co.uk/wp-content/uploads/2017/05/Autonomic-Dysreflexia.pdf

Neurogenic bowel dysfunction—spina bifida

Spina bifida is a congenital anomaly that can result in mobility issues and incontinence both bowel and bladder.

Causes

The cause of spinal bifida is where the structure of the neural tube of the spinal cord does not develop or close properly during the early stages of pregnancy. This in turn leads to defects in the spinal cord and vertebrae.

Symptoms

There are two main problems that can occur in spina bifida bowel dysfunction:
- Constipation and incomplete evacuation (inefficient emptying of the rectum)
- Faecal incontinence.

Assessment

Assessment will depend upon the problem and should include specific assessment for NBD (➔ p. 463). Additionally assessment should also be for faecal incontinence (➔ p. 448–9) or constipation (➔ p. 458–9).

Physical assessment is per faecal incontinence (➔ p. 449) or constipation (➔ p. 459).

Bowel management—spina bifida

Bowel management is based on the individual's symptoms and will include several factors to ensure success:
- Regular toileting and consistent toileting times because of the lack of sensation
- Keeping a regular stool consistency with adjustment of diet and fluids as per spinal cord injury advice (➔ p. 464)
- Toilet position (➔ p. 458 to constipation)
- Oral laxatives depending on need and to avoid constipation and impaction (➔ p. 458 to constipation)
- Enemas to keep the rectum empty
- If all the above measures do not adequately improve bowel dysfunction, TAI should be considered (➔ p. 448 to faecal incontinence).

Further reading

www.schn.health.nsw.gov.au/fact-sheets/spina-bifida-introduction-to-bowel-management-and-spina-bifida (Accessed 29/07/2019).

Neurogenic bowel dysfunction—cauda equina syndrome

Cauda equina syndrome is low spinal cord damage, for example injury, post-laminectomy, cord compression, or tumour.

Causes

In cauda equina syndrome, the sensory and motor functions of the lower bowel are partially or completely disrupted.

Assessment

Assessment will depend upon the problem and should include specific assessment for NBD (➲ p. 448–9). Additionally assessment should also be for faecal incontinence (➲ p. 448–9) or constipation (➲ p. 458–9).

Physical assessment is per faecal incontinence (➲ p. 449) or constipation (➲ p. 459).

Bowel management—cauda equina

Bowel symptoms are usually constipation; however, faecal incontinence can also occur because there is no anorectal sensation and poor control with a lax anus. It is difficult to balance constipation and faecal incontinence. However, the following may offer some predictability:

* Regular toileting and consistent toileting times because of the lack of sensation
* Keeping a regular stool consistency with adjustment of diet and fluids (➲ p. 464 to spinal cord injury)
* Toilet position (➲ p. 458 to constipation)
* Many patients may require digital removal of faeces
* If all the above measures do not adequately improve bowel dysfunction, TAI should be considered (➲ p. 448 to faecal incontinence).

Neurogenic bowel dysfunction—multiple sclerosis

Multiple sclerosis (MS) is a chronic, typically progressive disease involving damage to the sheaths of nerve cells (the insulating layer surrounding the neurones) in the brain and spinal cord. This can result in mobility issues and bowel dysfunction.

Causes

MS is an autoimmune condition.

Symptoms

As a consequence of the nerve damage, signals are interrupted and slower. This results in fewer contractions in the colon, which increases transit time and leads to constipation. At the same time, there is a reduced sensation of rectal filling and a weakness of the anal sphincter because of weak muscular contraction; as a consequence, the individual suffers with faecal incontinence.

Assessment

Assessment will depend upon the problem and should include specific assessment for NBD (⊃ p. 448–9). Additionally assessment should also be for faecal incontinence (⊃ p. 448–9) or constipation (⊃ p. 458–9).

Physical assessment is per faecal incontinence (⊃ p. 449) or constipation (⊃ p. 459).

Bowel management—multiple sclerosis

It is difficult to balance constipation and faecal incontinence, which often coexist and may be acute, chronic, or intermittent due to the fluctuating pattern in MS. However, the following may offer some predictability:
- Regular toileting and consistent toileting times because of the lack of sensation
- Keeping a regular stool consistency with adjustment of diet and fluids (⊃ p. 464 to spinal cord injury)
- Toilet position (⊃ p. 458 to constipation)
- Many patients may require digital removal of faeces
- If all the above measures do not adequately improve bowel dysfunction, TAI (⊃ p. 462) should be considered (⊃ p. 448 to faecal incontinence).

Further reading

www.mssociety.org.uk/about-ms/signs-and-symptoms/bowel/managing-bowel-incontinence (Accessed 29/07/2019).

Neurogenic bowel dysfunction— cerebrovascular accident/stroke

A stroke is when the blood supply is cut off from part of the brain that can cause paralysis and death or other symptoms such as reduced mobility.

Symptoms

Patients may also have bowel dysfunction, such as constipation and/or faecal incontinence. The reasons for bowel dysfunction can be neurogenic, due to immobility, loss of sensation, dependence, and/or medications.

Assessment

Assessment will depend upon the problem and should include specific assessment for NBD (**Ð** p. 448–9). Additionally assessment should also be for faecal incontinence (**Ð** p. 448–9) or constipation (**Ð** p. 458–9).

Physical assessment is per faecal incontinence (**Ð** p. 449) or constipation (**Ð** p. 459).

Bowel management—cerebrovascular accident

Bowel management is as per spina bifida (**Ð** p. 468 to spina bifida bowel management)

Further reading

www.stroke.org.uk/sites/default/files/continence_problems_after_stroke.pdf   (Accessed   online 30/07/2019).

Neurogenic bowel dysfunction— Parkinson's disease

Parkinson's disease is a progressive neurological condition affecting the brain. Constipation is the predominant factor in bowel dysfunction.

Assessment

Assessment will depend upon the problem and should include specific assessment for NBD (➲ p. 448–9). Additionally assessment should also be for faecal incontinence (➲ p. 448–9) or constipation (➲ p. 458–9).

Physical assessment is per faecal incontinence (➲ p. 449) or constipation (➲ p. 459).

Bowel management—Parkinson's disease

Bowel management is as per spina bifida (➲ p. 468 to spina bifida bowel management).

Further reading

www.parkinsons.org.uk (Accessed online 30/07/2019).

Surgery

Enhanced recovery after surgery—pre-operative care

There are a number of necessary steps to ensure that safe surgery is undertaken. These can be grouped under the topic of pre-operative elements of enhanced recovery; that include:

• Pre-admission information, education, and counselling.
• Pre-operative optimization—to include the use of a risk assessment tool. It is important to correct anaemia and improve nutritional status, such as malnutrition. Additionally, to encourage and support smoking cessation and stopping alcohol consumption for 4 weeks pre-operatively.
• Pre-habilitation—to improve general fitness prior to surgery.
• Pre-anaesthetic medication—is generally avoided.
• Bowel preparation—use is controversial: currently opinion is generally to avoid the use of bowel preparation in colonic surgery, although it might be beneficial for rectal surgery. There is some evidence for the use of oral antibiotics when bowel preparation is used.
• Avoidance of prolonged starvation—it is important to ensure no clear fluids for 2 h prior to surgery and no milk or food for 6 h prior to surgery. Carbohydrate loading is advocated prior to surgery, with a specially formulated clear oral drink. No prolonged starvation helps to avoid dehydration and electrolyte imbalance. The specially formulated carbohydrate drinks are consumed about 3 h before surgery: these are then quickly eliminated from the stomach so as to avoid the risk of aspiration during surgery

Nursing care

It is important to use appropriate language when speaking to patients. Give information to help allay anxiety and ↓ fear, including:

• Introduce the patient to the ward environment
• Explain the procedure and general anaesthetic
• Discuss pain relief
• Discuss the length of stay—often 2–4 days for colonic surgery
• Take bloods
• Monitor baseline observations
• Explain about anti-embolic stockings
• Being nil by mouth for 2 h for clear fluids and 6 h for solids and milk
• Explain bowel preparation—if needed
• Referral to a stoma care nurse—if appropriate for information and stoma siting.

Further reading

Gustafsson UO, Scott MJ, Hubner M, et al. (2018) Guidelines for perioperative care in elective colorectal surgery: Enhanced Recovery After Surgery (ERAS) Society recommendations: 2018. *World Journal of Surgery* 43:659–95.

Enhanced recovery after surgery—intra-operative care

There are a number of intra-operative elements related to colorectal surgery, including:
- Standardized anaesthetic protocol—this includes monitoring, such as cerebral function monitoring for high-risk patients. Avoidance of benzodiazepines is advocated and use of short-acting general anaesthetic agents, as well as opioid-sparing, enables rapid awakening as well as fewer residual effects.
- Intra-operative fluid and electrolyte therapy—should be given to avoid dehydration or fluid overload and excessive provision of sodium also needs to be avoided. Consider goal-directed fluid therapy in high risk patients
- Prevention of nausea and vomiting—for all patients with extra prophylaxis for high-risk patients
- Antimicrobial prophylaxis and skin preparation—use of intravenous (IV) antibiotics and skin cleansing prior to surgical incision
- Prevention of intra-operative hypothermia—this can include the use of warmed and humidified anaesthetic gases, warming IV fluids, and forced air warming
- Surgical access—minimally invasive surgery is the gold standard in many countries; including laparoscopic (including single-port surgery), robotic, and transanal surgery.
- Drainage of the peritoneal cavity and pelvis is not recommended routinely.

There are a number of ways in which the inside of the abdomen can be reached. This includes via a laparotomy, which is an incision into the abdomen, also termed open surgery, often the incision is in the midline. Laparoscopic surgery also comes under the terms minimally invasive surgery or keyhole surgery. Laparoscopic surgery often involves multiple small incisions, whereas single-port surgery is conducted through one single port in the abdomen. Robotic surgery is another form of minimally invasive surgery, using a robot controlled remotely by a surgeon. Transanal minimally invasive surgery (TAMIS) is technique using a single laparoscopic port that is inserted into the anal canal to remove benign rectal/sigmoid polyps and in some situations cancers; this results in no abdominal scars.

Further reading

Gustafsson UO, Scott MJ, Hubner M, et al. (2018). Guidelines for perioperative care in elective colorectal surgery: Enhanced Recovery After Surgery (ERAS) Society recommendations: 2018. *World Journal of Surgery* 43:659–95.

Enhanced recovery after surgery—post-operative care

There are a number of post-operative elements to enhanced recovery that include:

- No routine usage of a nasogastric tube post-operatively—unless a post-operative ileus occurs in which case it is advocated.
- Post-operative analgesia—this should be opioid-sparing and multimodal. Analgesia should include the use of paracetamol (➲ p. 406) which provides background pain relief and helps to enhance the effects of opioids, thus reducing the opioids required. Thoracic epidural analgesia (TEA) is advocated in open surgery. Non-steroidal anti-inflammatory drugs (NSAIDs) (➲ p. 406) are useful if not contraindicated. Other frequently used types of analgesia include transverse abdominis plane (TAP) blocks, spinal analgesia, and lidocaine infusion. Most non-oral routes of analgesia can be removed within a day or two of surgery
- Thromboprophylaxis is required during hospitalization to reduce the risk of blood clots in the form of well-fitting compression stockings and/or intermittent pneumatic compression while hospitalized and low molecular weight heparin, the latter at least during the time in hospital but for high-risk patients, such as people with cancer (➲ p. 352) or inflammatory bowel disease (IBD) (➲ p. 368–9), this might be advocated for 28 days after surgery.
- Careful use of post-operative fluids and electrolytes. Avoid IV fluids if able to consume adequate oral intake, usually possible by the day after surgery. If clinically indicated to use IV fluids, such as for a post-operative ileus, then use with caution, such as 25–30 ml/kg per day. Be careful not to give excessive daily sodium infusions but potassium supplements may be required. It is necessary to replace the losses from vomiting and/or high stomal output.
- Early removal of transurethral catheter is advocated—between 1and 3 days after surgery, based on risk factors, such as pelvic surgery.
- Fluid and diet should be resumed when nausea-free, usually the same day as the surgery. Consider oral nutritional supplements, as often insufficient diet is consumed while in hospital
- Early mobilization should be encouraged but the exact mobilization programme is poorly defined but includes walking on the day after surgery.
- Meeting defined discharge criteria, to include mobilization, dietary intake, and proficiency with stoma care (if applicable) is needed to ensure a safe discharge home.

Postoperative nursing care

It is important to:

- Monitor and assess observations regularly, as per policy to include blood pressure, pulse, respiration rate, temperature, and oxygen saturations.
- Observe for signs of bleeding, such as hypotension, tachycardia, pale, clammy, and cold.

- Observe for signs of an anastomotic leak, such as tachycardia, pyrexia, prolonged ileus, or sepsis with a rigid abdomen indicating peritonitis—consider a computed tomography (CT) scan and return to theatre for abdominal washout or defunction with a stoma.
- Observe for signs of a post-operative ileus, such as nausea, vomiting, abdominal distention, and no flatus/bowel function—consider decompression with a nasogastric tube and hydration with intravenous fluids. If symptoms last for 5 days consider parenteral feeding (➔ p. 312).
- Observe for signs of infection suggested by a low-grade fever: this can originate from the chest, urinary catheter, wounds, an anastomotic leak or collection, intravenous access site, or a deep vein thrombosis. Wounds may have a discharge.
- Monitor and assess pain requirements as per hospital policy
- Monitor intravenous access sites for signs of infection and leakage.
- Monitor wounds for signs of infection, bleeding, or dehiscence.
- Monitor drains (if used) for output, colour, and volume.
- Monitor stoma (➔ p. 507–24).
- Reintroduce diet and fluids as tolerated.
- Monitor urinary output and remove catheter when appropriate (consider risk factors for urinary retention): note that oliguria alone does not necessitate increase in IV fluids in the post-operative period if there are no other clinical indications.

Note that people with comorbidities such as diabetes, cardiac problems, circulatory problems, or respiratory problems are more likely to have post-operative complications. This can include infections or wound healing issues. The same applies to malnourished or undernourished people.

Discharge advice

Discharge advice includes:
- Follow-up is often 2–6 weeks after surgery with the surgeon
- No driving for about 6 weeks
- Caution with heavy lifting and return to work, usually 6–12 weeks after surgery to prevent the risk of hernia formation such as incisional (➔ p. 494) or parastomal (➔ p. 518)
- Wound care.

Further reading

Gustafsson UO, Scott MJ, Hubner M, et al. (2018). Guidelines for perioperative care in elective colo-rectal surgery: Enhanced Recovery After Surgery (ERAS) Society recommendations: 2018. *World Journal of Surgery* 43:659–95.

Abdominoperineal resection of the rectum

An abdominoperineal resection of the rectum (see Fig. 20.1) is also termed APER, APR, or APE, and there can be additional descriptions such as the surgical plane, for example, ELAPE (extralevator abdominoperineal excision). There will be incisions on the abdomen and the perineal area; in addition to the removal of the rectum, the anal canal and anus are also removed and the resulting wound is sutured shut. In addition, the sigmoid colon and some of the descending colon are also removed. Thus, to pass faeces and flatus, the colon is diverted to the abdominal wall and formed into a colostomy.

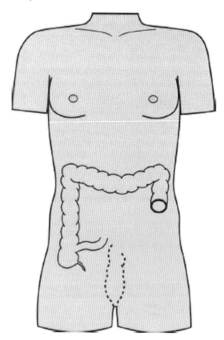

Fig. 20.1 Abdominoperineal excision of the rectum.
Reproduced with kind permission © Burdett Institute 2008.

Indications for surgery

An abdominoperineal resection of the rectum is most commonly performed for a low rectal cancer or an anal cancer than cannot be treated non-surgically.

Surgical complications
- Wound infection
- Perineal wound breakdown.

Nursing advice
The nurse needs to ensure that the patient has learnt to care for their colostomy (→ p. 504–5) prior to discharge home from hospital and has adequate colostomy appliances (→ p. 512–13). It is important for the patient to know what is normal and abnormal in respect of their healing wounds and their newly formed stoma.

There are risks of sexual dysfunction for both men and women after an abdominoperineal of the rectum. Men may be unable to attain an erection due to nerve damage, but with newer surgical techniques permanent nerve damage is often avoidable. For women the position of the vagina may alter once the rectum is removed resulting in changes in sensation and dyspareunia. The nurse can reiterate the surgeon's pre-operative discussion and suggest that further advice be sought from the surgeon at their clinic appointment.

Anorectal disorders

There are a number of surgical options for anorectal disorders, such as:

- An anal sphincterotomy is when an incision is made in the internal anal sphincter that lowers the pressure in the internal anal sphincter—used for an anal fissure (➔ p. 120–1).
- Laying opening is when the fistula tract is cut out/laid open to help heal an anorectal fistula (➔ p. 122–3).
- Drainage of sepsis +/− insertion of a seton stitch is the use of a stitch inserted into the anorectal fistula (➔ p. 122–3).
- An advancement flap is when the fistula is curetted and a flap of tissue is used to cover the wound defect for an anorectal fistula (➔ p. 122–3).
- LIFT (ligation of the intersphincteric fistula tract) is an incision made above the fistula, where the muscles are divided, the fistula tract cleaned, and the defect in the external sphincter muscle is repaired.
- VAAFT (video assisted anal fistula treatment) enables the fistula tract to be cleaned, prior to the internal fistula opening being sealed.
- Haemorrhoidectomy (➔ p. 492) is the removal of the haemorrhoidal pads—used for haemorrhoids (piles).
- Soave (see Fig. 20.2) is a pull-through procedure performed for Hirschsprung's disease (➔ p. 398–9).
- Seton stitch is the insertion of non-absorbable stitch into an anal fistula tract.
- Fibrin glue can be used to seal a fistula to encourage healing; it can be used for a simple fistula but is less effective than a fistulotomy.

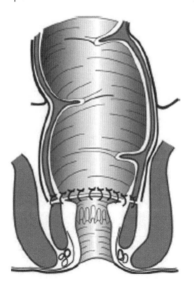

Fig. 20.2 Soave.
Reproduced with kind permission © Burdett Institute 2008.

Indications for surgery

There are a number of indications for surgery:

- An anal fissure may be required if conservative treatment fails.
- An anorectal abscess might need to be acutely treated if there is anorectal sepsis.
- An anorectal fistula may require treatment of sepsis.
- Haemorrhoids require surgery if painful or bleeding. Haemorrhoids may require acute surgery if they become strangulated or thrombosed.

Surgical complications

There are a number of complications so that can occur as a result of ano-rectal surgery, including:

- Infection
- Delayed wound healing
- Anal incontinence
- Recurrence of a fistula.

Nursing advice

It is ideal to advise patients to take laxatives, to prevent straining to pass a motion. Analgesia is often needed for a short period after anorectal procedures.

If there is a wound, this needs to be kept clean, such as daily showering. If the wound is laid open, the wound may require digitation. The nurse will use a gloved finger to break any healing that is not occurring from the wound base upwards. Healing may take months.

Anterior resection of the rectum

An anterior resection is the removal of part or most of the rectum and the distal colon with an anastomosis of the colon and remaining rectum (see Fig. 20.3). A more extensive version of this operation is a total mesorectal excision (TME), where the anterior resection is undertaken and in addition the area around the rectum, the mesorectum (→ p. 482) is also removed. If a TME is performed, there is usually a temporary loop ileostomy formed.

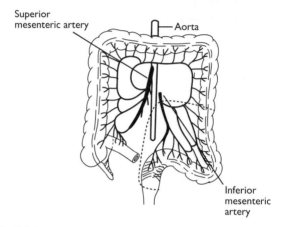

Superior mesenteric artery

Aorta

Inferior mesenteric artery

Fig. 20.3 Anterior resection.

Reproduced from Agarwal, AK et al, 'Colorectal surgery, appendix, and small bowel', in Greg R. McLatchie and David J. Leaper, *Operative Surgery, Second Edition*, p. 283, Figure 7.47 © Oxford University Press, 2006.

Indications for surgery

This operation is usually performed for a rectal cancer (→ p. 352).

Surgical complications

Potential surgical complications include:
• Wound infection
• Anastomotic leakage, about 10% risk for a TME.

Nursing advice

Depending on the amount of the rectum that is removed, there may be bowel dysfunction that includes frequency and urgency. The former refers to frequently returning to the toilet, often in the morning, whereas urgency refers to having to quickly reach the toilet. If unable to reach the toilet, there may be faecal incontinence (→ p. 448–9). This collection of bowel dysfunctions is often termed anterior resection syndrome and is more common, the lower the anastomosis is formed. The nurse also needs to advise that if an ileostomy is performed that it will need to be reversed at a later date, this might need to be after completion of chemotherapy.

Appendicectomy

Appendicectomy, also termed appendectomy, is the surgical removal of the appendix.

Indications for surgery

Suspected appendicitis.

Surgical complications

Potential surgical complications include:
- Wound infection
- Abscess formation.

Bariatric surgery

Bariatric surgery is a term for surgical treatment of obesity. There are a number of different operations (see Fig. 20.4) that can be performed, such as:

- Gastric banding—a small band is placed around the top of the stomach. This creates a small pouch which limits food intake (see Fig.20.4a).
- Gastric bypass (Roux-en-Y)—a small pouch is formed from the top of the stomach that restricts food intake. By 'bypassing' most of the stomach, duodenum, and upper small intestine there is reduced absorption of food (see Fig.20.4b). This is the most commonly performed weight-loss surgery performed
- Sleeve gastrectomy—the capacity of the stomach is reduced (through removal of the greater curve of the stomach) and gastric emptying altered (see Fig.20.4c).

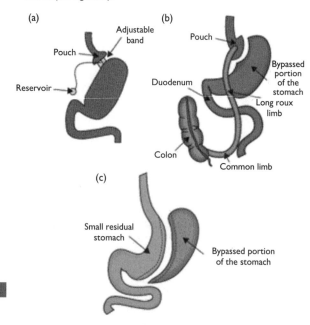

Fig. 20.4 Types of bariatric surgery (a) gastric banding (b) gastric bypass (c) sleeve gastrectomy.

Reproduced from Jolly, Elaine, Fry, Andrew, and Chaudhry, Afzal, *Oxford Specialty Training: Training in Medicine*, p. 304, Figure 7.62 © Oxford University Press, 2016.

Indications for surgery

Bariatric surgery is undertaken to aid weight loss if the body mass index (BMI) (€ p. 306) is over 40, or if over 35 and there are comorbidities, such as diabetes or cardiac disease, if other weight loss methods have failed.

Surgical complications

Complications can occur at home in the short term that require the patient to contact a healthcare professional:
- Abdominal pain that is not resolving or is worsening
- Tachycardia
- Pyrexia above 38°C
- Chest pain
- Shortness of breath
- Repeated vomiting +/- blood
- Melaena
- Wound infection—pain, erythema, swelling, and/or pus.

Complications that can occur in the longer term that require addressing:
- Intermittent abdominal pain
- Intermittent vomiting
- Indigestion
- Nocturnal cough
- Persistent nausea
- Persistent diarrhoea
- Flushed, sweaty, or feeling faint
- Excess skin folds after weight loss
- Dietary deficiencies in vitamins (€ p. 294) and minerals that probably will require life-long supplementation
- Gallstones (€ p. 198–9)
- Slippage of the gastric band.

Nursing advice

It is important for the nurse to assist in giving advice on diet. This is initially fluids only, building up to runny foods, soft food, and then a gradual return to a healthy diet. Additionally, it is important to eat slowly, chew food well, and to eat small amounts at a time. In addition to weight-loss surgery, it is also important to undertake exercise. It is important to advise patients that they need to have long-term follow-up with the GP to include:
- Blood tests—to check for vitamin and mineral deficiencies
- Check physical health
- Emotional and/or psychological support might be necessary
- Re-enforcement of the need for a healthy diet and exercise.

Cholecystectomy

Cholecystectomy is the surgical removal of the gall bladder ($\circlearrowright$ p. 14). A cholecystectomy is generally performed laparoscopically. Cholangiography might be performed during surgery to image and confirm the bile duct anatomy and presence of stones in the ducts.

Indication for surgery

A cholecystectomy is an elective procedure, which is seldom performed acutely, except if perforation of the gall bladder is suspected or seems imminent. If asymptomatic, surgery is usually only performed if the gallstones are located in the bile duct.

Surgical complications

There is a very low rate of bile duct injury and the conversion rate from laparoscopic to open surgery is <5%. A cholecystectomy is safe, even in elderly and infirm people, except if cirrhosis is also present.

Bile duct stricture—the main risk during a cholecystectomy is injury to the bile ducts, with subsequent stricture formation. Injury is often not noticed during surgery. A person with a bile duct stricture might present with:
• Jaundice—if the bile ducts are completely occluded
• Pain—if the bile duct is partially occluded.

Treatment of occlusion is usually with endoscopic balloon dilatation, endoscopic stent placement, or surgical reconstruction.

Post-cholecystectomy syndrome—is a variety of abdominal symptoms, including pain, bloating, nausea, and dyspepsia. These are often short-lived and resolve within a few months of having a cholecystectomy.

Nursing advice

Most patients recover and return to normal activity (including work) within 1 week. Use the surgical experience as an opportunity for patient education on modifying cholesterol intake and general health advice.

Colectomy

A colectomy is the removal of part or all of the colon, and usually the remaining parts of the bowel are joined (anastomosed). There are a number of terms within this category including:

- Sigmoid colectomy—removal of the sigmoid colon (● p. 11) +/-part of the descending colon (see Fig. 20.5)
- Left hemicolectomy—left half of the colon (descending colon) is removed (● p. 11)
- Extended left hemicolectomy—resection of the descending colon and part of the transverse colon (● p. 11)
- Transverse colectomy—removal of the transverse colon (● p. 11)
- Right hemicolectomy—right half of the colon (ascending) is removed (● p. 11)
- Extended right hemicolectomy—the ascending colon and part of the transverse colon are resected
- Subtotal colectomy—resection of most of the colon possibly leaving some sigmoid colon in situ
- Total colectomy—removal of all of the colon from the ascending to sigmoid colon inclusive. The ileum can then be formed into an ileostomy or joined to the rectum in an ileorectal anastomosis (see Fig. 20.6).

Indications for surgery

A colectomy might be required for:

- Cancer of the colon (● p. 352)—hemicolectomy or sigmoid colectomy
- Ulcerative colitis (UC) (● p. 370)—total colectomy
- Crohn's disease (● p. 377)—total colectomy, subtotal colectomy, or right hemicolectomy
- Familial adenomatous polyposis (● p. 92–3)—total colectomy.

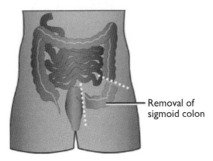

— Removal of sigmoid colon

Fig. 20.5 A diagrammatic representation of a sigmoid colectomy.
Reproduced with kind permission © Burdett Institute 2008.

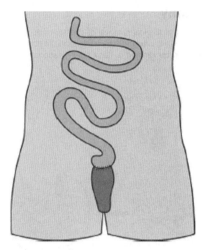

Fig. 20.6 Colectomy with ileo-rectal anastomosis.
Reproduced with kind permission © Burdett Institute 2008.

Surgical complications

Potential surgical complications include:
• Wound infection
• Anastomotic leakage, if there is an anastomosis.

Nursing advice

The more of the colon that is removed, the more the bowel function will alter. This is particularly the case for people having a total colectomy and subtotal colectomy where bowel function may be 4–6 times daily. There is likely a looser and more frequent bowel motion for people having an extended left or right hemicolectomy. Perianal skin care is important when bowels first begin to function and dietary advice can include reducing fibre levels, if loose bowel functions are encountered. A little more salt is needed each day in the diet, to replace the sodium lost in the loose faeces. Also, adequate volumes of oral fluids are advocated, such as 2 litres daily, for people with all or a large amount of their colon removed.

Gastrectomy

A gastrectomy is the surgical removal of the stomach, either a distal gastrectomy or a total gastrectomy, depending upon the position of the cancer. The operation can be termed a Roux-en-Y oesophagojejunostomy (see Fig. 20.7).

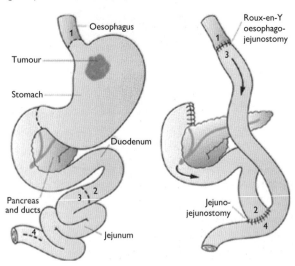

Fig. 20.7 Operative diagram of a total gastrectomy with a Roux-en-Y reconstruction.

Reproduced with permission from Callaghan C et al (2008) *Emergencies in Clinical Surgery*. Oxford University Press.

Indications for surgery

The most common indication for a gastrectomy is a gastric cancer. Other indications include:
• Obesity—life-threatening
• Oesophageal cancer
• Peptic ulcer.

Surgical complications

As people who undergo a gastrectomy are often malnourished preoperatively with other comorbidities, there is the risk of complications such as:
• Wound infection
• Chest infections.

Nursing advice

As the stomach is removed, there will be problems eating. In the short term, this can mean intravenous feeding (→ p. 337), whereas in the long term, it is advisable to have small frequent meals and likely vitamin supplementation.

There is also the risk of dumping syndrome, which occurs when certain foods are eaten, such as high levels of sugar or carbohydrates. As these food types pass into the small bowel, there can be a fall in blood pressure as fluids shift into the small bowel. This can cause:

• Fainting
• Sweating
• Palpitations
• Nausea
• Bloating
• Indigestion
• Diarrhoea.

To resolve these symptoms, it can be advised to:

• Eat slowly
• Eat small, frequent meals
• Avoid high sugar meals
• Avoid liquid type foods, such as soup
• Rest for up to 45 min after a meal.

Dietetic referral can be useful. Other problems can include vomiting and diarrhoea, the latter due to the damage to the vagus nerve and the former due to the reduced gastric capacity.

Haemorrhoid treatment

Treating haemorrhoids is the surgical removal of the haemorrhoidal pads. This can be performed in a number of ways:

- Rubber band ligation—bands are used at the base of the internal haemorrhoid
- Haemorrhoidal artery ligation—using stitches to occlude the blood supply to the haemorrhoids
- Injection sclerotherapy—injection of the haemorrhoids causing thrombosis and fibrosis
- Haemorrhoidectomy—surgical excision of the haemorrhoidal pads
- Stapled haemorrhoidopexy—part of the anorectum is stapled, meaning haemorrhoids are less likely to relapse secondary to reducing the blood supply and reduction in the haemorrhoids.

Indications for surgery

Second and third-degree haemorrhoids can be treated if medical management fails.

Surgical complications

There are a number of potential complications:

- Rubber band ligation—can be uncomfortable if not undertaken above the dentate line and risks include bleeding, pain, and sepsis.
- Haemorrhoidectomy—can result in anal stenosis, pain, bleeding, sepsis, and incontinence (flatus/faecal).
- Stapled haemorrhoidopexy—can result in faecal urgency, more risk of rectal perforation and severe sepsis, and there is the rare risk of a fistula between the rectum and vagina in women. There is a higher risk of recurrence than with a conventional haemorrhoidectomy.

Nursing advice

Having haemorrhoids removed is painful and requires analgesia. It is possible that treatment will be unsuccessful and may have to be repeated but it is successful in up to 80% of cases. Injection sclerotherapy is less effective than rubber band ligation and may require repeated injections. Stapling is less painful but more likely to be followed by recurrence compared to a haemorrhoidectomy.

Dietary advice can help prevent recurrence of haemorrhoids, such as suggesting a high fibre diet and not straining to pass a motion.

Hartmann's procedure

A Hartmann's procedure is the removal of the sigmoid colon and part of the rectum and descending colon. The two ends are not joined; the proximal end is formed into a colostomy (◑ p. 504–5); and usually the rectal stump is closed (see Fig. 20.8). Alternatively, the rectal stump can be formed into a mucus fistula (◑ p. 504–5).

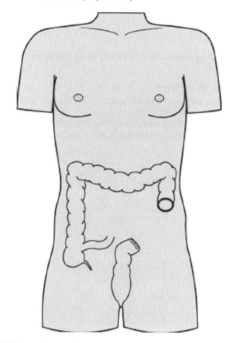

Fig. 20.8 Hartmann's procedure.
Reproduced with kind permission © Burdett Institute 2008.

Indications for surgery

The most common reason to perform a Hartmann's procedure is for perforated diverticular disease (◑ p. 90–1) in an emergency situation to resolve peritonitis (◑ p. 442).

Nursing advice

Training for stoma care and careful observation for wound breakdown is important in the post-operative period. Advice on the care of the colostomy is also needed (◑ p. 504–5).

Hernia repair

An abdominal hernia repair is the surgical repair of an organ pushing through a weak area of abdominal wall. There are a number of types of hernia (see Fig. 20.9) that include:

- Inguinal
- Epigastric
- Umbilical
- Femoral
- Incisional
- Parastomal.

Surgical repair is commonly performed using mesh to reinforce the abdominal wall.

Indications for surgery

If the hernia is causing problems, such as pain, it might be treated with elective surgical repair rather than conservatively with a support belt and analgesia. However, if the hernia becomes 'strangulated' then emergency surgery is required, as the bowel that is within the hernia sac may become gangrenous.

Nursing advice

It is important to provide advice on being careful when lifting.

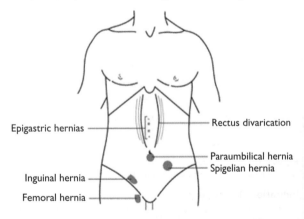

Fig. 20.9 Anterior abdominal wall hernia.

Reproduced with permission from Callaghan C (2008) *Emergencies in Clinical Surgery*. Oxford University Press.

Kock pouch

The Kock pouch or continent ileostomy is a surgical procedure that involves the removal of the colon, rectum, anal canal, and anus. The small bowel is then formed into a reservoir. The reservoir is attached to the abdominal surface with a channel that is created from the small bowel with a nipple valve to maintain continence. A flush stoma is formed from the channel on the abdominal surface. The pouch needs to be regularly emptied of the faeces that collect within it, using a medina catheter. Thus about 4–6 times daily the stoma needs to be intubated +/− irrigated to aid emptying and the pouch is emptied. A stoma cap is used to cover the pouch.

Kock pouch intubation

Collect the equipment for intubation:
- Medina catheter
- Lubricating gel
- Soft wipes
- Stoma cap
- Bladder syringe and water (if irrigation is undertaken).

Intubation is undertaken by removing the stoma cap, cleaning the stoma (if needed), lubricate the catheter, gently insert the catheter into the stoma, irrigate (if needed); occasionally change the position of the catheter until faeces have drained out. Clean the stoma and use a new stoma cap.

Indications for surgery

A Kock pouch is usually formed when surgery is required for UC or familial adenomatous polyposis.

Surgical complications

There are a number of complications that can occur for people with a Kock pouch. Initial complications include:
- Nipple valve necrosis—requires careful observation and surgical revision may be required
- Nipple valve ischaemia—requires careful observation and surgical revision may be required
- Pouch fistula—may require surgical revision
- Nipple valve stenosis—may require dilation or surgical revision
- Intubation difficulties—may require surgical revision
- Slipped nipple valve—may require surgical revision
- Pouch leakage—a stoma plug may be useful
- Prolapsed pouch—may require surgical revision.

Nursing advice

The nurse needs to advise that the new Kock pouch needs to be emptied regularly. Furthermore, food if not chewed well might block the catheter during intubation.

Pancreatectomy

There are a number of ways that the pancreas can be partially or completely removed.

- Distal pancreatectomy involves the removal of the tail and body of the pancreas. The operation may also include removal of the spleen, part of the stomach, small bowel, left adrenal gland, left kidney, and left diaphragm. Only 5% of people with cancer in the body or tail of the pancreas can undergo a distal pancreatectomy
- Total pancreatectomy involves the removal of the whole pancreas, bile duct, gallbladder, spleen, part of the small intestine, the surrounding lymph nodes, +/− part of the stomach.

Surgical complications

Complication rates are high after a distal or total pancreatectomy. Such as:

- Pancreatic fistula
- Abscess
- Anastomotic leak
- Pneumonia
- Pulmonary embolism
- Wound infection.

Nursing advice

After a distal pancreatectomy, some people need to replace pancreatic enzymes and some people may become diabetic. After a total pancreatectomy, the person will need to replace pancreatic enzymes and the person will also be a life-long diabetic. Removal of the spleen increases the risk of infections and affects blood clotting, necessitating regular vaccinations to prevent infections and life-long antibiotics.

Panproctocolectomy and end ileostomy

A panproctocolectomy or total proctocolectomy (Fig. 20.10) is the total removal of the rectum and colon, including the anus and anal canal. The faeces are re-routed to the abdomen and passed from an ileostomy (➲ p. 504–5) into a stoma appliance (➲ p. 512–13).

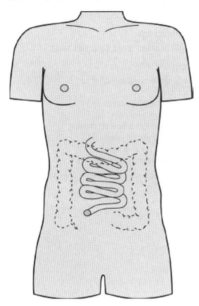

Fig. 20.10 Panproctocolectomy.
Reproduced with kind permission © Burdett Institute 2008.

Indications for surgery

A panproctocolectomy might be performed for UC (➲ p. 370), Crohn's disease (➲ p. 377), or familial adenomatous polyposis (➲ p. 92–3).

Surgical complications

Potential surgical complications include:
• Wound infection.

Nursing advice

The nurse needs to advise that bowel motion will be loose, often described as 'porridge-like' and will pass from the abdomen into an ileostomy appliance (➲ p. 512–13). Patients need to learn to care for their ileostomy prior to being discharged home from hospital. The perineal wound can take some time to heal and may require community nursing services to ensure healing occurs. More salt is needed each day to replace the sodium lost in the loose faeces and also adequate oral fluids such as 1.5–2 litres daily are required.

Pilonidal abscess

A pilonidal abscess is an infected pilonidal sinus in the natal cleft that may require incision and drainage. The wound is left open and dressed regularly. If there are recurrent pilonidal abscesses, then a flap may be required.

Indications for surgery

A pilonidal abscess that does not resolve with antibiotics.

Surgical complications

Not all wounds will heal and some abscesses recur.

Nursing advice

It is advisable while the wound is healing to:
- Keep the area clean
- Wear loose-fitting cotton underwear
- Avoid straining to pass a motion
- Eat a high-fibre diet to keep bowels moving
- Avoid heavy lifting for about week
- Avoid riding a bicycle for 6–8 weeks
- Avoid swimming until wounds are healed.

Many people have about 2 weeks off work after surgery.

Pylorus preserving pancreatic duodenectomy

Pylorus preserving pancreatic duodenectomy (PPPD) involves removal of the head of the pancreas, part of the duodenum, the gallbladder, and part of the bile duct. The tail of the pancreas is joined to the small bowel.

Surgical complications

Complication rates are high after a PPPD. Such as:
- Delayed gastric emptying
- Pancreatic fistula
- Wound infection
- Haemorrhage
- Pancreatitis.

Nursing advice

After a PPPD some people need to replace pancreatic enzymes. Also, people may become diabetic.

Rectal prolapse repair

A rectal prolapse (◉ p. 138–9) repair is a surgical procedure, and there are a number of options:

- Delorme's procedure—stripping of excess rectal mucosa and plication of the prolapsed rectal muscle wall; no resection is undertaken during this perineal approach
- Altemeier's procedure—involves opening the peritoneal cavity via the prolapse and resecting the rectosigmoid colon and performing an anastomosis
- Rectopexy—mobilization and straightening of the rectum, then fixing it onto the sacrum with sutures or a mesh, sometimes a resection is performed.

Indications for surgery

A surgical repair of a rectal prolapse is usually undertaken if conservative management fails or if people are symptomatic. A Delorme's procedure is used in frail people who need to have spinal rather than general anaesthetic.

Nursing advice

The nurse needs to give advice to help prevent the recurrence of the prolapse: this can include dietary advice and to not strain during defaecation. One in four people undergoing a Delorme's procedure can expect the condition to recur. An Altemeier's procedure has a lower rectal prolapse rate than a Delorme's procedure but a higher rate of anastomotic dehiscence and thus localized sepsis. A rectopexy has lower recurrence rates of the prolapse compared to a Delorme's procedure but there are higher subsequent rates of defaecatory disorders (◉ p. 500).

Restorative proctocolectomy

A restorative proctocolectomy is the removal of the rectum and colon but the anus and anal canal are retained meaning that passage of the faeces can be restored to pass from the anus. There are a number of terms used for a restorative proctocolectomy including an ileo-anal pouch, IPAA (ileo-pouch anal anastomosis), and J pouch. Often this procedure requires two or three operations. In the two-stage operation, the first operation includes a proctocolectomy (removal of the colon and rectum), and formation of the ileo-anal pouch and temporary loop ileostomy. The second operation is the reversal or closure of the loop ileostomy. The three-stage operation involves initially a colectomy and formation of an end ileostomy. The second stage is removal of the rectum, formation of the pouch, and formation of the loop ileostomy, and finally the stoma is reversed in the last operation.

Indications for surgery

A restorative proctocolectomy is usually performed for UC (➋ p. 370) or familial adenomatous polyposis (➋ p. 92–3).

Surgical complications

Potential surgical complications include:
• Wound infection
• Anastomotic leakage.

  Long-term complications include:
• Pouchitis—inflammation within the pouch causing symptoms similar to IBD (➋ p. 368–9). The aetiology is unknown, but pouchitis is more likely to affect people with UC. It affects 10–20% of all pouches and the incidence is over long-term follow-up. Treatment is antibiotic therapy.
• Cuffitis—inflammation of the columnar cuff, which is situated above the anal transition zone.
• Outflow problems—difficulty in evacuating: either incomplete emptying or inability to evacuate because of stenosis.
• Incontinence—usually passive (often nocturnal).
• Pouch vaginal fistula—associated with stapled surgical procedures.
• Pelvic abscess—because of delayed healing or long-term steroids before surgery.
• Retained rectal mucosa—poor surgical procedure, resulting in pouchitis-like symptoms.
• Perianal skin soreness—caused by a combination of frequency, leakage, and poor skin care.

Nursing advice

Bowel function will be looser and more frequent; often 4–6 motions will be passed daily. Perianal skin care is important when bowels first begin to function. Dietary advice can include reducing fibre levels, if loose bowel functions are encountered. More salt is needed each day to replace the sodium lost in the loose faeces and also adequate oral fluids such as 2 litres daily are required.

Small bowel resection

A small bowel resection is the surgical removal of a section of small bowel (➲ p. 10). Note that it is important after resection of the small bowel to know the amount of bowel remaining, as the initial length varies, rather than how much was removed.

Indication for surgery

There are different reasons that part of the small bowel might need to be removed such as:

- Small bowel Crohn's disease
- A bowel infarct.

Nursing advice

It is important to recognize that if certain areas of the small bowel are resected that these might have specific roles; for example, the terminal ileum is responsible for the absorption of vitamin B_{12}, thus if resected supplementation may be necessary. If the bowel function is loose after the resection, it is important to provide dietary advice or a dietetic referral to assist in bowel control. Perianal skin care is important when bowels first begin to function and dietary advice can include reducing fibre levels, if loose bowel functions are encountered. More salt is needed each day to replace the sodium lost in the loose faeces and also adequate oral fluids, such as 2 litres daily. Furthermore, if there is limited length of small bowel remaining after a resection, it is possible that the person will require nutritional support such as parenteral nutrition (➲ p. 312) if they have intestinal failure (➲ p. 70–3).

Stoma formation

A stoma is a surgical opening made through the abdominal wall to pass the bowel through to re-route the passage of faeces and flatus (colostomy or ileostomy) or a segment of bowel that is used as a conduit to pass urine (ileal conduit).

A colostomy is formed from the colon, commonly the sigmoid colon (➋ p. 2–3) or descending colon (➋ p. 2–3), but it could also be formed from the transverse colon (➋ p. 2–3). The ideal colostomy should be minimally raised about 5 mm above the abdominal wall.

An ileostomy is formed from the ileum (➋ p. 2–3), most commonly the end of the ileum that joins the caecum (➋ p. 2–3). The ideal length is '554' (see Fig. 20.11) to form a 25 mm spout that slightly points downwards.

A urostomy is formed from a small segment of ileum. One end of the ileum is closed shut, the two ureters are attached to this end of the urostomy, and the other end is formed into the stoma. The bowel ends are turned over and stitched to the abdominal wall with dissolvable sutures that stay in situ for about 6–8 weeks after the stoma formation.

A mucus fistula is formed from a distal segment of bowel; this is often the rectal stump after a colectomy is performed. A mucus fistula might pass a small amount of mucus or the mucus can be reabsorbed or passed from the anus. This is more likely to be formed if the patient is unwell.

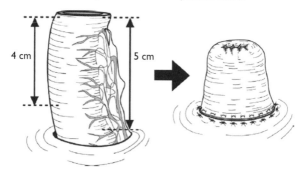

Fig. 20.11 '544' ileostomy.
Reproduced with kind permission © Burdett Institute 2008.

Indications for surgery

There are many operations that can or may result in the formation of a stoma, including:

- Abdominoperineal resection of the rectum (➋ p. 478–9)—permanent colostomy
- Hartmann's procedure (➋ p. 493)—temporary colostomy
- Ileo-anal pouch formation (➋ p. 376)—temporary ileostomy
- Anterior resection (➋ p. 482) +/- temporary ileostomy
- TME (➋ p. 482)—temporary ileostomy
- Panproctocolectomy (➋ p. 497)—permanent ileostomy.

There are a number of reasons that a stoma might be formed that includes:
- Colorectal cancer (→ p. 352)
- Crohn's disease (→ p. 377)
- UC (→ p. 370)
- Diverticular disease (→ p. 90–1)
- Trauma
- Bowel obstruction (→ p. 438–9).

Surgical complications

Potential surgical complications include:
- Wound infection
- Complications with the stoma (→ p. 516–18).

Nursing advice

It is important that the nurse ensures that prior to discharge home from hospital that the patient is able to independently care for their stoma. The patient also needs to know what is normal or abnormal, and who to contact in the case of problems with their stoma.

Stoma reversal

A temporary stoma (➲ p. 508) can be reversed or closed in an operation. The bowel is anastomosed and returned to the abdominal cavity and the abdominal wall and skin opening is closed.

Indications for surgery

A temporary stoma can be reversed, if the anal sphincter muscles are adequate to maintain anal continence.

Surgical complications

There is the risk of an anastomotic leak or damage to the perianal skin, when the stoma is reversed from the faecal output.

Nursing advice

Careful anal skin care (➲ p. 520–1) should be advised, to prevent perianal skin damage. Dietary advice can be given to assist bowel function (➲ p. 451). Pelvic floor and anal sphincter exercises (➲ p. 453) can be advised.

Whipple procedure

The Whipple procedure involves the removal of the head of the pancreas (➲ p. 14), the duodenum (➲ p. 10), gallbladder (➲ p. 14), and part of the bile duct +/– partial gastrectomy. The bile duct and pancreas are rejoined to the small bowel. A Whipple procedure is a long, complicated operation.

Indication for surgery

The Whipple procedure is the most common operation undertaken to treat pancreatic cancer.

Surgical complications

Complication rates are high after a Whipple procedure. Such as:
- Anastomotic leak
- Delayed gastric emptying
- Chyle leak
- Haemorrhage
- Chest infection
- Malabsorption
- Diabetes.

Nursing advice

After a Whipple procedure about 1 in 3 people need to replace pancreatic enzymes. Also, people may become diabetic.

Chapter 21

Stoma care

Types of stoma

There are three main types of output stoma: the colostomy, ileostomy, and urostomy (ileal conduit). Stoma is derived from the Greek word for mouth. A stoma can be temporary or permanent, an end stoma, loop stoma, or double-barrelled stoma.

Colostomy

A colostomy is formed from the colon, commonly the sigmoid or descending colon but also sometimes from the transverse colon. A colostomy will usually pass formed faeces and flatus each day. The appliance used is a colostomy appliance (➲ p. 512–13) that requires changing.

Ileostomy

An ileostomy is formed from the ileum, commonly the terminal ileum (end of the ileum). An ileostomy will usually pass loose faeces and flatus. An ileostomy appliance (➲ p. 512–13) is used to collect and contain the faecal output, and needs to be emptied and changed.

Urostomy (ileal conduit)

A urostomy is usually formed from a small segment of the small bowel that is used as a conduit to pass the urine, thus, it's termed an ileal conduit. The bowel will make mucus and thus a small amount of mucus will be passed with the urine. A urostomy appliance (➲ p. 504–5) is used to collect and contain the urine and requires emptying and changing.

Temporary stoma

A temporary stoma can be reversed or closed (➲ p. 506) after healing or chemotherapy, for example.

Permanent stoma

This stoma cannot be reversed and will be with the person for the rest of their life.

End stoma

The bowel is divided, and one end is formed into a stoma.

Loop stoma

A loop of bowel is split and both ends are formed into a stoma. One end (proximal) will be active, passing faeces and flatus. The other end (distal) will be inactive but might pass mucus from the distal section of the bowel.

Double-barrelled stoma

Two ends of bowel can be brought to the abdominal surface, with close together or apart and both formed into a stoma. One end (proximal) will be active, passing faeces and flatus. The other end (distal) will be inactive but might pass mucus from the distal section of the bowel.

Pre-operative stoma care

Prior to planned surgery, it is important to have information about the stoma. This includes what it will look like, how it will function, what a stoma appliance looks like, and how to care for the stoma. This list is not exhaustive and may also include what changes will occur as a result of the stoma and any changes to dietary intake.

Teaching the person on how to change the stoma appliance before surgery and following surgery will help the individual gain independence in their care. Assessing for any comorbidities, such as dexterity or dementia, prior to stoma formation will help with the post-operative phase. This is usually the remit of the stoma specialist nurse.

Stoma siting

Prior to a planned stoma formation, the stoma specialist nurse will site the stoma. Stoma siting means marking a place on the abdominal wall that is the best place for the stoma to be formed during the operation by the surgeon. A colostomy is usually sited in the left iliac fossa and the ileostomy and urostomy in the right iliac fossa. If two stomas are required these will be sited one in each iliac fossa and at dissimilar heights on the abdominal wall.

Postoperative stoma care

While in hospital after the stoma forming surgery, it is essential to train the person to be independent with their stoma. This includes practical care of the stoma, knowing what can be done and when, and who to contact if there is a problem with the stoma.

Postoperative stoma checks

It is important to check the stoma in the postoperative period to ensure that it is healthy. A stoma should be:
• Red or pink
• Warm to touch
• Moist.

Note that universal precautions should be taken by the nurse when touching bodily fluids, by wearing gloves. A patient does not need to wear gloves when caring for their stoma.

The skin around the stoma should appear the same as the rest of the abdominal skin and should not be broken or discoloured, although when the appliance is removed initially, the skin maybe slightly red.

Table 21.1 Stoma output

Output	Colostomy	Ileostomy	Urostomy
On leaving theatre	Nil +/− blood staining	Nil +/− blood staining	Urine, mucus +/ − blood staining
Initial output	Flatus, loose faeces	Flatus, loose faeces	Urine and small amounts of mucus
Output at discharge	Flatus and formed faeces	Flatus and porridge-like faeces	Urine and small amounts of mucus
Long-term output	Flatus and formed faeces	Flatus and porridge-like faeces	Urine and small amounts of mucus

Stoma appliance change

There are several variations to the stoma appliance change technique but in general this will include:

- Collecting all the equipment together (clean appliance, cleaning cloths, warm tap water, rubbish bag, measuring guide, scissors, pen, +/− any other stoma products used).
- Gently remove the appliance (emptying before if possible) from the abdominal skin
- Stick the two edges of the used appliance together and place in the rubbish bag.
- Clean and dry the skin using the cloths and warm water. Ensure all faeces/urine is removed from the skin; the stoma itself does not require cleaning and may bleed if cleaned too firmly.
- If within the first eight weeks of formation—the stoma size needs to be measured using the guide, marked with the pen and the aperture cut with the scissors—the ideal size is the same shape but 2–3 mm larger than the stoma.
- For stomas in the long term, the size should be checked periodically, such as if weight is lost or gained as this can affect the size of the stoma.
- The backing from the stoma appliance should be removed and the appliance should be placed over the stoma so that the whole stoma is enclosed within the aperture of the stoma appliance.
- The flange should be pressed with the fingers to ensure that it is well stuck to the abdominal wall and then held in place for about 30 seconds to enable it to adhere.
- Clinical waste should be disposed of as per local policy.

Patients should have the opportunity to practice their stoma care daily and whenever the appliance needs emptying or changing.

Stoma appliances and additional products

A stoma appliance is used to collect and contain the output from the stoma. A stoma appliance, also termed a stoma bag or a stoma pouch, is made from plastic, to enable to contents not to leak out. Usually there is an integral soft cover to help reduce sweating. The appliance adheres to the abdominal wall with an adhesive part termed a flange, baseplate, or faceplate. The flange is usually flat.

Convex appliances

There are stoma appliances available that have a dome-shaped flange that is used for a stoma that is retracted for example.

One-piece appliance

The collection part and the adhesive part of the stoma appliance are integral.

Two-piece appliance

The collection part and the adhesive part of the stoma appliance are two separate parts. These parts are joined together. There are a number of ways in which this can occur such as two locking rings or an adhesive surface on the collection part. Two parts means that the adhesive flange can be left in place on the abdomen and the collection part changed when necessary.

There are three main appliance types:
• Closed—used for a colostomy
• Drainable with a Velcro type fastening—used for an ileostomy
• Drainable with a tap or bung—used for a urostomy.

The appliances for a colostomy and an ileostomy have an integral filter to allow the flatus to leave the appliance, preventing ballooning but the odour stays within the appliance. A urostomy appliance has an integral internal mechanism that prevents the urine from flowing back up to the top of the appliance.

A colostomy appliance is not emptied. A colostomy appliance is on average changed once daily but this can vary from three times a week to three times a day.

An ileostomy appliance is emptied about 4–6 times daily and occasionally at night. An ileostomy is on average changed every 1–3 days.

A urostomy appliance is emptied about 4–6 times daily. At night it can be attached to a leg or night bag. A urostomy appliance is on average changed every 1–2 days.

Adhesive paste

There are stoma pastes that are used to provide additional adherence to a stoma appliance. The adhesive paste can be applied, sparingly, directly to the skin or to the adhesive part of the appliance. Some adhesive pastes contain alcohol and can sting broken skin.

Adhesive remover

To remove the adhesive of a stoma flange from the skin an adhesive remover can be used. Adhesive removers can be sprays or wipes. Adhesive removers can be used for people who have weak skin to prevent damage at appliance removal or for residual adhesive left on the skin when the appliance is replaced. The spray or wipe is used on the flange as it is removed or on the residual as part of the cleaning. Some adhesive removers can be slightly greasy and any residue may need to be removed before using the clean appliance.

Barrier film

A barrier film can be used to protect skin at risk of being damaged from the stoma output. A barrier film is available as a spray or wipe. After the skin around the stoma has been cleaned and dried, the barrier film is used prior to adhering the appliance.

Flange extenders

For people who require a little extra security, such as during sports, there are strips of adhesive tape that can be added to the outer edge of the flange once it is in situ on the abdominal wall. Flange extenders should not be used to cover a leak as this is likely to lead to painful, broken skin.

Protective paste

Protective paste is a greasy paste that is used to protect a wound such as in mucocutaneous separation (➔ p. 516). The paste should be used on areas that do not require the flange to adhere to. If the protective paste is on skin that requires something to adhere to it, it should be carefully removed from the skin.

Protective powder

Stoma powder is powdered hydrocolloid that is used on broken skin to help to heal the skin and provide a dry skin surface. It is applied sparingly to the skin after cleaning and drying. It is important to remove any excess powder as this can impair healing. There can be a stinging sensation for a very short period after application in some people.

Seals

A seal is usually a round-shaped, hydrocolloid that is used around a stoma to aid adhesion. The seal needs to be the size of the stoma and can be adhered directly to the skin or to the back of the stoma flange during the appliance change.

Discharge advice

It is imperative to ensure that the person with a newly formed stoma leaves the hospital during a carefully planned discharge. This includes ensuring that:

• The person can independently change their appliance.
• There are adequate stoma appliance stocks provided; usually two weeks of stock.
• The stoma is active to expected stoma output (➔ p. 510).
• The person is physically well enough.

It is imperative to ensure that the patient has been given advice on:

• Exercise
• Work
• Sexual activity
• Diet (➔ p. 515)
• Follow-up (➔ p. 522)
• Complications (➔ p. 516–18).

Exercise

Gentle exercise, such as walking, is a fundamental to postoperative care whilst in hospital. Once at home, walking needs to be continued and increased, as tolerated. It is important to not lift anything heavy for at least six weeks; however, this can depend upon the operation, recovery, and any comorbidities.

There is some evidence that wearing a support garment can help to reduce the risk of a parastomal hernia (➔ p. 518), when also used in conjunction with abdominal exercises.

Work

It is important to have a short period away from work; the duration of this will be guided by the type of occupation, the type of surgery, and any additional treatment such as chemotherapy. Most people would have six to eight weeks away from work and many undergo a phased return when possible. It is generally considered possible to undertake any occupation with a stoma.

Sexual activity

Most people after stoma forming surgery do not initially feel well enough to participate in sexual activities and some may notice changes in sexual function. Men are more at risk of sexual dysfunction, such as erectile problems (➔ p. 529) if they have radiotherapy or pelvic surgery; this is generally discussed with the surgeon pre-operatively. There are treatment options, such as medication, that can be explored with the GP if required. Women might have problems with dyspareunia (difficult or painful sexual intercourse) (➔ p. 528). This can be as a result of cancer treatment or removal of the rectum, which alters the internal anatomy.

Further reading

Association of Stoma Care Nurses (2016) *Stoma care nursing standards and audit tool.* ASCN UK. London.

Dietary advice

A balanced diet is central to help with recovery; however, there may be specific dietary changes required according to stoma type.

Colostomy—diet

People with a colostomy in hospital should start oral intake after their stoma formation with water, increasing as tolerated. Initially meals are usually better tolerated if they are small, frequent, and light. Often for the first few meals, fibre is taken with caution. By the time that people leave hospital, they should be eating normal food types but often in smaller quantities than usual.

Once at home, people with a colostomy should be encouraged to drink about 1.5 litres daily. Alcohol is allowed but within the limits. A normal diet can be resumed that should include a combination food. Some food is more likely to cause flatus to be produced, such as beans, and can be avoided if this causes a problem for an individual.

Ileostomy—diet

People with an ileostomy in hospital should recommence oral intake after their stoma formation with water, increasing as tolerated, and changing to other fluids. Initially small, frequent meals are better tolerated. Most people with an ileostomy avoid fruit and vegetables when in hospital. By the time that people are leaving hospital, they should be increasing the variety of foods taken but eating in smaller quantities than usual. It is important to encourage a little extra salt in the diet each day and to ensure that 1.5–2 litres daily are drunk. It is advisable for people with an ileostomy to carefully chew food for the first six to eight weeks as the ileostomy may still be swollen and there is a greater chance of a blockage occurring.

Once at home, people with an ileostomy should be encouraged to drink as before, alcohol is allowed within limits, but beer, lager, or cider may increase the ileostomy output. A normal diet can be slowly resumed to include a combination of food types. When recommencing high fibre food, it is ideal to try a small amount and chew it well. Often cooked or tinned fruit and vegetables are better tolerated than raw versions.

Urostomy—diet

People with a urostomy in hospital should recommence their oral intake with water, increasing the volume and variety of fluids taken. Initially meals are better tolerated if they are small, frequent, and light. By the time that people leave hospital, they should be eating normal food types but often in smaller quantities than usual.

Once at home, people with a urostomy should be encouraged to drink about 2 litres daily. Alcohol is acceptable but within the limits. A normal diet can be resumed that should include a combination food.

Stoma complications

There are a number of complications that can occur to the stoma. These can occur when in hospital after stoma forming surgery or once at home.

Necrosis

Necrosis is the result of reduced blood supply to the stoma and can result in a dark or black stoma as the tissue dies. Necrosis needs at initial presentation to be urgently referred to the surgeon as the person may need to return to theatre for resection of the necrotic tissue. In less severe cases the stoma should be regularly checked for warmth and colour: if the colour worsens or if the stoma loses blood perfusion then this needs urgent surgical review.

Bleeding

Small amounts of bleeding from the surface of the stoma are normal when cleaning, particularly in the first few weeks, due to the well-perfused bowel. Bleeding should spontaneously stop and advise the person to clean their stoma more gently. If bleeding persists, use light pressure onto the source of the bleeding. If bleeding is from the bowel lumen, this requires urgent surgical review.

Oedema

It is normal for a stoma to be oedematous initially as a result of the surgery. Oedema should settle within six to eight weeks. If the swelling increases, it is possible that there could be a postoperative complication and a surgical review is advocated.

Mucocutaneous separation

Mucocutaneous separation is when the join between the stoma and the abdominal wall becomes separated. This can be the result of tension on the sutures, poor wound healing factors, such as diabetes, or medication, such as steroids. Treatment will depend upon the extent of the separation and may include stoma powder or a dressing; as advised by the stoma specialist nurse. If the separation is deep on first presentation, this requires review by the surgeon as very infrequently treatment can be surgery.

Prolapse

A prolapsed stoma is when the bowel telescopes out of the body becoming longer. This can be cause by inadequate fixation during surgery or occasionally as a result of increased pressure, due to excessive coughing for example. A prolapse should be referred to the surgeon at first presentation. Treatment is usually only conducted by a doctor or the stoma specialist nurse and can include manipulation of the prolapse back into the abdomen, although this is not always possible. Some prolapses may require surgical revision. The nurse needs to reassure the patient and advise them that while the prolapse is present that care must be taken not to injure the prolapsed bowel and that the colour and temperature must be checked at each appliance change, looking for signs of damage.

Granuloma

A granuloma is a mass of granulation tissue often secondary to infection, inflammation, or a foreign body, such as a stitch, commonly seen at the junction of the stoma and the skin. The term over-granulation relates to excess granulation tissue that prevents healing by secondary intention. Treatment is often the use of silver nitrate for both problems. There is controversy about the use of silver nitrate for use in this situation.

Pre-existing skin conditions

Pre-existing skin conditions, such as psoriasis and eczema, can affect the adhesion of a stoma appliance. Treatment is usually topical, but caution should be used as greasy creams can affect stoma appliance adhesion.

Constipation

A person with a colostomy can become constipated. As the cause can be a diet low in soluble fibre, or lacking an adequate fluid volume (1.5 litres), or any other cause of constipation (→ p. 458), the cause of the problem should be addressed. If constipation occurs treatment can include laxatives (→ p. 422–3), suppositories, and enemas. The latter two are more prone to falling out of the colostomy because there are no sphincter muscles to retain them; the stoma specialist nurse can advise on ways to deliver these medications more effectively.

Ileostomy blockage

A person with an ileostomy may have a food bolus blockage of insufficiently chewed foods, this presents as no output from the ileostomy and possibly nausea or vomiting may occur. This is not to be confused with an ileostomy that is not working after surgery. Treatment at home can be to drink plenty to try and flush the blockage. If this fails, it is advisable to attend hospital, where it is likely that a nasogastric tube will be inserted and intravenous fluids given while waiting for the blockage to pass. It is likely that once the blockage passes that there will be a higher than usual output from the ileostomy.

Retraction

A retracted stoma is one that is pulled back into the body, caused by weight gain or a stoma that was not well mobilized in surgery, for example. Generally, if the stoma is active and the appliance adheres well there is no need for further treatment. The use of a convex appliance is may be necessary to help the appliance to adhere to the abdominal wall.

Stenosis

A stenosed stoma is one that is tight and does not expand to easily pass the output from the stoma, often the result of scarring that follows healing or extensive mucocutaneous separation. Treatment usually consists of dilation of the stoma, sometimes in theatre or possibly with the use of a dilator. Guidance of its use is advised and care must be taken not to cause damage to the surrounding skin as this might result in further scarring.

Caput medusae

Caput medusae is the formation of small blood vessels under the skin near the stoma, usually as a result of liver damage. These blood vessels can bleed, and can be alarming and potentially life-threatening. Treatment is to stop the bleeding, possibly through pressure or surgery. To reduce the risk of bleeding, the underlying cause of liver damage needs to be treated.

Parastomal hernia

A parastomal hernia presents as a bulge around the stoma as a result of the bowel pushing into the weakened abdominal wall. The bulge can cause discomfort, often described as a dragging sensation. Treatment is prevention through the use of a support garment and abdominal exercises. If a hernia is present, treatment remains the same. For an extensive or a problematic hernia, it is possible to have a surgical repair, but it is highly likely to recur. It is important to inform people that they need to check the stoma at each appliance change to ensure that the blood supply is not compromised: if this occurs, hospital attendance is urgently required. If the bowel stops working, it is also possible that it has twisted, again requiring hospital attendance.

Peristomal skin complications

There are two main categories for peristomal skin complications that have evolved from tissue viability. These are PMASD (➲ p. 520–1) and PMARSI (➲ p. 520–1).

PMASD

Peristomal moisture associated skin damage (PMASD) is most frequently caused by the output from the stoma touching the abdominal wall and breaking down the skin surface. PMASD can occur in the initial period in hospital. It is commonly seen in the first eight weeks while the stoma oedema reduces where resizing of the appliance aperture is unchanged, causing the output from the stoma to touch and damage the skin. Treatment can be as simple as carefully cleaning and drying the skin and then ensuring that the stoma appliance aperture is cut to the correct size, about 2–3 mm larger than the stoma and the same shape. If the skin surface is broken the sparing use of stoma powder (➲ p. 512–13) might be advocated.

Irritant contact dermatitis

Irritant contact dermatitis is under the category of PMASD (➲ p. 520) and is the result of the output from the stoma touching the skin around the stoma which results in dermatitis, usually seen as erythema (red skin) in a mild case, progressing to broken skin and ulceration in more severe cases. Treatment is to prevent the cause of the stoma output touching the skin.

PMARSI

The term peristomal medical adhesive related skin injury (PMARSI) relates to conditions of the peristomal skin that are a result of the stoma appliance adhesive. There are a number of types of skin problem that are within this category and treatment will depend upon cause.

Skin stripping

Skin stripping is within the category of PMARSI (➲ p. 520–1) and is when the top layer of skin is removed as a result of the adhesive during an appliance change. In more severe cases, this can remove several layers of the skin surface and cause bleeding. The cause in this situation is forceful removal of the stoma appliance or friable skin. Treatment is to ensure that the individual is more careful during the removal process or the use of an adhesive remover (➲ p. 513).

Maceration

Maceration can be seen to be within the category PMARSI (➲ p. 520–1) and is the softening of skin tissues as a result of prolonged exposure to moisture, such as the stoma output, that is trapped under the adhesive flange. Maceration is usually seen as paler tissues immediately around the stoma. These tissues are easily damaged and removed when cleaning which can be painful or result in bleeding. Treatment is to reduce the contact between the skin and the stoma output and resolution usually occurs quickly, often by resizing the hole in the appliance aperture. If not treated, maceration can progress to erosion of the skin.

Folliculitis

Folliculitis is within the category of PMARSI (➔ p. 520–1) and is a common skin condition where the hair follicles become inflamed, with red or white raised areas around the hair follicles under the stoma appliance. The cause is often an infection either bacterial or fungal, seen when these hairs are either inadvertently pulled out when the appliance is removed or when they are shaved. Treatment can range from nothing to the use of stoma powder (➔ p. 513) or topical treatment.

Fungal infection

Fungal infections are within the category of PMARSI (➔ p. 520–1) and seen in the skin around the stoma, for example, thrush, but this is less common in the UK compared to warmer countries. Treatment is often sparingly used topical treatment for thrush, applied under the flange during an appliance change. Be cautious of using too much cream as this can adversely affect appliance adhesion.

Allergic dermatitis

Allergic dermatitis is within the category of PMARSI (➔ p. 520–1) and this can present as erythema (red skin) that is in the shape of the stoma adhesive and can be itchy. The cause is an allergy to something within the ingredients of the flange. Treatment is usually to stop using that appliance and choose one from another manufacturer. It should be noted that a true allergy is rarely seen, but sensitivities are more common. Treatment is the same but often the appliances can be rotated so that when the sensitivity occurs with one, another is used.

Tension blisters

Tension blisters can occur when the skin is stretched by distension, for example, and the appliance adhesive pulls the skin surface resulting in a blister. Care of the intact or burst blister is needed and prevention is ideal.

Follow-up care

Follow-up care of a person with a stoma will be with the stoma specialist nurse. This might include visits at home, but more commonly visits to a clinic. During these appointments, the nurse may check the skin, the stoma, and how well the person is coping physically and emotionally. This is also an opportunity to undertake further teaching/reminders about diet, exercise, and resuming work.

It is ideal to have a review with the stoma specialist nurse once a year to check the stoma, the stoma products used, and how the person is coping. It is also important to assess people to see if the person with a stoma requires any further assistance.

Living with a stoma

A person with a stoma might have concerns about how they look, such as will others be able to see their stoma appliance. In general, the nurse can advise that if the appliance is well adhered and that it is emptied and/or changed regularly that it is not likely that others will know that they have a stoma.

Bathing and showering

It is possible to bath or shower with a stoma. The appliance is waterproof and requires drying after surgery. It is possible to bathe without the appliance on but there is a chance that the stoma will be active while bathing, although it is not unsafe to do so.

Exercise

It is possible to undertake exercise after stoma formation. It is ideal to walk initially and gradually build up strength and stamina. Seeking advice about progressing onto more vigorous exercise from the surgeon is advisable. Consideration needs to be made to prevent the formation of a peristomal hernia; this is possible by wearing an abdominal support belt each day in conjunction with undertaking abdominal exercises to strengthen the abdominal muscles.

Sexual relations

It is usually possible to have sexual intercourse and to have children after stoma forming surgery. If the nerves are damaged, such as with radiotherapy, then an erection may not be possible. Highlighting concerns and raising issues regarding sexual function with the surgeon after stoma forming surgery will help recovery and onward referral for further treatment.

Support groups

There are support groups available that can assist people with a stoma:
  Colostomy—Colostomy UK: www.colostomyuk.org
  Ileostomy—Ileostomy & Internal Pouch Association: www.iasupport.org
  Urostomy—Urostomy Association: www.urostomyassociation.org.uk

Stoma reversal/closure

A stoma reversal or stoma closure is performed as part of surgery. Following reversal, bowel movements may be more frequent with looser stools. Location of toilets during this period is crucial for the patient managing independently. Additionally, as the sphincter muscles (➔ p. 11–12) have not been used for several months they may not work as effectively as they did previously.

The nurse can advise that the bowel function should settle down after about six to twelve weeks. If it does not, the person should be advised to speak to their surgeon as they may require additional assistance, depending on their symptoms there may be constipation (➔ p. 458–9), anal incontinence (➔ p. 448–9), or faecal incontinence (➔ p. 448–9).

Other issues in gastrointestinal care

Body image

Body image refers to a person's perception of their own physical appearance, although it also comprises emotional attitudes and beliefs about bodily characteristics. The importance of physical appearance as a feature of individuality is very closely connected with the view of who we are as people. Body image carries significant meaning, and is consistent with self-concept, self-esteem, and identity. Body image perceptions adapt to the naturally changing events in life such as puberty, pregnancy, and ageing. However, unpredictable or unavoidable alterations to body image sometimes yield long-term consequences.

Body image can be significantly affected by illness of any nature and certainly by surgery, which as a result may adjust the appearance of the body, and how it may be perceived and function for the individual. Common factors associated with body image may include cancer, violation of body integrity, i.e. stoma, scars, inflammatory bowel disease (IBD), and bowel dysfunction. This type of body image is generally considered as an effect as a precursor to life experience, medical condition or treatment. On the other hand, there are some disorders where body image is the cause rather than the effect, which include anorexia nervosa and bulimia.

Encountering body image concerns is a relatively common experience, although is not classed as a mental health problem in itself. However, there is a suggestion that the higher the concern with body image, the more chance of there being a connotation with reduced quality of life and psychological disturbance. As a result, this then has an impact on well-being, affects sense of identity, and reduces participation in social/everyday activities, which as a result may develop into depression and/or anxiety.

Causes

- Experiences of chronic illness, particularly those where the effects are physically visible, have been linked with greater body image concerns, for example cancer, IBD, bowel dysfunction, surgery, and stoma formation.
- Surgery—scars
- Changes in body weight.

Nursing interventions

Recognising the perceived alteration in body image is important in planning care with the following as suggested interventions that can be addressed by the nurse:

- Note feelings of frustration, anger, withdrawn behavior, and denial.
- Help to identify positive behaviours that can aid recovery.
- Assist the patient to incorporate actual changes to activities of daily living, social life, interpersonal relationships, and occupational activities.
- Be realistic and positive during treatments, avoid giving false reassurance.
- Provide positive reinforcement of progress and encourage patient to set and achieve goals.
- Provide information for support groups if required.
- Identify ways of coping.
- Onward referral may be necessary for specialist support as follows.

Specialist intervention/treatment

Specialist support is often required when adjusting to any changes in physical appearance and function:
- Discussion of the side effects of treatments and how this may have the potential to impact on sexuality and sexual function
- Cognitive behavioural therapy (CBT) and psychotherapeutic interventions as well as support for educational approaches for improving body image.

Further reading

Bolton MA, Lobben I, Stern TA (2010). The impact of body image on patient care. *Primary Care Companion to the Journal of Clinical Psychiatry* 12(2): PCC.10r00947. https://www.ncbi.nlm.nih.gov/pmc/articles/PMC2911009/ (Accessed 24/0/2019)

https://www.mentalhealth.org.uk/publications/body-image-report (Accessed 13/06/2019).

https://nurseslabs.com/disturbed-body-image/#Nursing-Interventions (Accessed 24/06/2019)

Sexual dysfunction

Sexual dysfunction refers to a problem that may occur at any phase during the sexual response cycle. There is some suggestion that sexual dysfunction is common, although it is a topic that many people are tentative about discussing.

The sexual health needs of patients require assessment and treatment at all stages of care. When sexual issues are not addressed, it can have a significant negative impact on the quality of life and not only affect the patient, but their partners as well.

Types of sexual dysfunction

Sexual dysfunction is generally classified into four categories:
- Desire disorders—lack of sexual desire or interest in sex
- Arousal disorders—inability to become physically aroused or excited during sexual activity
- Orgasm disorders—delay or absence of orgasm
- Pain disorders— pain during intercourse (vaginismus).

Causes

There can be physical or psychological causes for sexual dysfunction:

Physical causes
- Hormonal imbalance/treatments
- Psychotropic medications
- Surgery
- Changes in weight following surgery and/or other treatments
- Tumours
- Pelvic floor dysfunction
- Neurological conditions, i.e. spinal cord injury, multiple sclerosis.

Psychological causes
- Stress
- Anxiety
- Depression
- Concerns about body image
- Relationship.

Interventions/treatment

- CBT and psychotherapeutic interventions as well as educational/informational support
- Discussion of the side effects of treatments and how this may have the potential to impact on sexuality and sexual function
- Medication such as Viagra for men, and hormone treatments for women
- Mechanical aids for men—vacuum devices, penile implants
- Mechanical aids for women—vaginal dilators
- Sex therapy (counselling)
- For women, lubrication or a change in position can assist with pain.

Further reading

https://my.clevelandclinic.org/health/diseases/9121-sexual-dysfunction (Accessed 24/06/2019)

Erectile dysfunction

Erectile dysfunction in men is also known as impotence, which is the inability to get and/or maintain an erection.

Causes

Erectile dysfunction can have a range of causes, both physical and psychological.

Physical

- Narrowing of the blood vessels going to the penis—commonly associated with hypertension, high cholesterol, or diabetes
- Hormonal problems
- Surgery
- Injury
- Obesity
- Multiple sclerosis
- Medication
- Tobacco use
- Treatments for prostate cancer or enlarged prostate
- Surgeries or injuries that affect the pelvic area or spinal cord.

Psychological

- Anxiety
- Depression
- Relationship problems
- Poor communication.

Intervention/treatment

Erectile dysfunction is largely treated by tackling the cause of the problem, whether this is physical or psychological.

- CBT and psychotherapeutic interventions as well as educational/informational support
- Discussion of the side effects of treatments and how this may have the potential to impact on sexuality and sexual function
- Medication such as Viagra
- Mechanical aids—vacuum devices, penile implants
- Sex therapy (counselling).

Further reading

https://www.mayoclinic.org/diseases-conditions/erectile-dysfunction/diagnosis-treatment/drc-20355782 (Accessed 24/06/2019)

Index

Note: Tables, figures, and boxes are indicated by an italic *t*, *f*, and *b* following the page number.

U

ulcerative colitis (UC)
  acute abdominal pain 433
  cause 372
  colorectal cancer
    surveillance 377
  definition 370
  endoscopic trading 370t
  incidence 373
  investigations 374
  medical treatment 375
  perforation 440, 441
  severity, assessment of 370t
  surgical treatment 376
  symptoms 371
ultrasound
  abdominal 227
  endoanal 228
undernutrition 302
unsaturated fatty acids 290, 291
urge resistance 453
urostomy (ileal conduit)
    504–5, 508
  diet 515
  stoma appliances 512
  stoma output 510t
  support group 523
ursodeoxycholic acid 428
uveitis 393

V

vanadium 295
vancomycin 408
variceal balloon tamponade
    276–7, 276f
varices 55, 443
vegetables see fruit and
    vegetables
video assisted anal
    fistula treatment
    (VAAFT) 480–1
virtual colonoscopy (VC) 229
visceral peritoneum 5
vitamins 294
  A 294
  B_1 (thiamine) 294
  B_2 (riboflavin) 294
  B_6 294
  B_{12} 294
    deficiency 79
  C (ascorbic acid) 294
  D 294
  E 294
  K 294
volvulus 116, 404
vomiting see nausea and
    vomiting

W

warts, anal (condylomata
    acuminata) 124
weight, and nutritional
    requirements 285
Wernicke–Korsakoff
    syndrome 350
Whipple procedure
    189–90, 506
white cell scan 226
Wilson's disease 178–9
wind (flatus) 94
  incontinence 448–9
withholding and
    withdrawing nutrition
    support 314–15
work see employment
World Health Organization
    Dioralyte 426

X

X-ray
  abdominal 230
  transit 231

Z

Zinc 295